AMA
AMERIC
MEDIC
ASSOCIAT

Guides to the Evaluation
of
DISEASE AND INJURY
Causation

EDITORS

J. Mark Melhorn, MD
William E. Ackerman, III, MD

Vice President, Business Products: Anthony J. Frankos
Director, Editorial: Mary Lou White
Director, Production and Manufacturing: Jean Roberts
Senior Acquisitions Editor: Barry Bowlus
Developmental Editor: Lisa Chin-Johnson
Copy Editor: Claudia Appledorn
Director, Marketing: Pam Palmersheim
Marketing Manager: Erica Duke
Senior Production Coordinator: Boon Ai Tan
Senior Print Coordinator: Ronnie Summers

www.ama-assn.org

This book is intended for information purposes only. It is not intended to constitute legal advice.
If legal advice is desired or needed, a licensed attorney should be consulted.

Additional copies of this book may be ordered by calling 800 621-8335 or from the secure
AMA Book Store web site at www.amabookstore.com. Refer to product number OP230107.

Library of Congress Cataloging-in-Publication Data

Guides to the evaluation of disease and injury causation / editors, J. Mark Melhorn,
William E. Ackerman III.
   p. ; cm.
 Includes bibliographical references and index.
 Summary: "This book is intended as a guide to help bridge the gap between occupational
and non-occupational evidence based causation"-- Provided by publisher.
 ISBN 978-1-57947-945-9 (alk. paper)
 1. Disability evaluation. 2. Occupational diseases--Etiology. I. Melhorn, J. Mark. II.
Ackerman, William E. III. American Medical Association.
 [DNLM: 1. Occupational Diseases--etiology. 2. Disability Evaluation. 3. Evidence-Based
Medicine--methods. 4. Occupational Exposure. WA 400 G9469 2008]

 RC963.4.G82 2008
 616.07'5--dc22
                                                  2007042396

The authors, editors, and publisher of this work have checked with sources believed to be reliable in their efforts
to confirm the accuracy and completeness of the information presented herein and that the information is in
accordance with the standard practices accepted at the time of publication. However, neither the authors nor
the publisher nor any party involved in the creation and publication of this work warrant that the information
is in every respect accurate and complete, and they are not responsible for any errors or omissions or for any
consequences from application of the information in this book.

Although we believe the authors to be experts in their fields, the ideas and opinions expressed in this book do not
reflect the views or official policy of the American Medical Association (unless otherwise specifically indicated).
The ideas and opinions provided in this book are intended to provide guidance only and should not be used as a
substitute for independent medical judgment and/or examination. It is the responsibility of the attending physician
or other health care professional, to rely on their independent experience and knowledge of their patient or
individual being evaluated, to determine the best treatment or evaluation course for their patient or individual.
The field of medicine and the area of causation is constantly changing and the reader should update their
knowledge and understanding with current best science. The American Medical Association, editors, and authors
do not assume any responsibility for any loss, injury, and/or damage to cases, persons, or property arising out of
or related to any use of the material contained in this book.

ISBN 1-57947-945-9
BQ77: 07-P-033:12/07

This book is dedicated to my patients and family, who have taught me the need for understanding and compassion when dealing with people. This has developed my desire to improve the quality of life for my patients as they struggle with their injuries and illnesses.

– JMM

This book is dedicated to my loving wife, Carrie and my family for their patience and understanding for the many hours that I spent on this book.

– WEA

CONTENTS

CHAPTER

Introduction   1

J. Mark Melhorn, MD, and William E. Ackerman III, MD

CHAPTER

Understanding Work-Relatedness   13

J. Mark Melhorn, MD, William E. Ackerman III, MD,
Lee S. Glass, MD, and David C. Deitz, MD, PhD

CHAPTER
Causal Associations and Determination of Work-Relatedness   33

Kurt T. Hegmann, MD, MPH and **Steven J. Oostema, MS**

CHAPTER
Methodology   47

J. Mark Melhorn, MD, and **Kurt T. Hegmann, MD, MPH**

CHAPTER

Apportionment   61

Charles N. Brooks, MD, and J. Mark Melhorn, MD

CHAPTER

The Causality Examination   73

Ian Blair Fries, MD

CHAPTER

Report Writing   103

Paul F. Waldner, JD, and Gary Freeman, MD, JD

CHAPTER
Spinal Disorders Causation   113

Donald Krawciw, MD, CCFP, Dip Sports Med

CHAPTER
Upper Limb   141

**J. Mark Melhorn, MD, Douglas Martin, MD,
Charles N. Brooks, MD, and Shirley Seaman, PAC-C**

CHAPTER

Lower Limb   203

Kenneth P. Subin, MD, MPH, and Christopher R. Brigham, MD

CHAPTER

Musculoskeletal Disorders   221

William Edward Ackerman, III, MD, and J. Mark Melhorn, MD

CHAPTER

Causation in Common Cardiovascular Problems   237

Elizabeth Genovese, MD and **Mark H. Hyman, MD**

CHAPTER

Causation in Common Pulmonary Problems   263

Elizabeth Genovese, MD, and **Mark H. Hyman, MD**

CHAPTER

Genitourinary Problems   347

Fred Kuyt, MD, William Ackerman, MD and **Mark H. Hyman, MD**

CHAPTER

Causation in Common Gastrointestinal Problems   357

Elizabeth Genovese, MD, and **Mark H. Hyman, MD**

CHAPTER

Causation in Ear, Eye, Nose, and Throat Disorders and Sun Exposure   371

William Edward Ackerman, III, MD, Roger M. Belcourt, MD, and **Marc T. Taylor, MD**

CHAPTER

Causation Related to Gender and Sex, Leukemia Related to Radiation, and Occupational Skin Lesions   387

William Ackerman, MD, and **Laurie Massa, MD**

FOREWORD

THERE PRESENTLY IS A DISABILITY epidemic in the United States. Disability is so rampant, and the psychosocial implications so pervasive that Dr. David Randolph, past president of the American Academy of Disability Evaluating Physicians, has termed disability a disease in and of itself. The number of workers on disability or "light duty" is growing faster than the population. Despite millions of dollars being spent on studying and improving ergonomics in the work place, disability from back "injuries" has continued to increase, not decrease, as it should if bad ergonomics were the cause. Needless to say, this is a very timely book.

The list of "diseases" and "conditions" that have been inappropriately attributed to the workplace environment goes on and on. Carpal tunnel caused by typing, chronic back pain caused by minor trauma, depression caused by the stress of going to work, CRPS (formerly called reflex sympathetic dystrophy) and fibromyalgia are but a few examples. There is ample evidence now that there is a strong psychosocial component to these conditions. By far, the majority of workers on disability from chronic back pain have a diagnosable psychological condition, and the evidence shows that that diagnosis pre-existed the onset of the chronic back pain. Many of these disabled workers sustained childhood abuse. In one study of lumbar fusions, almost no patients who had sustained childhood abuse had a good result.

There have been numerous studies defining the true etiology of many of these conditions. Twin studies have demonstrated that degenerative disc disease is much more related to genetic makeup of a person than to the type of work that person did. When one identical twin had a light job and the other a heavy job, requiring a lifetime of heavy lifting, there was no difference in the amount of DJD. There is no scientific evidence, for instance, that working on a railroad all your life causes any more deterioration of the lumbar spine than would have occurred from that natural history. In addition, the so-called cumulative trauma disorders have more to do with genetic makeup and anatomical variations rather than workplace injuries.

The country of Sweden was nearly rendered monetarily insolvent by disability payments and would have been had they not seen the light and changed the laws

xvi Guides to the Evaluation of Disease and Injury Causation

making chronic back pain less compensable. The United States cannot compete in the global market if we continue to render our workers disabled for conditions that have more to do with a worker's anatomy and psychological makeup than they do with actual on the job injuries.

Even worse than the monetary problems caused by our disability epidemic is the psychological trauma of taking a worker off work. The Canadian study demonstrated a doubling of the mortality rate in workers who are retired or are taken off work. And even if the worker doesn't die, it has been shown that there is no enjoyment of life. The worker is taken out of his/her social environments. Disabled workers do not enjoy life. Many are left acting sick to justify their disability. Illness behavior has been shown to be self-predicting. The sicker a worker acts, the sicker he/she becomes.

Well meaning plaintiff attorneys are also to blame and need to be educated. The plaintiff attorney's job in workers compensation cases is to protect the worker and get for him or her fair compensation for missing work, for medical expenses and for any true residual impairment that the worker incurred. The attorneys need to understand that by encouraging the worker to remain off work rather than getting back into the work place, they are actually doing damage to their client. Returning to work is beneficial and is often an essential part of a rehabilitation program.

In the past, many physicians have left the determination of causation to the legal system. Since treating and evaluating physicians rarely have the ability to investigate a case in detail, it has been easier to "go along" with the patient who claims that his/her condition started at the workplace. The data on the etiology of low back pain and other conditions has been scant and was often supportive of a workplace origin. More recently, however, there is ample data to prove that many of the conditions we previously attributed to the workplace have other etiologies.

The solution to this problem will take a massive educational effort. Physicians need to learn to return the worker to the job if at all possible, employers need to learn that it is better to have a worker at work, even on limited duty, rather than at home, attorneys and union officials need to understand that to encourage their clients to stay off work is actually doing the worker harm, and insurance companies need to learn that it is less expensive to have a worker at work than to incur indemnity payments.

This book is a first step. It will serve as a resource to all stakeholders in this monumental education effort that many of us feel is essential.

Robert H. Haralson III, MD, MBA, FAAOS, FAADEP
Medical Director, American Academy of Orthopaedic Surgeons

ABOUT THE EDITORS

J. Mark Melhorn, MD, FAAOS, FAADEP, FACS, is an occupational orthopaedic physician that specializes in the hands and upper extremities. He received his BS from McPherson College and his MD from the University of Kansas. Dr. Melhorn is board certified in orthopedic surgery, with added qualifications in surgery of the hand. In addition to his practice of orthopaedics at The Hand Center in Wichita, Kansas, Dr. Melhorn is a Clinical Assistant Professor, Section of Orthopaedics, Department of Surgery, University of Kansas School of Medicine, Wichita. He has authored over 350 articles, chapters, and publications about his research of workplace injuries and illnesses; return to work options; impairment and disability; and prevention of musculoskeletal pain in the workplace. He has lectured extensively to physicians, employers, insurers, administrators, and legislators on industrial musculoskeletal, upper extremity disorders, and prevention of musculoskeletal pain (MSDs) in the workplace. He is currently the program director for the American Academy of Orthopaedic Surgeons continuing education course on "Occupational Orthopaedics and Workers' Compensation: A Multidisciplinary Perspective" and for the American Academy of Disability Evaluating Physicians on "Annual Scientific Meeting," serves on the Board of Directors for the American Academy of Disability Evaluating Physicians, the Committee for Occupational Health for the American Academy of Orthopaedic Surgeons, Industrial Injuries and Prevention Committee for the American Society for Surgery of the Hand, Return to Work Committee and the Evidence Based Practice Committee for the American College of Occupational and Environmental Medicine, lead contributor section of Upper Extremities for the American Medical Association's 6th Edition of *Guides to the Evaluation of Permanent Impairment* and 5th edition chapter reviewer, co-section editor for musculoskeletal area of the Medical Advisory Board for Medical Disability Advisor—Disability Duration Guidelines and the Official Disabilities Guidelines (ODG) of the Work Loss Data Institute, Editorial Board of APG Insights Newsletter (designed as supplement, interpretation and application of the ACOEM Clinical Practice Guidelines), previous member of the Ergonomic Committee for the American College of Occupational and Environmental Medicine, past president of the Kansas Orthopedic Society, Continuing Medical Education committee for AAOS, a Musculoskeletal chapter-reviewer for the American Medical Association's 5th Edition of *Guides to the Evaluation of Permanent Impairment*, and previous faculty for continuing education courses by SEAK and American Board of Independent Medical Examiners.

Dr. Melhorn is the co-editor of the text "A Physicians' Guide to Return to Work" AMA Press (2005) and is the lead author for the Upper Extremity chapter in the 6th Edition of the AMA *Guides to the Evaluation of Permanent Impairment.*

William E. Ackerman III, MD, FAADEP, is a fellowship-trained, American Board of Anesthesiology certified anesthesiologist with added qualification in Pain Medicine. He has years of experience in pain medicine doing research and teaching as well as years of experience in the diagnosis and treatment of occupational pain disorders. He is a graduate of Spring Hill College, the University of Louisville, School of Medicine and was selected chief resident at the University of Kentucky when he was a resident in anesthesiology. He did a pain medicine fellowship at the Texas Tech Health Sciences Center. Dr. Ackerman has an extensive academic career and is now in private practice as a medical director of pain medicine at a private hospital. Dr. Ackerman has been and is still involved in medical research and he has presented the results of his scientific research at international and national scientific meetings. He has been a guest speaker at medical school department meetings and academic symposiums throughout the country. Dr. Ackerman has published over one hundred scientific journal articles and has published over one hundred scientific abstracts. He has authored multiple chapters in medical textbooks and has been lead author on two previously published textbooks. He has been nominated previously for the Southern Medical Society Research Award as well as the Bristol-Meyers Squibb Award for distinguished Achievement in Pain Research.

ACKNOWLEDGMENTS

I would like to thank my office staff at The Hand Center who continue to share my passion for patient care; the medical librarians at Via Christi Regional Medical Center and Wesley Medical Center, who continue to obtain references for me; Barry Bowlus, Lisa Chin-Johnson, and the AMA Business Products Staff; and Shirley Seaman PA-C who has read the book to enhance its readability.

– JMM

A book such as this is in reality a bringing together of ideas of colleagues and experts in the different fields discussed in this book. I would like to thank Dr. Scott Carle for his suggestion for the need of a book of this type, which addresses occupational causation. I would also like to thank the many adjusters and case workers and my patients that I have interacted with over the years, whose questions and comments inspired many of the topics in this book.

—WEA

The authors would like to thank Jim Talmage MD, Barry Bowlus, Lisa Chin-Johnson, and the AMA Business Product Staff for their dedication and efforts to bring this book to completion.

CONTRIBUTORS

1 Robert J. Barth, PhD
   Chattanooga, TN and Birmingham, AL

2 Roger M. Belcourt, MD, MPH, FACOEM
   Reno, Nevada

3 Christopher R. Brigham, MD, MMS, FAADEP, FACOEM
   President
   Brigham and Associates, Inc.
   Portland, Maine

4 Charles N. Brooks, MD
   Bellevue, Washington

5 Albert J. Carvelli, MD
   Clinical Assistant Professor Dept. of Anesthesiology
   University of Pittsburgh, School of Medicine
   Pittsburgh, Pennsylvania

6 Brian Cicuto, DO, PT
   Assistant Professor Pain Medicine
   University of Pittsburgh Medical Center
   Pittsburgh, Pennsylvania

7 David C. Deitz, MD, PhD
   National Director Liberty Mutual
   Boston, Massachusetts

8 Gary Freeman, MD, JD
   Gulf Freeway Orthopaedic
   Houston, Texas

9 Ian Blair Fries, MD, FACS, FAAOS
   Bone, Spine, and Hand Surgery, Chartered
   Brick, New Jersey
   Vero Beach, Florida

10 Elizabeth Genovese, MD, MBA, FACOEM, FAADEP
   Occupational Medicine/Internal Medicine
   Bala Cynwyd, Pennsylvania

11   Lee S Glass, MD, JD
     Medical Director
     Washington State Department of Labor & Industries
     Olympia, Washington

12   Kurt Hegmann, MD, MPH
     Dept of Family and Preventive Medicine
     The University of Utah
     Salt Lake City, Utah

13   Mark H. Hyman, MD, FACP, FAADEP
     Associate Clinical Professor of Medicine
     University of California, Los Angeles
     Los Angeles, California

14   Fred S. Kuyt, MD, MS
     Clinical Instructor, University of Southern California
     Keck School of Medicine
     Attending, Cedars-Sinai Medical Center
     Century Urology Medical Group
     Los Angeles, California

15   Donald Krawciw, MD, CCFP, Dip Sports Med
     Occupational Physician
     WorksafeBC
     Victoria, Canada

16   Gideon Letz, MD, MPH
     San Francisco, CA

17   Douglas Martin, MD, FAADEP, FACOEM, FAAFP
     Medical Director
     St. Luke's Center for Occupational Health Excellence
     Sioux City, Iowa

18   Laurie Massa, MD
     Dermatology Associates of Kentucky, P.S.C.
     Lexington, Kentucky

19   Shirley Seaman, MSA, PA-C
     Wichita, Kansas

20   David Silver, MD
     Associate Clinical Professor of Medicine
     UCLA School of Medicine
     Former Clinical Chief of Rheumatology
     Cedars Sinai Medical Center

21   Kenneth P. Subin, MD, MPH
     Senior Physician Consultant
     Brigham and Associates, Inc.
     Portland, Maine

22   Paul F. Waldner, JD
     Vickery & Waldner, LLP
     Houston, Texas

CHAPTER 1
Introduction

J. Mark Melhorn, MD, and William E. Ackerman III, MD

Purpose

Health care providers are often asked whether a condition is work-related or attributable to a specific event. It is incumbent on clinicians to give an opinion based on a careful review of three critical pieces of information:

1. Individual clinical findings
2. Individual workplace exposures
3. The literature linking (or not linking) the exposure of concern and the condition in question

This book is designed to assist health care providers, ancillary service providers, attorneys, and legislative agencies in using this information, in conjunction with individual clinical and exposures data, to make an evidence-based decision about whether a person's medical condition is work-related or attributable to a specific event or exposure.

Background

There is a large body of literature about the causal relationship between non–work-related factors (e.g., genetic, dietary, age-related, anthropomorphic, and environmental) and disease. The evidence basis used to determine causation as it relates to these factors has generally already been well characterized, with the strengths and limitations of available evidence well appreciated by experts in the relevant medical specialties.

This book will fill the void by examining the evidence-based literature available to better understand the relationship between selected medical conditions and exposure to physical and environmental factors that occur in the workplace or as a result of a specific exposure. Specific attention is given to analyzing the weight of the evidence for the strength of the association between these medical conditions and work factors commonly referred to as occupational exposure. Because the relationship between exposure to physical work factors and the development and prognosis of a particular illness, disorder, or medical condition may be modified by preexisting conditions and biopsychosocial factors, the literature concerning non-occupational risk factors and biopsychosocial factors and their impact on symptoms will also be reviewed. Understanding the interaction of these associations and relating them to the cause of symptoms is critical. Because the final determination of work relatedness is established by legal definitions, a discussion of jurisdictional statutes is included.

The US Congress recognized that statistics on workplace injuries and diseases were essential to an effective national program of occupational disease prevention. Therefore, when the Occupational Safety and Health Administration

(OSHA) Act was passed in 1970 (Code of Federal Regulations, Title 29, Chapter XVII, Part 1910), employers were required to maintain records on workplace injuries and illnesses using the OSHA 200 or 300 logs. The act delegated responsibility to the Bureau of Labor Statistics (BLS) for collecting statistics on occupational injuries and illnesses. To comply with the OSHA Act, the BLS conducts an annual survey of occupational injuries and illnesses in the United States.[1] The survey compiles the OSHA 300 logs from more than 200,000 establishments grouped by industry codes established by the BLS in the North American Industry Classification System (http://www.bls.gov/bls/naics.htm).

Exact figures for occupational injuries and illnesses are not available. The best data for the United States are provided by the Annual Survey of Occupational Injuries and Illnesses by the BLS, US Department of Labor.[1] To understand the data, it is important to know the definitions for injuries and illnesses. According to OSHA, an occupational *injury* is any injury such as a cut, fracture, sprain, or amputation that results from a work accident or from a single instantaneous exposure in the work environment.[2] An occupational *illness* is any abnormal condition or disorder, other than one resulting from an occupational injury, caused by exposure to environmental factors associated with employment. Occupational illnesses include acute and chronic illnesses or diseases that may be caused by inhalation, absorption, ingestion, or direct contact.[2]

To properly interpret BLS data, it is important to understand OSHA's record-keeping requirement. Employers are required to record workplace injuries and illnesses in their OSHA 300 logs. According to OSHA, a *workplace injury* is a cut, fracture, sprain, amputation, or other injury that results from a single instantaneous exposure in the work environment.[2] *Minor injuries* are defined as injuries requiring only first-aid treatment (e.g., not involving medical treatment, loss of consciousness, restricted work, or transfer to another job) and are not recorded in the logs. On the other hand, all occupational illnesses are recordable.

Known limitations of BLS data include the following: The survey estimates of occupational injuries and illnesses are based on a scientifically selected probability sample rather than a census of the entire population. Because the data are based on a sample survey, the injury and illness estimates probably differ from the figures that would be obtained from all units covered by the survey. Also, the survey measures the number of new work-related illness cases that are recognized, diagnosed, and reported during the year. Some conditions (e.g., long-term latent illnesses caused by exposure to carcinogens) are often difficult to relate to the workplace and are not adequately recognized and reported. These long-term latent illnesses are believed to be understated in the survey's illness measures. In contrast, the overwhelming majority of the reported new illnesses are those that are easier to track (e.g., contact dermatitis and carpal tunnel syndrome).

Although they are one of the best sources for benchmarking occupational disease, BLS data markedly underreport the extent of the problem. Not all injuries and illnesses are reported by the employer because of fear of retaliation,[3] administrative obstacles,[4] and efforts by OSHA to use these data to target on-site inspections. (Having only a few entries on the OSHA 300 logs may limit the frequency and extent of OSHA workplace inspections)

It is important to understand that the OSHA definition for work-relatedness is more inclusive than most definitions. Injuries and illnesses also occur at work that do not have a clear connection to a specific work activity, condition, or substance that is peculiar to the employment environment. For example, an employee may trip for no apparent reason while walking across a level factory floor, be sexually assaulted by a coworker, or be injured accidentally as a result of an act of violence perpetrated by one coworker against a third party. In these and similar cases, the employee's job-related tasks or exposures did not create or contribute to the risk that such an injury would occur. Instead, a causal connection is established because the injury would not have occurred but for the conditions and obligations of employment that placed the employee in the position in which he or she was injured or made ill.[5]

In 2005, nonfatal workplace injuries and illnesses numbered 4.2 million, of which 4.0 million (approximately 95%) were injuries, resulting in an occurrence rate of 4.6 cases per 100 equivalent full-time workers among private industry employers.[6] This rate was a decline from the rate of 4.8 reported for 2004.[7] Incidence rates for injuries and illnesses combined declined in 2005 for most case types, with the exception of 2.2 million cases with days away from work, transfer to another job, or restricted duties. The rate for days away from work was 1.4 cases per 100 workers and for job transfer or restriction, 1.0 case per 100 workers.[7]

Statistics for nonoccupational injuries and illnesses are not as easily determined. There is not a specific agency that tracks these injuries and illnesses. Determining statistics for this group of injuries and illnesses is further complicated by the fact that the injuries and illnesses may occur with the responsibility attributable to the person affected or to someone else. When responsibility is attributable to another person, *tort law* may be involved. A *tort* is a civil, not criminal, wrong or an injury against a person or property, with the exception of breach of contract. Tort is derived from the Latin word *tortus,* which was changed to *tortious* in English, and which means twisted. *Tort law* is the body of the law that permits an injured person to recover compensation from the injuring party, which may occur when one person injures another, intentionally or by negligence. A court may award money damages to the injured party as compensation for the injury. The requirement to establish responsibility in tort law is a major reason that health care providers are asked to provide an opinion concerning causation. The costs associated with torts are significant.

Several sources provide injury and cost data: the Centers for Disease Control and Prevention (http://www.cdc.gov), the National Safety Council (http://www.nsc. org), the National Library of Medicine at the National Institutes of Health (http:// www.nlm.nih.gov), insurance providers, and the World Wide Web. By using these sources, several key documents were identified, as follows: *The Economic Costs of Injuries,*[6] Summary Health Statistics for the US Population: National Health Interview Survey, 2002,[7] and 2007 edition of *Injury Facts.*[8]

The total cost of nonoccupational injuries and illnesses often labeled as unintentional in 2005 was $625.5 billion. Of this $625.5 billon, 50% was assigned to wage and productivity losses, 18% to medical expenses, 18% to legal and administrative costs, 10% to property damage, and 4% to uninsured costs. No data were available for costs of punitive damages associated with unintentional injuries, when applicable.

Overview

Occupational exposures and their association with or causation of injuries and illnesses are often debated. Because a determination for association or causation is required to determine eligibility for compensation and, therefore, financial responsibility for workers' compensation or tort cases, debates and disputed legal cases often ensue. The significance of such disputes is underscored by the reported direct health care costs for the nation's work force of more than $418 billion and indirect costs of more than $837 billion. Reducing the more than $1.2 trillion workers' compensation costs[9] and the $625.5 billion non-occupational costs[8] has become a national priority. Even though the reported incidence of work-related injuries and illnesses is slowly decreasing, the direct and indirect costs, which include indemnity associated with the injuries and illnesses, are increasing, especially in the illness group commonly described as musculoskeletal disorders such as carpal tunnel syndrome.[10]

Although described as a single system, workers' compensation is a complex set of judicial and legislative rules and regulations that is different for each state and territory, with separate systems for state and federal employers; railroad employers; and along-shore and harbor workers. The causation threshold requirement varies from "one iota to a more probable than not" contribution. In other words, many injuries and illnesses are considered work-related and, therefore, work compensable even if the workplace risk factors contributed little to the causation. On the other end of the spectrum, some states have legislated certain medical conditions as not compensable, despite multiple scientific reviews linking the conditions to workplace exposures.

The tort law system is even more varied. Because each state establishes case precedents, the approach from state to state can widely vary in what is considered acceptable evidence and how the evidence is to be applied.

Fraud

Statistics for fraud (defined in the broadest sense as deception made for personal gain) are difficult to determine and measure. Fraud can be intentional or unintentional and can be committed by the employee, employer, physician, insurer, and others. Therefore, the estimates provided by insurance companies are general. The insurance fraud industry estimates that nearly a quarter of all workers' compensation claims filed involve some degree of fraudulent activity.[11] Of the 25% suspected fraudulent claims, most involve some type of malingering in which the claimant may extend time off even though the injury has healed sufficiently for return to work. Malingering is an abuse of the system and is fraud, but little time is spent investigating it because of limited resources.[11] The types of workers' compensation claims that are usually investigated involve injuries that did not occur at work and claimants working while collecting benefits. These types account for about 10% of all compensation claims filed.[11]

Fraud can also occur when the claimant tries to mislead the physician. One study reported that 42% of subjects were not truthful on a test of memory. The authors concluded that exaggeration of cognitive symptoms is widespread in disability-related evaluations.[12] It would be unwise to accept self-reported memory complaints at face value. Criteria-normalized symptom validity testing should be done to rule out symptom exaggeration.[12] A physician can also contribute to fraud when granting unnecessary time off work or, possibly, based on a misguided sense of social justice, attributing causation when causation does not exist.[13-19]

Definitions

The remainder of this chapter contains definitions used throughout the book.

Evidence-based medicine has become the standard for determining appropriate medical care. The most common definition was provided by Sackett et al[20]: *Evidence-based medicine is the conscientious, explicit, and judicious use of current best evidence in making decisions about the care of individual patients . . . integrating individual clinical expertise with the best available external clinical evidence from systematic research.* Unfortunately, controlled, randomized clinical studies are uncommon and difficult to perform in the workplace. Therefore, most of the information available is from epidemiologic studies. Although epidemiologic studies can *disprove* an association, they cannot *prove* an association.[21]

Epidemiology is the biomedical discipline focused on the distribution and determinants of disease in groups of people who happen to have some characteristics, exposures, or diseases in common. Viewed as the study of the distribution and societal determinants of the health status of populations, epidemiology is the basic scientific foundation of public health.[22] The goal of epidemiologic studies is to identify factors associated (positively or negatively) with the development or recurrence of adverse medical conditions. For this book, a search strategy of bibliographic databases was used to identify epidemiology literature that addresses causation related to specific medical conditions as outlined in Chapter 4, Methodology.

Medical conditions are injuries or illnesses that meet the standard criteria for a diagnosis in the *International Classification of Diseases, Ninth Revision.*[23]

Disability is the alteration of a person's capacity to meet personal, social, or occupational demands or statutory or regulatory requirements because of impairment. Disability is a relational outcome, contingent on the environmental conditions in which activities are performed.[24]

Impairment is a loss, loss of use, or derangement of any body part, organ system, or organ function.[24]

Occupational exposures and physical factors at work are identifiable occupational exposures to possible exuberating or aggravating agents. Examples of physical factors for the musculoskeletal system are often described in terms of repetition, force, posture, vibration, temperature, contact stress, and unaccustomed activities.[25,26] For hearing, sound levels are often measured in decibels; for radiation, exposure levels in millirad; and for chemical, exposure levels in milligrams per cubic meter or parts per million.

Nonoccupational exposures include individual risk characteristics such as age, sex, hand preference, comorbid medical conditions such as diabetes, body mass index, depression, and hobbies.

Work environment is defined by OSHA in paragraph 1904.5(b)(1), as the establishment and other locations where one or more employees are working or are present as a condition of their employment.[27] The work environment includes not only physical locations, but also the equipment or materials used by the employee during the course of work.[5]

Aggravation occurs when a preexisting injury or illness that has been significantly aggravated, for purposes of OSHA injury and illness record keeping, when an event or exposure in the work environment results in any of the following[5]:

1. Death, provided that the preexisting injury or illness would likely not have resulted in death but for the occupational event or exposure;
2. Loss of consciousness provided that the preexisting injury or illness would likely not have resulted in loss of consciousness but for the occupational event or exposure;
3. One or more days away from work, days of restricted work, or days of job transfer that otherwise would not have occurred but for the occupational event or exposure; or
4. Medical treatment in a case in which no medical treatment was needed for the injury or illness before the workplace event or exposure or a change in medical treatment was necessitated by the workplace event or exposure.

This definition of aggravation is similar to that in the American Medical Association *Guides to Evaluation of Permanent Impairment*, fifth edition: A factor(s) (e.g., physical, chemical, biological, or medical condition) that adversely alters the course or progression of the medical impairment. Worsening of a preexisting medical condition or impairment (p. 599).[24]

Exacerbation is a transient worsening of a prior condition by an injury or illness, with the expectation that the situation will eventually return to baseline or pre-worsening level.[28]

Recurrence is similar to exacerbation, but it generally involves the reappearance of signs or symptoms attributable to a prior injury or illness with minimal or no provocation and does not necessarily occur related to work activities.[28]

Apportionment represents a distribution or allocation of causation among multiple factors that caused or significantly contributed to the injury or disease and resulting impairment. The factor could be a preexisting injury, illness, or impairment.[24]

Summary

What is a cause? Rothman[29] defined a cause as "an event, condition or characteristic that plays an essential role in producing an occurrence of the disease." There is causation, in other words, only when one factor necessarily alters the probability of a second. Causality is the relating of causes to the effects they produce. Most of epidemiology concerns causality, and several types of causes can be distinguished. It must be emphasized that epidemiologic evidence by itself is insufficient to establish causality, although it can provide powerful circumstantial evidence.

What is risk? Risk is the probability that an event will occur. In epidemiology, it is most often used to express the probability that a particular outcome will follow a particular exposure. A *risk factor* is an environmental, behavioral or biologic factor confirmed by temporal sequence, ideally in longitudinal studies, that, if present, directly increases the probability a disease will occur, and, if absent or removed, reduces that probability. Risk factors are part of the causal pathway or expose the host to the causal pathway.[30]

Precisely which factors predominate in the etiology of work-related medical conditions is the subject of ongoing debate. Often a specific diagnosis has a multifactorial etiology and a single cause cannot be identified. Multiple risk factors are occupational and non-occupational. Furthermore, the presence of one risk factor does not negate other pathways with other causal roles. Causal models are complicated by differences in personal susceptibility (it is unlikely that all people have equal susceptibility to any disorder) and genetic disposition, repeated exposures to low levels of the suspected causal agent(s) (risk factors), and a latency period that varies with individual susceptibility and severity of exposure. Several different risk factors may be in play in any given case, combining and interacting in ways that are difficult to study and to understand. It is necessary to distinguish between factors that aggravate the symptoms of the condition and factors actually responsible for the development of the condition.

Disagreement then centers on the relative importance of the multiple causal risk factors and whether these risk factors are occupational or nonoccupational and to what degree. The data presented in this text explore the science to determine work-relatedness in an individual case, the science needs to be applied by using the six parts of assessment described by the National Institute for Occupational Safety and Health and detailed in Chapter 4, Methodology.

We thank Thomas Hales, MD, MPH, senior epidemiologist at the National Institute for Occupational Safety and Health, Robert Taft Lab, Cincinnati, Ohio, for review and contributions to this chapter.

References

1. US. Department of Labor. *Workplace Injuries and Illnesses in 2005*. Washington, DC: Bureau of Labor Statistics; 2006:1-29.
2. US Department of Labor. *Recordkeeping Guidelines for Occupational Injuries and Illnesses*. Washington, DC: US Dept of Labor; 1996:1-200.
3. Pransky G, Snyder T, Dembe A, Himmelstein J. Under-reporting of work-related disorders in the workplace: a case study and review of the literature. *Ergonomics.* 1999;42:171-182.
4. Azaroff LS, Lax MB, Levenstein C, Wegman DH. Wounding the messenger: the new economy makes occupational health indicators too good to be true. *Int J Health Serv.* 2004;34:271-303, 2004.
5. US Department of Labor. Occupational Safety and Health Administration. http://www.osha.gov/pls/oshaweb/owadisp.show_document?p_table=FEDERAL_REGISTER&p_id=16312, published 01-19-2001. Accessed May 15, 2007.
6. Centers for Disease Control and Prevention. *The Economic Costs of Injuries.* Washington, DC: National Center for Injury Prevention and Control; 2007.
7. Centers for Disease Control and Prevention. *Summary Health Statistics for the US Population: National Health Interview Survey, 2002.* Washington, DC: US Dept of Health and Human Services; 2004:1-110.
8. National Safety Council. *Injury Facts.* Itasca, IL: National Safety Council; 2007.
9. Brady W, Bass J, Royce M, et al. Defining total corporate health and safety costs: significance and impact. *J Occup Environ Med.* 1997;39:224-231.
10. Feuerstein M, Miller VL, Burrell LM, Berger R. Occupational upper extremity disorders in the federal workforce: prevalence, health care expenditures, and patterns of work disability. *J Occup Environ Med.* 1998;40:546-555.
11. Workers Compensation Research Institute. Cambridge, MA: Workers Compensation Research Institute; 2007. http://www.wcrinet.org/result/BMcscope_CA_result.html. Accessed July 21, 2007.
12. Richman J, Green P, Gervais R, et al. Objective tests of symptom exaggeration in independent medical examinations. *J Occup Environ Med.* 2006;48:303-311.
13. Bonzani PJ, Millender LH, Keelan B, Mangieri MG. Factors prolonging disability in work-related cumulative trauma disorders. *J Hand Surg [Am].* 1997;22A:30-34.
14. Deyo RA. Pain and public policy. *N Engl J Med.* 2000;342:1211-1213.
15. Hadler NM. If you have to prove you are ill, you can't get well: the object lesson of fibromyalgia. *Spine.* 1996;21:2397-2400.
16. Melhorn JM. Rediscovering occupational orthopaedics for the next millennium. *J Bone Joint Surg Am.* 1998;81A:587-591.
17. Melhorn JM. Workers' compensation: avoiding the work-related disability. *J Bone Joint Surg Am.* 2000;82A:1490-1493.
18. Melhorn JM. Impairment and disability evaluations: understanding the process. *J Bone Joint Surg Am.* 2001;83A:1905-1911.
19. Wynia MK, Cummins DS, VanGeest JB, Wilson IB. Physician manipulation of reimbursement rules for patients: between a rock and a hard place. *JAMA.* 2000;283:1858-1865.

20. Sackett DL, Rosenberg WM, Gray JA, Haynes RB, Richardson WS. Evidence based medicine: what it is and what it isn't. *BMJ.* 1996;312:71-72.
21. Hadler NM. *Occupational Musculoskeletal Disorders.* Philadelphia, Pa: Lippincott Williams & Wilkins; 1999:1-300.
22. Melhorn JM. Epidemiology of musculoskeletal disorders and workplace factors. In: Mayer TG, Gatchel RJ, Polatin PB, eds. *Occupational Musculoskeletal Disorders Function, Outcomes, and Evidence.* Philadelphia, PA: Lippincott, Williams & Wilkins; 1999:225-266.
23. American Academy of Orthopaedic Surgeons. *Orthopaedic ICD-9-CM Expanded.* Rosemont, IL: American Academy of Orthopaedic Surgeons; 1996:1-107.
24. American Medical Association. *Guides to the Evaluation of Permanent Impairment.* Chicago, IL: AMA Press; 2001:1-613.
25. CtdMAP. Workplace activity risk factors. In: *CtdMAP Occupational Health Intervention Technologies.* Wichita, KS: MAP Managers; 2006.
26. Melhorn JM. Upper-extremity cumulative trauma disorders on workers in aircraft manufacturing [letter]. *J Occup Environ Med.* 1998;40:12-15.
27. Occupational Safety and Health Administration. *MSDs: Frequently Asked Questions.* Washington, DC: Occupational Safety and Health Administration;2002:1-5.
28. Talmage JB, Melhorn JM. *A Physician's Guide to Return to Work.* Chicago, IL: AMA Press; 2005.
29. Rothman KJ. *Modern Epidemiology.* Boston, MA: Little Brown & Co; 1986:51-76.
30. Burt B. *Definitions of Risk.* Ann Arbor, MI: University of Michigan; 2001.

CHAPTER

2 Understanding Work-Relatedness

J. Mark Melhorn, MD, William E. Ackerman III, MD, Lee S. Glass, MD, and David C. Deitz, MD, PhD

Prevalent Perceptions of Work-Relatedness

It is important that common perceptions or popular opinions of causation be based on the best available scientific evidence. For example, the speculation that carpal tunnel syndrome is related to arm use is widely accepted but unproven. Many published studies have implicated occupation, wrist position, vibration, cold temperature, and repetitive motion.[1-15] Because this proposed linkage is appealing and pervasive and seems to make sense, the lay press has advanced this association despite several quality scientific investigations that found little or no relationship between carpal tunnel syndrome and occupation or hand use.[16-19] Furthermore, several studies have implicated inherent genetic factors.[20-32] This does not mean that future quality studies will not establish a relationship; medicine has been wrong in the past, as in its rejection of the Hippocratic humoral theory to explain health and illness.

Therefore, this book is devoted to how to blend the advances in the medical and scientific understanding of causation with the law. Medical evidence is drawn from observation, and medical conditions are multifactorial and more likely to be controlled by probability than by a single cause or event. In contrast, in law, the finding of causal connection between a wrongful act and harm is essential to the attribution of legal responsibility. This difference in perspective often results in dissatisfaction of litigants, uncertainty for judges, and friction between health care professionals and their legal counterparts.

Determining whether a symptom, injury, or illness is factually and legally due to employment conditions is important to the individual patient (employee), the employer, and other workers who may be exposed to similar conditions. This determination has two applications: the first relates to the primary prevention of injuries and illnesses and, therefore, to public health; the second addresses work-relatedness and workers' compensation, which is linked to the employer's potential liability for the costs associated with the symptoms, injury, or illness. The concept of work-relatedness is complex and may not be intuitively obvious. Although by definition work-related disorders affect workers, the disorder may not necessarily have been caused by work.[33]

Work-relatedness, in the context of industrial injuries, involves concepts of medical and legal causation. The two may be mutually exclusive. Definitions of medical causation and legal causation arise from different sources—one from science and the other from the desire for social justice. For physicians treating injured workers, understanding the differences between the two concepts is essential.

Similarly, specific injuries or illnesses that did not occur as a direct result of the workplace (tort cases) can create the same demands of health care providers for determinations of causation. Although this chapter addresses primarily work-relatedness, the same approach can be applied to many tort cases.

Medical causation deals with scientific cause and effect. For example, a physician may conclude, based on well-accepted principles of science, that exposure to smoke in a workplace is likely to have been the cause of a patient's squamous cell carcinoma. A different physician who questions whether a particular microbe is the cause of a patient's disease might apply the various tests of the Koch postulates. An ambiguity or inconsistency in the test results may cause the physician to conclude that the microbe might not be the cause of the patient's disease. In both cases, the physicians made cause-and-effect determinations that were based solely on scientific principles. Presumably, any challenge to the physicians' conclusions would similarly be rooted in science.

The courts did not have their origins in science, and, therefore, the laws developed are not scientifically derived. The courts were, in the greater part, institutions of the church, and their function was to promulgate, not to discern order. That a chasm will always exist between science and religion—i.e., between why things are and how things ought to be—should not come as a surprise. Nor should it be a surprise that causation in law is not the same as in science.

In a causation analysis, the law considers two separate and distinct components: cause in fact and proximate (or "legal") cause. Workers' compensation adjudicators must consider both components, and it is important that both be understood by physicians involved in the adjudication of industrial-insurance claims.

Cause in Fact

If one event brings about another, the former can be considered the *cause in fact* of the latter, regardless of the number of events involved. For example, many physical and chemical reactions occur between the squeeze of a trigger and the bullet's impact with its intended target, but the pressure on the firing mechanism would indisputably be a *cause in fact* of the target being hit.

To establish medical causation, there must be a cause-and-effect association between the outcome and the postulated cause. Such an association may be direct or indirect. A *direct* causal association exists only when the event is necessary for the outcome to have occurred. Permanent brain damage can be caused solely by severe blunt trauma to a person's head; the trauma is the direct cause because no other variables are required for the damage to occur. An *indirect* causal association exists when the event produces the outcome that occurred only in the presence of other contributing factors. Poverty itself does not cause disease, but when combined with inadequate nutrition and sanitation and lack of access to health care, disease can occur.

A non-causal relationship can also exist between two factors. A non-causal relationship—a *correlation*—exists when a factor other than the event in question is responsible for a medical outcome. For example, people with gray hair may have a higher incidence of myocardial infarction than people with black hair. However, gray hair does not—by itself or with other factors—provide a biologically plausible explanation for the occurrence of a myocardial infarction. There is a non-causal relationship between hair color and myocardial infarction: the presence of gray hair and the incidence of myocardial infarction both increase with age, for unrelated reasons.

Causal fallacies exist, and at least one of them requires attention here. *Post hoc ergo propter hoc* (after this, therefore because of this) occurs when a causal relationship is asserted based on this false reasoning. It is a fallacy to conclude that one event followed by a second necessarily demonstrates a causal relationship between the events.[34] A collision that occurs minutes after a black cat crosses a person's path does not establish a causal relationship between the encounter and the collision because the cat did not cause the accident. When assessing the possibility of a relationship between events, it is important to consider and correctly apply the distinct concepts of cause and correlation.

Proximate Cause

In the reasoning of the law, a potential liability of intolerable magnitude would exist if cause in fact were the only issue in a causal analysis. Some philosophers believed that all events in our universe were connected, although the threads were more gossamer in some instances than others. If cause in fact were the only consideration, we would refer to a "web" of rather than a "chain" of causation, which would have made it impossible to go through life without continually becoming ensnared in the web.

The second part of causation analysis seeks to determine whether two events that are linked *in fact* should also be linked *in law*. This second test is referred to as *proximate cause* or *legal cause*. In essence, the question is whether the two events are so closely linked that liability should be attached or assigned to the first event for producing the second event, the harm. For example, if two coworkers met and became attracted to one another in the workplace but close contact was solely outside the workplace and one became infected with tuberculosis, a physician would likely find that the sustained physical proximity between the coworkers was the medical cause of disease transmission. It is likely that a court, however, would find that proximate cause has not been established because of the minimal connection to the workplace.

The accepted wisdom of justice and fair play that underlie the concept of proximate cause are subject to many different interpretations in workers' compensation law. Within broad limits, each state may determine for itself what constitutes proximate cause. Such determinations may be made by legislatures or by the courts (an independent branch of government). Although all states might agree that liability should be attached when a person deliberately discharges a firearm with the intent to kill another, not all states would agree that the weapon's manufacturer was the proximate cause of the resulting harm.

Judges and legislatures have the power to substitute convenience for science. One common method for doing so in workers' compensation cases is the establishment, by legislative or judicial decree, of presumptions that institutionalize societal choices. For example, a state, through its legislature or the State Supreme Court, might create a presumption that links a particular illness to a particular type of employment. Under this presumption, some states have created a compensable nexus between cardiovascular disease and employment as a fire fighter. Presumptions may be rebuttable or irrebuttable. A rebuttable presumption shifts the burden of proof to the party against which the presumption applies. Typically, the party must then introduce sufficient evidence to overcome the presumption if that party is going to successfully avoid an adverse result such as being liable for damages. In many states, the opinion of a treating physician is officially deemed to have presumptively greater credence than that of any other physician. Legally, it is possible, albeit usually difficult, for an insurer to rebut such a presumption, and, in such situations, the courts are under no obligation to apply medical evidence-based principles.

An irrebuttable presumption, on the other hand, essentially establishes a legal conclusion, ie, once the necessary facts have been established. A firefighter who is sheltered under the protection of an irrebuttable presumption that his myocardial infarction was caused by employment need not fear a denial of benefits because the myocardial infarction occurred while he was on vacation or worry that proof of a strong family history of heart disease, a long-standing diagnosis of untreated hypercholesterolemia, and a several-packs-per-day smoking habit will allow his workers' compensation insurer to avoid payment of benefits. Our system of checks and balances applies to presumptions; judicially created presumptions can be abolished by legislatures, and legislatively adopted presumptions can be made ineffectual by judicial decree. Presumptions vary widely from state to state, and neighboring states may reach different conclusions from the same set of facts solely by virtue of the differences in the presumptions that might apply.

Whether the presence of a risk factor will be relevant to the determination of an outcome in a workers' compensation case depends on a number of different factors. Generally, workers' compensation systems are a genuine "no-fault" form of insurance. For that reason, the presence of a risk factor, which might increase the odds that an injury may occur, is not taken into consideration. Risk factors for osteoporosis and, in fact, osteoporosis itself, would generally not be considered factors in determining whether medical payments or time-loss benefits apply to a lifting-induced vertebral compression fracture. An assessment of the causal relationship of a risk factor and a medical condition is more likely to be necessary if the condition might logically have been caused by virtue of the risk factor or a contended industrial injury. An assessment of the risk factors for carpal tunnel syndrome and their relationship to the numbness and tingling in the hands of a pregnant typist might be determinative in the adjudication of her workers' compensation claim. This type of causation considerations would apply when a causal relationship between a risk factor and a condition must be made.

Epistemology

Epistemology, the study of knowledge, is one of the four main disciplines of philosophy. Epistemology can be translated into "What we know and how we know it." For medical causation (cause in fact), this requires a basic understanding of biostatistics and probability.[35,36]

A risk factor for a particular illness or injury, by definition, increases the probability that an exposed person will, at some point, experience the illness or injury in question. For many occupational risks, this can be difficult to prove. Because workers are usually exposed to many risks simultaneously, statistical analysis is used to analyze whether differences between people with a given outcome might have occurred by chance. Most medical studies refer to results as statistically significant when there is a less than 5% chance that a given result could have resulted by random variation (results indicated as $P < .05$) with some studies reporting other probabilities when it is even less likely that chance alone could account for observed results. Note that statistical significance does not prove an outcome or association beyond all doubt. Most epidemiologists are comfortable only when studies of causation are large, carefully controlled for all possible risk factors, and, ideally, repeated with similar findings.

Even small differences in risk may be statistically significant without being clinically meaningful and, as noted, not all risk factors will be taken into consideration in a workers' compensation claim. Nevertheless, risk factors, which produce large differences in outcomes between exposed and non-exposed populations, such as coal miners' exposure to dusts, will typically be considered in evaluating causation claims.

Definition of Terms

Sensitivity, specificity, and other statistical measures are used to identify the diagnostic discrimination of tests. Table 2-1 identifies the factors involved in positive and negative risk factors. The lowercase labels for true- and false-positives and true- and false-negatives are used in the equations in the following definitions.

TABLE 2-1 Sensitivity and Specificity 4 × 4 Table

Positive Risk Factor	True-Positives (a)	False-Positives (b)
Negative Risk Factor	False-Negatives (c)	True-Negatives (d)
	Sensitivity (true positive/ sum of true positive and false negative)	Specificity (true negative/ sum of true negative and false positive)

Sensitivity is defined as true-positives divided by the sum of true-positives and false-negatives. In a 2 × 2 grid, sensitivity is represented by the following equation:

$$a/(a + c)$$

Specificity is defined as true-negatives divided by the sum of true-negatives and false-positives. In a 2 × 2 grid, specificity is represented by the following equation:

$$d/(b + d)$$

Positive predictive value is defined as true-positives divided by the sum of true-positives and false-positives and, in a 2 × 2 grid, it is represented by the following equation:

$$a/(a + b)$$

Negative predictive value is defined as true-negatives divided by the sum of true-negatives and false-negatives, as represented by the following equation in a 2 × 2 grid:

$$d/(c + d)$$

Positive and negative predictive values are not absolute attributes of test results; rather, they are attributes of results obtained from testing a specific population. Positive and negative predictive values depend on the prevalence of the disease in the population, which may differ from study to study.

The *likelihood ratio* (LR) is a statistical expression that describes how likely it is that a given test result would occur when a disease or condition is present compared with the likelihood that the same result would occur when the disease or condition is not present. Likelihood ratios are calculated by using the reported sensitivity and specificity. The LR for a positive result (positive LR) is the sensitivity divided by 1 minus specificity. The LR for a negative result (negative LR) is 1 minus sensitivity divided by the specificity.

Likelihood ratios of more than 1 increase the probability that the target disorder is present; the higher the LR, the greater the probability. Conversely, LRs of less than 1 decrease the probability that the target disorder is present; the smaller the LR, the greater the decrease in that probability. A positive LR tells us how much to increase a prediction of the probability of disease if the test result is positive, whereas a negative LR tells us how much to decrease a prediction if the test result is negative. A positive LR corresponds to the clinical concept of "ruling in" disease, and a negative LR corresponds to the clinical concept of "ruling out" disease. Calculations are as follows:

For tests:

LR, the chance that the test result is positive in people with the condition divided by the chance that the test result is positive in people without the condition:

$$[a/(a + c)]/[b/(b + d)]$$

Negative LR, the chance that the test result is negative in people with the condition divided by the chance that the test result is negative in people without the condition:

$$[c/(c + d)]/[d/(d + c)]$$

For subjects:

Positive LR, the chance of having the condition if the test result is positive divided by the chance of having the condition if the test result is negative:

$$[a/(a + b)]/[c/(c + d)]$$

Negative LR, the chance of not having the condition if the test result is positive divided by the chance of not having the condition if the test result is negative:

$$[b/(a + b)]/[d/(c + d)]$$

The following is a rough guide for LRs:
- More than 10.0 or less than 0.1 generate large, and often conclusive changes from pretest to posttest probability
- 5.0 through 10.0 and 0.1 through 0.2 generate moderate shifts in pretest to posttest probability
- 2.0 through 5.0 and 0.5 through 0.2 generate small (but sometimes important) changes in probability
- 1.0 through 2.0 and 0.5 through 1.0 alter probability to a small (and rarely important) degree

κ *(kappa or kappa statistic)* is a measure of the influence of chance in the agreement of two or more test results. Ideally, a "gold standard" is desirable in assessing whether a test accurately measures the presence or absence of a variable of interest. Historically, the gold standard for many diagnostic tests for cancer is a tissue diagnosis, established via surgical biopsy (or autopsy). In the real world, many variables of interest have no gold standard to determine their presence or absence. In such cases, two or more tests might be used to assess the presence or absence of the variable based on the assumption that the *agreement* or similarity between the test results increases the validity of the conclusion that the variable is present or absent. The kappa statistic is one measure of the correctness of such an assumption. It measures the extent to which the level of agreement of two or more test results is not attributed to chance. A kappa value of more than 0.6 is good agreement, and a kappa value of more than 0.8 indicates excellent agreement.

The *P value* is a measure of type I or alpha error. It measures the number of chances a positive result is actually a false-positive result. In a 2 × 2 grid, it is represented by b/(b + d). A *P* value of less than .05 is usually accepted as statistically significant, meaning that the study's result would occur by chance only 5 times in every 100 trials.

The β *(beta)* is a measure of the chance of a type II error or a false-negative result. It measures the number of chances a negative result is actually a false-negative result. In a 2 × 2 grid, it is represented by c/(c + a). Statisticians accept a beta error rate of approximately 20 % (β ~ .20), which corresponds to a power of 80% (Power = 1 − β).

Absolute risk is the ratio of people in whom the condition developed divided by the number of people in whom the condition potentially could have developed. In a 2 × 2 grid, it is represented by a/(a + b).

Relative risk compares the outcome if the risk factor is present with the outcome if the risk factor is not present. It is the risk of the outcome in the intervention group compared with the risk of the outcome in the control group. Relative risk is calculated by dividing the former with the latter. In a 2 × 2 grid, it is represented by (a/a + b)/(c/(c + d). Relative risk is usually calculated in treatment studies.

Relative risk reduction is defined as the proportion of the baseline risk removed or decreased by the intervention being evaluated. Mathematically, it is *1 minus the relative risk.*

The *odds ratio* compares the odds of having the risk factor if the condition is present with the odds of having the risk factor if the condition is absent. In a 2 × 2 grid, it is represented by (a/c)/(b/d). The odds ratio is usually calculated in prospective cohort or case-control epidemiologic studies on causation. In most medical trials, the odds and risks are approximately equal. Unfortunately, many authors calculate the odds ratio but report their findings as "calculated risks."

Effect size is defined as the difference in outcomes between the intervention and control groups divided by the standard deviation. It summarizes the number of standard deviations between the intervention and the control groups. Investigators can then calculate a weighted average of effect sizes. It is used extensively in meta-analyses.

Study Types

The best scientific evidence usually comes from randomized controlled trials, in which study groups are evaluated before exposure (prospectively), assigned randomly to different groups, and reevaluated following exposure. In practice, such studies are difficult and often impossible to perform on employed populations; hence, the relationship between occupational risk and illness or injury must be studied by using other methods. The methodological approach that allows causation inferences to be drawn from these studies will be discussed in Chapter 4. Nevertheless, it is important to recognize that inferences must be drawn with great care from studies in which risks are not controlled and the exposed and non-exposed populations may differ.

In many cases, a particular pattern of illness or injury is observed to be associated with a particular occupation or group of employees. Studying all patients with a given injury as the injuries occur is referred to as a *case series*. Studies of such cases can generate hypotheses for testing, but by themselves, these cases cannot prove that a risk factor is the cause of an injury or illness. A more rigorous design, the *case-control study*, is often used to evaluate occupational risk. In this design, patients with the injury or illness to be studied (cases) are matched according to age, sex, and exposure to other known risk factors for the illness with at least one (and usually two or more) subjects who are comparable but do not have the condition being studied (controls). Case-control studies typically allow researchers to determine whether a given risk has a statistically significant association with an illness and, sometimes, to evaluate how strong the risk seems to be (odds ratio, see the "Definition of Terms" section). Nevertheless, because association cannot definitively establish causation, other studies are usually necessary. Case-control studies are also retrospective, which means that cases are not enrolled in the study until after the illness or injury of interest has already occurred. This design may create unforeseen biases because researchers are unable to study patients before the illness or injury.

Cohort studies allow for prospective study of potential patients and, thus, offer better assurance that the differences between people who sustain injury or illness and people who do not are accounted for. Nevertheless, cohort studies require enrolling and following up on a large number of people over time, sometimes years, which is a disadvantage in the modern workplace. For example, people may change jobs before completion of the study. If done properly, however, cohort studies are probably second only to randomized, controlled trials for providing evidence for causation.

Some studies of one or a few cases may be published because the illness and/ or its treatment are new or unusual. Although these studies can be valuable scientific communications (e.g., the first reports of infection with the human immunodeficiency virus were published as case reports), they serve more to raise scientific interest than to answer questions and cannot establish causation or provide scientific evidence of treatment efficacy.

Because studies of uncommon injuries or illnesses can be difficult and expensive to perform, researchers often attempt to sift available published evidence as much as possible to evaluate information on risk factors and/or treatment efficacy. A *systematic review* is an attempt to compile all available evidence on a clinical question and then critically assess such factors as how studies were conducted and whether the conclusions reached can be applied to other employee groups. Studies included in a systematic review may differ in design, hypotheses, groups included or excluded, and other important characteristics. It is important, however, that authors of such reviews have used acceptable comprehensive methods to locate all published studies on a particular topic, or other biases may be introduced. A more rigorous attempt to pool study results from multiple studies is referred to as a *meta-analysis*. Usually, only studies with similar methods and designs can be pooled, and researchers generally try to establish rigorous criteria for including or excluding data before performing the analysis to reduce the chances of introducing additional biases. Although systematic reviews and meta-analyses may allow new conclusions to be reached, they cannot generate new information and are subject to additional levels of error and uncertainty. Compiling several small, poorly executed, randomized, controlled trials into a larger, conclusive data table does not automatically convert poor evidence into good evidence, but it may suggest that a larger study should be performed.

Level of Certainty Needed to Establish Causation

For an opinion about causation to be admitted into evidence, the person offering the opinion needs to attest that he or she holds the opinion with some level of certainty. On a spectrum, the level of certainty might range from "completely uncertain" to "certain beyond any doubt." Administrative tribunals and courts will not accept opinions based on the lower level of certainty, and, in complex areas of medicine, physicians do not often offer opinions at the lower end of the certainty spectrum.

In our federal system, each state is free to adopt statutes and regulations that govern its workers' compensation systems in almost any way it decides. Similarly, the federal government can adopt rules and policies for the various industrial insurance programs that it provides or regulates. Relevant to the issue of causation, each workers' compensation system may adopt its own rules for the level of certainty that must accompany an opinion about causation before the opinion can be admitted into evidence.

There has been no previous effort to summarize the requirements imposed by the various states on the mandated level of certainty attached to medical opinions about causation. Table 2-2 provides jurisdiction-specific information in this regard. Table 2-2 was compiled by using a variety of sources, including physicians, defense and plaintiff attorneys, insurance carriers, and state workers' compensation departments. The data were accurate when the table was prepared, but readers are encouraged to verify data because changes might have occurred as a result of legislation, regulation, or judicial interpretation.

Type of Evidence That Must Be Introduced to Prove Causation

Most causation thresholds, to a greater or lesser extent, are based on the concept of "an injury that arises, in whole or in significant part, out of or in the course and scope of employment" (Melhorn 2000).[37] Often, evidence sufficient to prove causation may range from an injury that may be related solely to an event that occurred in the course of employment to a preexisting condition that was unrelated to employment but was aggravated to some extent by an occupational event.

Generally, all states require that a relationship between the injured worker's condition and his or her employment be on a more-likely-than-not basis. In most states, that general causation threshold may be modified by state-specific presumptions. For example, a myocardial infarction occurring in policemen in many jurisdictions is considered to be due to the "stress" of the job and is compensable regardless of the circumstances (i.e., an irrebuttable presumption).

Some states allow aggravation or exacerbation of a preexisting condition to meet the work-compensability causation threshold. Kansas and a number of other states have a liberal aggravation rule. For example, California has a "1% rule": if an employee's asthma is made worse by work by 1%, it may become compensable; Texas has a 3% threshold. Other states have unique aggravation rules that require "objective" evidence of aggravation from occupational trauma.

North Carolina has a pending Supreme Court case that will decide how easily the aggravation standard will be met. Maryland and Virginia have unique twists: In Maryland, single trauma injuries are treated as a relationship of more-likely-than-not. However, for "repetitive trauma" injuries, the occupational connection must be the sole and exclusive cause. In Virginia, only some repetitive trauma injuries are compensable, whereas others are not. For example, carpal tunnel syndrome is compensable, but epicondylitis is not. The distinctions are purely arbitrary.

The terms *aggravation* and *exacerbation* may not always be used interchangeably. In Texas, for example, an aggravation that leads to a permanent worsening of an underlying or preexisting condition may be a compensable, work-related injury. An exacerbation, however, is interpreted as a temporary worsening of symptoms, such as pain, that does not change an individual's underlying condition; an exacerbation alone may not always be deemed compensable, even if it is caused by work. When giving opinions around the issue of causation, it is important for physicians to be aware of such jurisdictional nuances.

To carry legal weight for the causation threshold, a physician's opinions or conclusions must generally be expressed in terms of probability that a given condition has or has not arisen in the course and scope of employment (i.e., *is* or *is not* work-related). The courts usually prefer expression related to the 50% threshold, which may involve phrasing such as "more likely than not." However, the required terminology is often jurisdiction-specific. Table 2-2 includes some common terms used by various jurisdictions in the United States.

TABLE 2-2   States Causation Threshold Definitions for Work-Relatedness

Jurisdiction	Causation Threshold
Federal	
Federal Black Lung Program	RDOMC
Federal Employees Compensation Act	MPTN
Federal Employers Liability Act	MPTN in federal court or applicable phrase in state court
Jones Act	Any of the definitions
Longshore and Harbor Workers' Compensation Act	MPTN

TABLE 2-2 States Causation Threshold Definitions for Work-Relatedness (continued)

Jurisdiction	Causation Threshold
State	
Alabama	RDOMP
Alaska	RDOMP
Arizona	
Arkansas	RDOMC and RDOM
California	RDOMP
Colorado	Medically probable
Connecticut	Any of the definitions
Delaware	RDOMC
District of Columbia	More likely than not
Florida	RDOMC, and the work injury must be the major contributing cause of the condition (ie, >50% contributory). There must be significant objective findings (by physical examination and diagnostic studies) causally related to the injury.
Georgia	RDOMC
Hawaii	Any of the definitions
Idaho	Any of the definitions
Illinois	RDOMC
Indiana	RDOMC
Iowa	RDOMC
Kansas	RDOMP
Kentucky	Arising out of and in the course of employment that is the proximate cause producing a harmful change in the human organism evidenced by objective medical findings

TABLE 2-2 States Causation Threshold Definitions for Work-Relatedness (continued)

Jurisdiction	Causation Threshold
Louisiana	RDOMP
Maine	MPTN
Maryland	RDOMP
Massachusetts	RDOMC
Michigan	Any of the definitions
Minnesota	RDOMC
Mississippi	RDOMC
Missouri	Any of the definitions
Montana	MPTN
Nebraska	RDOMC
Nevada	MPTN
New Hampshire	RDOMC
New Jersey	RDOMP
New Mexico	MPTN
New York	Any of the definitions
North Carolina	RDOMC
North Dakota	With medical certainty and by objective medical evidence
Ohio	More likely than not/RDOMC determined by nonmedical means
Oklahoma	RDOMC, modifying legislation
Oregon	MPTN
Pennsylvania	RDOMC
Rhode Island	RDOMC
South Carolina	RDOMC
South Dakota	RDOMP

TABLE 2-2 States Causation Threshold Definitions for Work-Relatedness (continued)

Jurisdiction	Causation Threshold
Tennessee	Any of the definitions
Texas	RDOMP
Utah	Unable to determine
Vermont	MPTN
Virginia	RDOMC
Washington	MPTN
West Virginia	Unable to determine
Wisconsin	Any of the definitions
Wyoming	RDOMC

Abbreviations: MPTN, more probable than not, includes states using a "probability > 50%" standard; RDOMC, reasonable degree of medical certainty; RDOMP, reasonable degree of medical probability.

Summary

Injuries and illnesses must be shown to have a sufficient relationship with employment for workers' compensation benefits to be made available. Just what type of relationship must exist and just what level of causal certainty must exist before benefits will be awarded varies from jurisdiction to jurisdiction. In every state, two elements of causation must be shown for benefits to be awarded: (1) medical cause and (2) proximate cause. The medical cause deals with factual cause and the proximate cause with legal cause. The burden of proving causation may be eliminated or complicated by judicial or legislative presumptions.

A physician offering an opinion about causation should be familiar with the level of certainty required for the opinion to be admitted as evidence, the various statistical and epidemiologic concepts that relate to issues of causation, and the terminology used to communicate such concepts. Being able to interpret studies relevant to causation may be critical to the task of assessing whether work-relatedness exists in any given case and to explain an opinion to a court or board.

Chapter 3 discusses causal associations in detail, and Chapter 4 provides insight into six parts of assessment to determine work-relatedness for individual cases using inductive and deductive reasoning.

References

1. Atterbury MR, Limke JC, Lemasters GK, et al. Nested case-control study of hand and wrist work-related musculoskeletal disorders in carpenters. *Am J Ind Med.* 1996; 30:695-701.
2. Bahou YG. Carpal tunnel syndrome: a series observed at Jordan University Hospital (JUH), June 1999-December 2000. *Clin Neurol Neurosurg.* 2002; 104:49-53.
3. Barnhart S, Demers PA, Miller M. Carpal tunnel syndrome among ski manufacturing workers. *Scand J Work Environ Health.* 1991; 17:46-52.
4. Cannon LJ, Bernacki EJ, Walter SD. Personal and occupational factors associated with carpal tunnel syndrome. *J Occup Environ Med.* 1981;23:255-258.
5. Chiang HC, Chen S, Yu H, Ko Y. The occurrence of carpal tunnel syndrome in frozen food factory employees. J Med Sci. 1990;6:73-80.
6. Feldman RG, Travers PH, Chirico-Post J, Keyserling WM. Risk assessment in electronic assembly workers: carpal tunnel syndrome. *J Hand Surg [Am].* 1987; 12A:849-857.
7. Franklin GM, Haug J, Heyer N. Occupational carpal tunnel syndrome in Washington State, 1984-1988. *Am J Public Health.* 1991; 81:741-745.
8. Koskimies K, Farkkila M, Pyykko I, et al. Carpal tunnel syndrome in vibration disease. Br J Ind Med. 1990;47:411-416.
9. Loslever P, Ranaivosoa A. Biomechanical and epidemiological investigation of carpal tunnel syndrome at workplaces with high risk factors. *Ergonomics.* 1993; 36:537-554.
10. Maizlish N, Rudolph L, Dervin K, Sankaranarayan M. Surveillance and prevention of work-related carpal tunnel syndrome: an application of the Sentinel Events Notification System for Occupational Risks. *Am J Ind Med.* 1995; 27:715-729.
11. Ruess L, O'Connor SC, Cho KH, et al. Carpal tunnel syndrome and cubital tunnel syndrome: work-related musculoskeletal disorders in four symptomatic radiologists. *AJR Am J Roentgenol.* 2003; 181:37-42.
12. Silverstein BA, Fine LJ, Armstrong TJ. Occupational factors in carpal tunnel syndrome. *Am J Ind Med.* 1987; 11:343-358.
13. Tang X, Zhuang L, Lu Z. Carpal tunnel syndrome: a retrospective analysis of 262 cases and a one to one matched case-control study of 61 women pairs in relationship between manual housework and carpal tunnel syndrome. *Chin Med J (Engl).* 1999;112:44-48.
14. Wieslander G, Norback D, Gothe CJ, Juhlin L. Carpal tunnel syndrome (CTS) and exposure to vibration, repetitive wrist movements, and heavy manual work: a case-referent study. Br J Ind Med. 1989; 46:43-47.
15. Yagev Y, Carel RS, Yagev R. Assessment of work-related risks factors for carpal tunnel syndrome. *Isr Med Assoc J.* 2001;3:569-571.
16. Clarke Stevens J, Witt JC, Smith BE, Weaver AL. The frequency of carpal tunnel syndrome in computer users at a medical facility. *Neurology.* 2001; 56:1568-1570.
17. Nathan PA, Meadows KD, Doyle LS. Occupation as a risk factor for impaired sensory conductions of the median nerve at the carpal tunnel. *J Hand Surg [Br].* 1988; 13B:167-170.

18. Nathan PA, Takigawa K, Keniston RC, Meadows KD, Lockwood RS. Slowing of sensory conduction of the median nerve and carpal tunnel syndrome in Japanese and American industrial workers. *J Hand Surg [Br]*. 1994; 19B:30-34.

19. Ring D. Carpal tunnel syndrome causation. Paper presented at: 74th Annual Meeting of the American Academy of Orthopaedic Surgeons; February 16, 2007; San Diego, CA and Rosemont, IL, American Academy of Orthopaedic Surgeons 1-2, 2007.

20. Becker J, Nora DB, Gomes I, et al. An evaluation of gender, obesity, age and diabetes mellitus as risk factors for carpal tunnel syndrome. *Clin Neurophysiol.* 2002; 113:1429-1434.

21. Bland JD, Rudolfer SM. Clinical surveillance of carpal tunnel syndrome in two areas of the United Kingdom, 1991-2001. *J Neurol Neurosurg Psychiatry.* 2003; 74:1674-1679.

22. Bleecker ML, Bohlman M, Moreland R, Tipton A. Carpal tunnel syndrome: role of carpal canal size. *Neurology.* 1985;35:1599-1604.

23. Boz C, Ozmenoglu M, Altunayoglu V, Velioglu S, Alioglu Z. Individual risk factors for carpal tunnel syndrome: an evaluation of body mass index, wrist index and hand anthropometric measurements. *Clin Neurol Neurosurg.* 2004; 106:294-299.

24. DeKrom M, Kester ADM, Knipschild PG, Spaans F. Risk factors for carpal tunnel syndrome. *Am J Epidemiol.* 1990; 132:1102-1110.

25. Ettema AM, Amadio PC, Zhao C, Wold LE, An KN. A histological and immunohistochemical study of the subsynovial connective tissue in idiopathic carpal tunnel syndrome. *J Bone Joint Surg Am.* 2004; 86A:1458-1466.

26. Gelberman RH, Hergenroeder PT, Hargens AR, Lundborg G, Akeson WH. The carpal tunnel syndrome: a study of carpal canal pressures. *J Bone Joint Surg Am.* 1981;63A:380-383.

27. Geoghegan JM, Clark DI, Bainbridge LC, Smith C, Hubbard R. Risk factors in carpal tunnel syndrome. *J Hand Surg [Br]*. 2004;29:315-320.

28. Hakim AJ, Cherkas L, El Zayat S, MacGregor AJ, Spector TD. The genetic contribution to carpal tunnel syndrome in women: a twin study. *Arthritis Rheum.* 2002; 47:275-279.

29. Jinrok O, Zhao C, Amadio PC, et al. Vascular pathologic changes in the flexor tenosynovium (subsynovial connective tissue) in idiopathic carpal tunnel syndrome. *J Orthop Res.* 2004;22:1310-1315.

30. Karpitskaya Y, Novak CB, Mackinnon SE. Prevalence of smoking, obesity, diabetes mellitus, and thyroid disease in patients with carpal tunnel syndrome. *Ann Plast Surg.* 2002;48:269-273.

31. Schottland JR, Kirschberg GJ, Fillingim R. Median nerve latencies in poultry processing workers: an approach to resolving the role of industrial "cumulative trauma" in the development of carpal tunnel syndrome. *J Occup Environ Med.* 1991; 33:627-630.

32. Vessey MP, Villard-Mackintosh L, Yeates D. Epidemiology of carpal tunnel syndrome in women of childbearing age findings in a large cohort study. *Int J Epidemiol.* 1990;19:655-659.

33. Chapell RW, Bruening W, Mitchell MD, Reston JT, Treadwell JR. Diagnosis and treatment of worker-related musculoskeletal disorders of the upper extremity. Rockville, MD; Agency for Healthcare Research and Quality; 2003. Evidence Report/Technology Assessment 62.

CHAPTER 2

34. Talmage JB, Melhorn JM. *A Physician's Guide to Return to Work.* Chicago, IL: AMA Press; 2005.

35. Guyatt G, Rennie D. *User's Guides To The Medical Literature A Manual for Evidence-Based Clinical Practice.* Chicago, IL: AMA Press; 2002:1-736.

36. Spindler KP, Kuhn JE, Dunn W, et al. Reading and reviewing the orthopaedic literature: a systematic, evidence-based medicine approach. *J Am Acad Orthop Surg.* 2005; 13:220-229.

CHAPTER

Causal Associations and Determination of Work-Relatedness

Kurt T. Hegmann, MD, MPH and Steven J. Oostema, MS

Causation of musculoskeletal disorders (MSDs) has been controversial, in large part owing to numerous weaknesses in the available, quantitatively large but qualitatively relatively sparse epidemiologic literature. These sparse data are in contrast with extensive, large-scale studies on other disorders such as neoplasms and cardiovascular disease. The differences are in large part attributable to disproportionate funding of research into fatal outcomes. In the case of MSDs, there are few prospective cohort studies, samples are small, exposures are not well measured in many studies, biases are not insignificant, and confounders are generally only partially controlled.

Epidemiologic vs. Individual Causal Assessments

Causal assessments are typically performed in two major realms. The first is an epidemiologically based causal assessment to evaluate whether a purported "risk factor," (e.g., force, repetition, obesity, or diabetes mellitus) is truly a disease determinant rather than merely an associated factor. If the factor is causal, then elimination of the risk factor *must* result in fewer cases of the particular disease.

The second type of causal assessment requires application of the aforementioned evaluation on an individual basis (e.g., assessment of whether a side effect is from a therapeutic modality, linkage of a disorder with an accident, or determination of work-relatedness of disease). For determinations of work-relatedness of disease, the evidence from the clinical evaluation, which includes the history, physical examination and possible supporting testing, and studies of a patient, is assessed to determine whether work is a significant factor in the development, material aggravation, or persistence of the condition. Therefore, the assessment of work-relatedness of a disease for any one individual necessarily relies on the causal epidemiologic association. A comprehensive review of the history and development of the science of causal inference follows this short discussion of causal association.

Epidemiologically Based Causal Associations

Epidemiologically based causal associations involve six main steps (Table 3-1). Each step is discussed in the following text.

Literature Review

The initial step in determining whether a causal association exists is collection of all epidemiologic studies on a subject through exhaustive literature searches. Although the accidental omission of some studies may not be fatal to the conclusions, omission of better designed studies (e.g., omitting prospective cohort studies rather than cross-sectional studies) substantially increases the probability of an error.

TABLE 3-1   *Steps for Concluding a Causal Association Exists*

---

1. Collect all epidemiologic literature on the disorder

2. Identify the design of each study

3. Assess the methods of each study
   a. Exposure assessment methods and potential biases
   b. Disease ascertainment methods and potential biases
   c. Absence of significant uncontrolled confounders; consideration of residual confounding
   d. Addressing of other potential biases
   e. Adequacy of biostatistical methods and analytic techniques

4. Ascertain statistical significance and the degree to which chance may have produced the results

5. Assess the studies using the Updated Hill Criteria; apply the criteria to individual studies (especially 5a-5c) and to the studies as a whole (5a-5l)
   a. Temporality
   b. Strength of association
   c. Dose-response relationship
   d. Consistency
   e. Coherence
   f. Specificity
   g. Plausibility
   h. Reversibility
   i. Prevention/elimination
   j. Experiment
   k. Analogy
   l. Predictive performance

6. Conclusion about the degree to which a causal association is or is not present

---

CHAPTER 3

Identification of Study Design

The second step in ascertaining causal association is the identification of epidemiologic study designs. The relative value of various study designs has been recognized for many years and has been incorporated in prior formal literature assessments.[1-7] The study design pyramid (Figure) may be used to rank the relative value of various types of study designs. In general, the prospective cohort study is the strongest epidemiologic study design for most exposures and is assumed to have better characteristics than the other designs. However, the hierarchy of studies in the design pyramid is not definitive because it is possible to have a poorly conducted cohort study but a well-conducted case-control study. Still, in the absence of evidence to the contrary, these rankings are assumed to hold true. Determination of the type of study design should be done independent of the author's statement in the methods section of the research report because the study design identified in the report might be inaccurate.

Study Design Pyramid

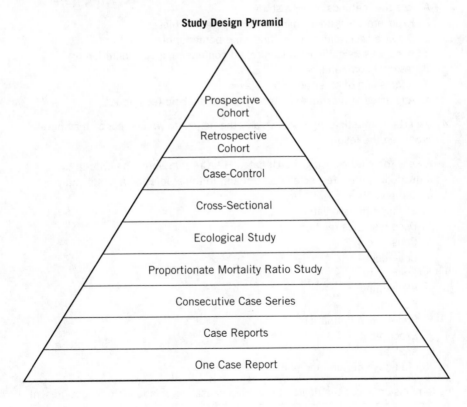

Prospective Cohort

Retrospective Cohort

Case-Control

Cross-Sectional

Ecological Study

Proportionate Mortality Ratio Study

Consecutive Case Series

Case Reports

One Case Report

Assessment of Study Methods

In this step, the methods of each study are critiqued for strengths and weaknesses. Biases need to be carefully considered because even one major uncontrolled bias may be a potentially fatal study flaw. The three major areas for biases to exert their effects are in the measurement of (1) exposure, (2) disease, and (3) confounders. Some of the more common exposure-related biases include selection bias (differential selection of people with and without the exposure for inclusion in the study), information bias (different exposure information obtained for the groups for comparison), recall bias (differential rates at which exposure is recalled, typically such that those with disease recall more exposure than those without disease, sampling bias (different probabilities of including subjects with and without exposure), and interviewer bias (researcher-based bias, such as a different degree of questioning based on researcher knowledge of the exposure status of individual subjects). Exposure measurement is ideally performed in a blinded manner. If measurement is not blinded, the concern is increased that job exposure measurements are artificially increased in the jobs the researcher believes have produced injuries.

Frequently, research reports do not include exposure measurements because most studies have relied on job titles for classification of exposure.[8] Another problem with exposure measurement is the lack of clarity about the validity and reliability of the methods used.[9] When evaluating a study, it is important to analyze the methods section of the study to ascertain the degree to which these factors are reported. For example, if the study only reports exposures by job categories, then it should be viewed as hypothesis-generating. Furthermore, the study should also be accorded a lower level of assurance that it represents the truth. If a study reports detailed exposure-metrics that one could duplicate in a local study, then there is more assurance that the exposure aspects are valid and reliable.

Disease status is susceptible to biases that include selection, information, recall, interviewer, and sampling. These biases are parallel with those for exposure measurement described previously. Measurement of disease status is ideally blinded from exposure. In addition, because there is much variability in diagnoses, an independent, standardized measurement is the ideal but rarely performed approach.[8-9]

Adequate case definitions in epidemiologic studies are rare. Considerations include consistency of symptoms, distribution of symptoms for inclusion, absence of confounding clinical conditions, physical examination findings, and, when relevant, confirmatory testing (e.g., imaging or electrodiagnostic studies).

All potential disease confounders should be addressed in a well-designed study. Addressing confounders can be particularly problematic in a disorder such as carpal tunnel syndrome for which there are at least 50 reported "risk factors." Objective measurements of the potential confounders are best, when possible, and reduce the probability of residual confounding.

Other potential biases may include the healthy worker effect, publication, lead time, and length. The healthy worker effect involves better health status among the employed than the underemployed, so any study that involves a comparison between an employed population and the general population that includes the underemployed is prone to an inherent bias, with different background rates of disease. Publication bias involves the greater probability to be published if the findings are positive, rather than negative. Lead time bias involves disease surveillance and the tendency for people to be diagnosed earlier, but the overall lifespan is not changed, thus there is an appearance that the surveillance successfully increased lifespan when in fact there was no impact. Length bias involves the fact that surveillance and subsequent follow-up may be biased by not having the short term cases or deaths to be included in the initial surveillance or screening interval. A consideration for proper statistical techniques is additionally required, including whether the correct statistical test was selected and whether multivariate models were properly constructed.

Ascertainment of Statistical Significance

In this step, the overall study results are assessed for statistical significance, and an overall assessment is made of whether the statistical methods selected were appropriate. The goal is to identify whether a study used appropriate statistical methods, whether findings are considered statistically significant, and the role that chance may have had in the results of each study. Although Hill argued that, "(b)eyond that (tests of significance) . . .contribute nothing to the 'proof' of our hypothesis,"[10(p299)] it is clear, particularly with the advent of multivariate regression and survival analysis techniques, there are many additional considerations at this step that were not present in the mid-1960s. Such considerations include appropriateness of the statistical tests selected, strengths and weaknesses of those tests, as well as problems with multiple comparisons which increase the probability of finding statistically significant, but non-causal associations by chance alone.

Assessment Using the Updated Hill Criteria

The next step in the assessment of a causal association is to evaluate the body of epidemiologic literature with respect to various factors. Although previously referred to as the Hill Criteria for Causation[10] these have been updated and expanded by numerous authors (See Table 3-1). The factors used to evaluate the epidemiologic literature include temporality (the exposure must precede the disease), strength of association (the higher the relative risk or odds ratio, the more likely the association is causal), dose-response relationship (more exposure results in more disease), and consistency (the same results are found in different populations with the same or similar exposure and the same disease, using different study designs and different methods).

Coherence requires that other collateral information is supportive of an association (e.g., lung cancer occurred in more men in the 1960s and men had started smoking to a far greater degree than women earlier in the 20th Century). Specificity is another measure of the effectiveness of a test or the selectiveness of the link or association (e.g., a physical factor or chemical causes either one disorder or a limited number of disorders, rather than multiple disparate conditions). Plausibility implies that the association being considered makes biological sense or is reasonable to support an exposure-response association. Reversibility considers that if the inciting stimulus is removed the disease or condition improves or regresses. Prevention/elimination is similar to reversibility in that if the exposure can be prevented or eliminated from a population, the development of the disease or condition does not occur. Experimental evidence includes potential animal and/or human laboratory experiments that may lend support to the purported association (e.g., for musculoskeletal disorders, it may include estimated human shoulder strength capabilities from laboratory studies). Analogy involves whether there is an analogous exposure-response relationship known to which the current purported relationship is similar (e.g., herpes simplex virus may be teratogenic, as may be zoster infection which is from the same virus family). Predictive performance suggests that the purported dose-response relationship could be used to predict the morbidity in another location, thus testing the accuracy of the proposed association.

Conclusions about Causal Association

The final step is the overall assessment of whether a causal association is likely to exist. Because this step requires substantial judgment, it also requires that the person(s) evaluating the body of evidence make statements of how sure they are that there is or is not a causal association. For example, if all steps are addressed with multiple, well-designed studies and all criteria are addressed, the causal association may be said to be concluded with a high degree of certainty. Alternatively, if there are some statistically positive studies on a disorder, few cohort studies, some conflicting results, and only a few criteria that are consistently addressed, it may be accurate to state that although there is some evidence, a causal association cannot be concluded. Finally, in situations in which there is no epidemiologic evidence, it should be apparent that a discussion of causal relationships (either the body of evidence on the topic, or an individualized work-relatedness determination) cannot begin and any such discussions are speculative.

Determination of Work-Relatedness of Disease

There are several steps for the determination of work-relatedness of a patient's disease, including the MSDs. Although different methods have been reported, perhaps the most commonly used is that developed by the National Institute for

Occupational Safety and Health (NIOSH)[8] and further adapted by the American College of Occupational and Environmental Medicine (ACOEM).[11] Because this may be the most common structured method used and it does not seem to have major weaknesses, it is the method outlined in this chapter used herein. Table 3-2 lists the steps of the NIOSH/ACOEM method for determining the work-relatedness of a disease. Because these are steps, they must be performed in order, and the failure of a step should stop the process of further evaluation.

TABLE 3-2   National Institute for Occupational Safety and Health/ American College of Occupational and Environmental Medicine Steps for the Determination of Work-Relatedness of a Disease*

---

1. Identify evidence of disease

2. Review and assess the available epidemiologic evidence for a causal relationship

3. Obtain and assess the evidence of exposure

4. Consider other relevant factors

5. Judge the validity of testimony

6. Form conclusions about the work-relatedness of the disease in the person undergoing evaluation

---

*Adapted from Kusnetz and Hutchison Eds. DHEW, CDC, NIOSH, Pub. No. PB298-561; 1979 and Occupational Medicine Practice Guidelines, 2nd Ed., ACOEM OEM Press, 2004.

Identify Evidence of Disease

The first step involves the evidence for or against the presence of a particular disorder, including symptoms, physical examination findings, confirmatory testing (e.g., nerve conduction study), and exclusion of other potential diagnoses. For example, is the distribution of tingling characteristic of a specific peripheral nerve distribution? Is there corroborating evidence from an electrodiagnostic study? Are other disorders in the differential diagnosis eliminated from consideration, or are major alternative diagnostic considerations considered unlikely to be present? If the evidence does not support a particular disorder, the assessment process ceases, and work-relatedness of the disorder is unlikely.

Review and Assess the Available Epidemiologic Evidence

The second step is the epidemiologic consideration. To have a scientific basis for the determination that a condition is work-related, there must be epidemiologic support for the condition to have an occupational basis. Unfortunately, this step is rather difficult with some MSDs because of conflicting epidemiologic evidence or owing to unclear attributable proportions of occupational and non-occupational factors. This step incorporates all steps in the prior section on a comprehensive evaluation of the epidemiological evidence. What study designs have been utilized? Have biases and confounders been adequately addressed? How well does the body of evidence support the causal criteria?

Obtain and Assess the Evidence of Exposure

Consideration of the evidence of exposure is the third step. There is a hierarchy of exposure data (Table 3-3). The highest quality data are measurements of the tasks of the worker. The least reliable level of exposure evidence is the worker's job title or self-report of exposure. Typical practitioners do not have experience in the assessment of these data and necessarily rely on others for the information, not unlike the reliance on industrial hygienists for chemical exposure measurements for toxicologic problems.

TABLE 3-3   Hierarchy of Exposure Data*

Type of Data	Approximation to Actual Exposure
1. Quantified personal or individualized measurement	Best
2. Quantified surrogate of exposure (another worker used to infer all workers' exposures doing same job)	↑
3. Quantified pseudosurrogates of exposure (another worker used to infer all workers' exposures doing similar jobs)	
4. Employment in a defined job category	
5. Employment in a defined job trade	
6. Employment in a plant or obtained from the employer	Worst

*Adapted from Niewenhuijsen MJ. (Ed). *Exposure Assessment in Occupational and Environmental Epidemiology.* Oxford (2003).

CHAPTER 3

Consider Other Relevant Factors

In the fourth step, multiple categories of such factors—risk factors, covariates, prior injuries, psychological factors, other diseases, disorders, and efficacy of treatments—need to be considered. Are there prior injuries, diseases or other exposures that cause or contribute to this condition? Are there risk factors that explain the person's condition irrespective of other exposures? How strongly are those factors associated with that disorder? Underlying the other factors are the epidemiologic underpinnings of the factors as *risk factors* for the disorder. Does the epidemiologic evidence support the listed factors as risk factors for the condition? How strongly have those studies adequately addressed confounders?

Judge the Validity of Testimony

The fifth step is the consideration of the validity of testimony. This step involves two main issues. One is information that may suggest to the provider that there is a conflict regarding some important aspect, such as date of injury, mechanism, or prior injury status. The other may deal with broader issues, such as opinions given that are not evidence-based or whether analyses and/or tests performed were appropriate. Often, there is no information available to the practitioner, even if it does exist, that suggests a problem with the patient's history, another's credentials, or analyses. Occasionally, the practitioner is the sole source of such information (e.g., the practitioner is the first to learn that the problem began at work or outside of work) and it is then incumbent on the practitioner to properly record such factors. In circumstances where the practitioner is knowledgeable about the truth or has a strong basis for an opinion (e.g., knowledge that the person is capable of performing work despite statements to the contrary), then such opinions should be stated and written. However, the step to document such incidents can be quite complex. For example, in cases where the examiner is not knowledgeable if an exposure occurred, the proper protocol is to record what is known or believed, qualify all statements appropriately by noting a lack of knowledge and/or certainty, and leave the remainder to a trier of fact.

Conclusions about Work-Relatedness

The last step involves reassessment of data obtained in the entire series of steps while taking into account the legal jurisdiction in which the action is occurring. The practitioner should know the definitions that determine whether the disorder is work-related. The determination should follow logically from each of the aforementioned steps. For example, a worker with a lower back injury, who experienced pain shortly after a manual patient transfer, has a condition that is associated with that exposure—whether they have nonoccupational conditions or not—is a straightforward case. In such instance, appropriate and supportive documentation should facilitate rapid treatment and finally, recovery under workers compensation. Conversely, if a 50-year old worker has a rotator cuff tear without a clear accident or injury, it can be said that the epidemiologic knowledge of his condition is poor. Hence, in this incident, there are no significant occupational exposures and other factors may be present, which makes it unlikely that the patient has a work-related condition regardless of a verbal claim to the contrary.

References

1. Canadian Task Force guide to Clinical Preventive Health Care. November 2000. http://www.ctphc.org/guide.htm. Accessed May 15, 2007.
2. United States Preventive Services Task Force. January 2007. Agency for Healthcare Research and Quality. Rockville, MD. http://www.ahrq.gov/clinic/uspstfab.htm. Accessed May 15, 2007.
3. The Cochrane Collaboration. Evidence Based Healthcare. http://www.cochrane.org/docs/ebm/htm. Accessed May 15, 2007.
4. Williams JK. Understanding evidence-based medicine: a primer. *Am J Obstet Gynecol.* 2001;185:275-278.
5. Feinstein AR. Efficacy of different research structures in preventing bias in the analysis of causation. *Clin Pharmacol Ther.* 1979;26:129-141.
6. Feinstein AR. Scientific standards vs statistical associations and biologic logic in the analysis of causation. *Clin Pharmacol Ther.* 1979;25:481-492.
7. National Research Council and the Institute of Medicine. *Musculoskeletal Disorders and the Workplace: Low Back and the Upper Extremities.* Washington, DC: National Academies Press; 2001.
8. National Institute for Occupational Safety and Health, Musculoskeletal Disorders and Workplace Factors: A critical review of epidemiologic evidence for work-related musculoskeletal disorders of the neck, upper extremity, and low back. Bernard B, Ed. US Dept. Health and Human Services, 1997.
9. Niewenhuijsen MJ. (Ed). Exposure Assessment in Occupational and Environmental Epidemiology. Oxford University Press: Oxford 2003.
10. Hill AB. The environment and disease: association or causation. *Proc R Soc Med.* 1965; 58:295-300.
11. Occupational Medicine Practice Guidelines, 2nd Ed.,ACOEM (Glass LS, Ed) OEM Press, 2004.

CHAPTER 3

Bibliography

Bailey L, Gordis L, Green M. Reference guide on epidemiology, V: the role of epidemiology in proving individual causation. In: Federal Judicial Center. *Reference Manual on Scientific Evidence.* Washington DC: Federal Judicial Center; 1994:167-170.

Buechley RW. A formulation of some logical problems in epidemiology. *Am J Epidemiol.* 1978;107:265.

Doll R, Hill AB. Mortality in relation to smoking: ten years' observations of British doctors. *Br Med J.* 1964;1:1399-1410.

Gelbke P. Comments to 'Can we reverse the burden of proof?' *Toxicol Lett.* 1997;90:233-234.

Goldsmith DF. Importance of causation for interpreting occupational epidemiology research: a case study of quartz and cancer. *Occup Med.* 1996;11:433-449.

Hansson SO. Can we reverse the burden of proof? *Toxicol Lett.* 1997;90:223-228.

Harber P, Shusterman D. Medical causation analysis heuristics. *JOEM.* 1996; 38:577-586.

Holland PW. Statistics and causal inference. *J Am Stat Assoc.* 1986;81:945-960.

Kusnetz S, Hutchison MK. *A Guide to the Work-Relatedness of Disease. Revised Edition.* Cincinnati, OH: US Dept of Health, Education, and Welfare, Public Health Service, Centers for Disease Control, National Institute for Occupational Safety and Health; 1979. DHEW (NIOSH) publication 79-116.

Maclure M. Popperian refutation in epidemiology. *Am J Epidemiol.* 1985;121:343-350.

Miettinen OS. Causal and preventive interdependence: elementary principles. *Scand J Work Environ Health.* 1982;8:159-168.

Muir DCF. Cause of occupational disease. *Occup Environ Med.* 1995;52:289-293.

Poole C, Rothman K. Our conscientious objection to the epidemiology wars. *J Epidemiol Community Health.* 1998;52:613-614.

Renton A. Epidemiology and causation: a realist view. *J Epidemiol Community Health.* 1994;48:79-85.

Riegelman R. Contributory cause: unnecessary and insufficient. *Postgrad Med.* 1979;66:177-179.

Rothman KJ. Synergy and antagonism in cause-effect relationships. *Am J Epidemiol.* 1974;99:385-388.

Rothman KJ, Poole C. Science and policy making. *Am J Public Health.* 1985;75: 340-341.

Samet JM, Lee NL. Bridging the gap: perspectives on translating epidemiologic evidence into policy. *Am J Epidemiol.* 2001;154(suppl):S1-S3.

Samet JM, Schnatter R, Gibb H. Invited commentary: epidemiology and risk assessment. *Am J Epidemiol.* 1998;148:929-936.

Shy CM. The failure of academic epidemiology: witness for the prosecution. *Am J Epidemiol.* 1997;145:479-484.

Susser M. Invited commentary on "Causation and disease: a chronological journey: the Thomas Parran Lecture." *Am J Epidemiol.* 1995;142:1125.

Szklo M. The evaluation of epidemiologic evidence for policy-making. *Am J Epidemiol.* 2001;154(suppl):S13-S17.

CHAPTER 3

US Department of Health, Education and Welfare. Criteria for judgment. In: US Department of Health, Education and Welfare, Public Health Service. *Smoking and Health: Report of the Advisory Committee to the Surgeon General of the Public Health Service.* Washington DC: US Dept of Health, Education and Welfare; 1964:19-21. DHEW publication (PHS) 1103.

Walker AM. "Kangaroo court": invited commentary on Shy's "The failure of academic epidemiology: witness for the prosecution." *Am J Epidemiol.* 1997;145:485-486.

Weed DL. Epidemiologic evidence and causal inference. *Hematol Oncol Clin North Am.* 2000;14:797-807.

Weed DL. On the use of causal criteria. *Int J Epidemiol.* 1997;26:1137-1141.

CHAPTER 3

CHAPTER 4
Methodology

J. Mark Melhorn, MD, and Kurt T. Hegmann, MD, MPH

Methods for Determining Work-Relatedness

Criteria to evaluate scientific evidence for the work-relatedness of various health conditions and effects have been accepted by epidemiologic and public health organizations. Epidemiologic surveillance provides aggregate information about occupational risk and the development of specific medical conditions. Physicians are often asked to provide an opinion for a specific case in which the workplace factors may be the only identifiable cause, one among several contributing causes, or one of several possible causes, each of which could independently produce the condition.

In general, a disease or an injury is considered occupational if the following criteria are met:

1. The medical findings of disease or injury are compatible with the effects of a disease-producing agent or an injury producing event to which the worker has been exposed;
2. Sufficient exposure is present in the worker's occupational environment to have caused the disease; and
3. The weight of evidence supports the disease as having occupational rather than nonoccupational origin.

The need to identify whether the criteria are met led to development of six parts of assessment for the six steps determining work-relatedness by the National Institute for Occupational Safety and Health[1] that were modified by Glass.[2]

1. Evidence of disease. What is the disease? Is the diagnosis correct? Does the evidence (e.g., history, physical examination findings, and results of diagnostic studies) support or fail to support the diagnosis?
2. Epidemiologic data. What is the epidemiologic evidence for the disease or condition? Do the data support a relationship with work?
3. Evidence of exposure. What evidence, predominantly objective, is there that the level of occupational environmental exposure (e.g., frequency, intensity, and duration) could cause the disease?
4. Other relevant factors. What other relevant factors are present in this case? Are there individual risk factors other than the occupational environmental exposure that could contribute to the development of the disease? For example, if the diagnosis is carpal tunnel syndrome, is the worker pregnant, obese, or diabetic?
5. Validity of evidence. Are there confounding or conflicting data to suggest that information obtained in the assessment is inaccurate?
6. Evaluation and conclusions. Do the data obtained in the preceding assessment support the presence of a work-related disease?

Study Design

One purpose of this book is to describe the literature basis for assertions about the causal relationship between work-related (or putatively work-related) exposures and identifiable anatomic and/or physiologic alterations leading to disease or dysfunction. The literature on industrial causation (occupational exposure) is relatively sparse.

In contrast, there is a large body of literature on causal relationships between non–work-related factors (e.g., genetic, dietary, age-related, anthropomorphic, and environmental) and disease. The evidence basis used to determine causation as it relates to these factors has generally been well-characterized, with the strengths and limitations of available evidence well appreciated by experts in the relevant medical specialties. Therefore, the literature on the causal relationships between nonoccupational factors and diseases was not rated. For each chapter that deals with specific medical diagnoses, determinations as to strength of the association with causation reflects expert opinion on the overall scientific merit based on the scientific validity of the current body of literature. Each conclusion is supported by references.

The literature on the causal relationship between industrial disease and occupational factors was obtained and reviewed in depth. When insufficient literature was available to evaluate factors and exposures to make a determination, the conclusions reflect our opinions. The basis for these conclusions is explicitly described and often reflects extrapolations from available literature, analyzed in the context of the anatomy and physiology of the organ system or body part putatively affected by the exposure. Research activities or study outcomes that allow for further clarification of causation in relation to the conditions discussed are described as well.

When sufficient occupational-exposures literature is available for evaluation, we propose the following five-step method as a guide for analyses. The term, *study* (any published article included in the relevant analysis) may be interchanged with the term *article*.

CHAPTER 4

Quality Scoring for Epidemiologic Studies on Musculoskeletal and Other Occupational Disorders

Step 1

A thorough literature search is performed to collect all peer-reviewed publications on a relevant topic using specific search criteria (Table 4-1). Review articles and meta-analyses are included for a comprehensive literature search.

Step 2

Each original study is submitted to a panel of three raters who are physicians or hold doctoral degrees and have experience in occupational epidemiologic studies (or equivalent). Each article is evaluated by a quality scoring scale, from 0 to 140 points (Table 4-2). The quality score for a given article is submitted to an independent staff member who compiles the quality scores for each of the three raters. If the range of quality scores is more than 20 points, the article will be discussed in a meeting or teleconference. If necessary, the article will be re-rated to obtain the mean rating, which will be the final quality score for the article. If the range of quality scores is less than 20 points, the mean score will be the final quality score for the article.

Step 3

Each article is also reviewed by a panel of at least three raters to identify the most appropriate study design classification. If there is not complete agreement on the study-design classification, the design would be discussed in a meeting or teleconference. If agreement is still not reached, the majority opinion will be used to determine the classification of the study.

Step 4

Each article quality score is multiplied by a weight factor (Table 4-3) to obtain the final impact rating (Table 4-4).

Step 5

To determine the strength of evidence for causation for a specific topic or diagnosis, the final impact ratings for all relevant studies are summed. It is unrealistic to expect that every possible occupational exposure risk will have been studied. Therefore, there might be no scientific evidence for some medical conditions and their causation. When possible, the conclusion of causal associations and determination of work-relatedness are based on multiple, high-quality studies, making it necessary to combine the quality ratings of individual studies into an aggregated rating that characterizes the body of evidence on which the conclusion is based. The evidence in the literature for a relationship between workplace factors and the development of a specific medical condition is classified into the categories shown in Table 4-5.

TABLE 4-1 Search Criteria

Database	Terms of Search	No. Found	No. Reviewed in Detail	No. Accepted
PubMed				
AHRQ				
CINAHL				
Cochrane Register				
EMBASE				
EMB Online				
MEDLARS				

Abbreviations: AHRQ, Agency for Healthcare Research and Quality; CINAHL, Cumulative Index of Nursing and Allied Health Literature; EMB, EMB is an evidence-based medicine database; EMBASE, EMBASE is a biomedical and pharmacological database; MEDLARS, MEDLARS is used for preparing publications like Index Medicus®.

CHAPTER 4

TABLE 4-2 Quality Scoring Scale*

Criteria	Range of Scores	Rating Anchor	Explanation of Rating Anchors
Clearly defined groups	0-10	0	Study lacks clearly defined groups or reports such groups, but subsequent analyses of data suggest groups were not clearly defined
		5	Clearly defined groups mentioned, but descriptions incomplete; or other questions about adequacy of study group identification cannot be adequately addressed
		10	Clearly defined groups specifically stated; reported data show well-defined groups
Exposure measurements	0-10	0	No mention of how exposures were measured
		2.5	Exposure measurement by job classification or questionnaires given to subjects; or assessment methods unclear
		5	Mixture of objective and subjective measures and lack of clarity and completeness about how measures were done; individualized assessment required for rating of 5 or higher
		7.5	Measures mostly objective and individualized; few questions about how exposure assessments were accomplished
		10	Exposures objectively measured and individualized; exposure assessments well described
Participation and dropout rates	0-10	0	Participation rate less than 50% or not mentioned (for cohort studies, annual dropout rate of 40% or higher)

TABLE 4-2 Quality Scoring Scale* (continued)

Criteria	Range of Scores	Rating Anchor	Explanation of Rating Anchors
		2.5	Participation rate of 50% to 59% (for cohort studies, annual dropout rate of above 30%)
		5	Participation rate of 60% to 69% (for cohort studies, annual dropout rate of 20%-29%)
		7.5	Participation rate of 70% to 79% (for cohort studies, annual dropout rate of 10%-19%)
		10	Participation rate of 80% or more (for cohort studies, annual dropout rate of less than 10%)
Blinding of exposure measurements	0-10	0	No mention of how measurements were blinded; measurement methods unlikely to result in blinding; or measurement relied on subjects' perceptions of exposure
		2.5	Some mention of blinding, but significant questions remain; complete blinding unlikely
		5	Mention of blinding; questions remain about adequacy of blinding
		7.5	Blinding procedures carried out; minor questions remain about adequacy of procedures
		10	Blinding procedures described that would result in exposure assessments being blinded
Health outcomes measurements	0-10	0	No mention of how health outcomes were assessed
		2.5	Measurement by administrative data-bases; or methods unclear or would result in substantial misclassifications

CHAPTER 4

TABLE 4-2 Quality Scoring Scale* (continued)

Criteria	Range of Scores	Rating Anchor	Explanation of Rating Anchors
		5	Measurement by individualized assessments of complete population; questions remain about adequacy of assessments or objective measures not used
		7.5	Measurement mostly objective; few questions about how outcome assessments were accomplished
		10	Health outcomes individually measured on all subjects; the most objective methods used; health outcomes assessments well described
Frequency of health outcomes assessments	0-10	0	Only one assessment
		2.5	More than one assessment but annually or less frequently; or more frequent assessments that do not include entire study population
		5	Health outcomes assessments of population at least every 6 months
		7.5	Health outcomes assessment of population at least quarterly
		10	Health outcomes assessments of population at least monthly
Blinding of health outcomes assessments	0-10	0	No mention of how health outcomes assessments were blinded; or methods unlikely to result in blinding
		2.5	Some mention of blinding; significant questions remain; complete blinding unlikely
		5	Mention of blinding; questions remain about adequacy of blinding

TABLE 4-2 Quality Scoring Scale* (continued)

Criteria	Range of Scores	Rating Anchor	Explanation of Rating Anchors
		7.5	Blinding procedures carried out; minor questions remain about adequacy of procedures
		10	Blinding procedures described that would result in health outcomes assessments being blinded
Comparable groups adjustment for confounders	0-20	0	Major confounders (individual risk factors, e.g., age, sex, obesity, diabetes mellitus, tobacco, or trauma) unaddressed; or statistical control procedures inadequate to control for confounders
		5	Some control for major confounders; significant questions remain; complete control for confounders unlikely
		10	Confounders addressed; attempts made to control for confounders; questions remain about adequacy of control for confounders
		15	Confounders addressed; adequate control procedures likely used; minor questions remain about adequacy of procedures used or minor confounders uncontrolled
		20	All major and minor confounders addressed; control procedures used; no remaining questions about adequacy of control for confounders; confounders measured objectively when possible
Bias	0-10	0	Significant biases (not coded else-where) possible that are uncontrolled and may have influenced the study's results

TABLE 4-2 Quality Scoring Scale* (continued)

Criteria	Range of Scores	Rating Anchor	Explanation of Rating Anchors
		5	Some biases present and reported but not controlled for; therefore results less likely to have been influenced by the biases in section O.
		10	Only minor biases or biases that are well controlled methodologically and unlikely to have influenced the study's results
Temporality	0-10	0	No description of how exposure preceded outcomes; or methods used could not address temporality
		5	Mention of exposure preceding outcomes; questions about whether methods could adequately address temporality
		10	Exposure preceded outcome; prospective cohort study; methods would result in assurance of temporality for inclusion in the study
Dose-response gradient	0-10	0	Dose-response assessment not possible (e.g., only two categories of exposure); or no gradient across categories
		5	Dose-response gradient assessed but not statistically significant
		10	Statistically significant dose-response gradient identified
Strength of association	0-10	0	No association between exposure and disease
		2.5	Non–statistically significant positive association
		5	Some strength of association with a statistically significant association of 2.0- to 3.9-fold risk

TABLE 4-2 Quality Scoring Scale* (continued)

Criteria	Range of Scores	Rating Anchor	Explanation of Rating Anchors
		7.5	Strong association with measure of effect of 4.0- to 7.9-fold risk
		10	Very strong evidence of association with a measure of effect (relative risk or odds ratio) of at least 8-fold risk
Psychosocial factors	0-10	0	No mention of psychosocial factors
		3	Some evaluation and control in one of the two domains (occupational and nonoccupational factors)
		5	Moderate evaluation and control in each of the two aforementioned domains
		7	Advanced evaluation and control methods in at least one domain and moderate evaluation and control methods in the other
		10	In-depth evaluation and control in both domains and few minor questions about adequacy of control

* Raters may select any integers (positive whole numbers) between 0 and 10 or 0 and 20 for the rating anchors. The integers provided should be used as guides and not absolutes for determining the appropriate value within the available range.

TABLE 4-3 Study Design Weighting Factors*

Study Design	Weighting Factor
Prospective cohort	1.0
Retrospective cohort	0.60
Case-control	0.30
Cross-sectional	0.15
Ecologic	0.05

*Each study design will be reviewed regardless of original author's statements about the design and will be assigned a weighting factor by the panel member rating the study.

TABLE 4-4	Final Study Impact Rating*
Article Title	**Final Study Impact Rating**
Sum	

*For each article, the average quality score as determined by using the quality scoring scale (Table 4-2) is multiplied by the weighting factor (Table 4-3) to obtain the final study impact rating. The final study impact ratings for all accepted articles are summed to determine the strength of evidence for a specific topic or diagnosis.

TABLE 4-5	Strength of Evidence of Causation in Epidemiologic Studies
Evidence	**Point Value**
Very strong	>500
Strong	300-500
Some	100-299
Insufficient	<100

Limitations and Other Considerations

Epidemiologic surveillance studies and aggregate information about occupational risk and the development of specific medical conditions are commonly confounded by psychosocial factors. Strength of evidence (determined by the quality score multiplied by the weighting factor) is used to rate the quality of the body of evidence. The body of evidence (the sum of the strength of evidence values for all studies reviewed) is determined by using the strength of evidence values shown in Table 4-5, providing a final conclusion for a causation relationship. Furthermore, study outcomes should be consistent with each other or the conclusions should be similar (implying minimal variance) and the study data groups should be similar (implying minimal variance, that is comparing apples to apples).

Psychosocial factors are addressed separately in Table 4-2. Unlike the more finite (and generally more familiar) range of physical factors (e.g., force, repetition, and posture), psychosocial factors includes a vast array of conditions that usually fall within two separate domains:

1. Factors associated with the job and work environment (occupational factors), and
2. Factors associated with the non-job environment, including the characteristics of individual workers (nonoccupational factors).

Interactions among factors within each of these domains constitute as a "stress process," the results of which are thought to affect health status and job performance.[3-6]

Included in the occupational domain are a host of environments, sometimes referred to as "work organization factors," that include various aspects of job content (e.g., repetition, force, posture, vibration, job control, mental demands, and job clarity); organizational characteristics (e.g., tall vs. flat organizational structures and communications issues); interpersonal relationships at work (e.g., supervisor-employee relationships and social support); temporal aspects of the work and task (e.g., cycle time and shift work); financial and economic aspects (e.g., pay, benefit, and equity issues); and community aspects (e.g., occupational prestige and status).[3,7-9] These occupational factors are often thought of as demands, or "risk factors," that may pose a threat to health.

Non-occupational factors typically include factors associated with demands arising from roles outside of work, such as responsibilities associated with a parent, spouse, children, hobbies, and/or interests. Individual worker factors correspond to three types of factors: genetic (e.g., sex and intelligence); acquired (e.g., social class, culture, and educational status); and dispositional (e.g., personality traits and characteristics and attitudes such as life and job satisfaction).[3]

Employees who are committed to remain at work will try to overcome limitations (physical or mental) resulting from (real or perceived) work intolerance by adapting or changing work tasks to fit their physical and mental abilities. Employees who experience job-related dissatisfaction are less likely to look for ways to match their physical abilities to the physical and mental demands of the job.

CHAPTER 4

Summary

This chapter provides the framework for determining causation for specific activities, conditions, or events. This approach can be applied to a specific case or to groups of workers. By using this scientific method, reasonable decisions about work-relatedness of various health conditions can be obtained from the current epidemiologic surveillance literature.

This chapter is copyrighted by Dr Melhorn. Drs Melhorn and Hagemann have decided to offer this chapter as "in the public domain and may be freely copied or reprinted" if appropriate acknowledgment of this reference source is used.

References

1. National Institute for Occupational Safety and Health. *A Guide to the Work Relatedness of Disease (Revised).* Washington, DC: US Department of Health, Education, and Welfare; 1979.
2. Glass LS. *Occupational Medicine Practice Guidelines ACOEM: Evaluation and Management of Common Health Problems and Functional Recovery in Workers.* 2nd ed. Beverly Farms, MA: OEM Press; 2004.
3. Melhorn JM. Epidemiology of musculoskeletal disorders and workplace factors. In: Mayer TG, Gatchel RJ, Polatin PB, eds. *Occupational Musculoskeletal Disorders Function, Outcomes, and Evidence.* Philadelphia, PA: Lippincott Williams & Wilkins;1999:225-266.
4. Bongers PM, de Winter CR, Kompier MAJ, Hildebrandt VH. Psychosocial factors at work and musculoskeletal disease. *Scand J Work Environ Health.* 1993;19.
5. The Joint International Labour Organization / World Health Organization on Occupational Health. *Psychosocial Factors at Work: Recognition and Control.* Geneva, Switzerland: International Labour Office; 1986.
6. Sauter SL, Swanson NG. Psychological aspects of musculoskeletal disorders in office work. In: Moon S, Sauter SL, eds. *Psychosocial Factors and Musculoskeletal Disorders.* London, England: Taylor and Francis: 1998.
7. US Department of Health and Human Services. *Musculoskeletal Disorders and Workplace Factors: A Critical Review of Epidemiologic Evidence for Work-Related Musculoskeletal Disorders of the Neck, Upper Extremity, and Low Back.* Cincinnati, OH: National Institute for Occupational Safety and Health: 1997;Bernard,BP, editor. National Institute for Occupational Safety and Health Cincinnati, OH: 1-500.
8. World Health Organization. Work with visual display terminals: psychosocial aspects of health. *J Occup Environ Med.* 1989;31:957-968.
9. J. J. Hurrell and L. R. Murphy. Psychological job stress. In: Environment and occupational medicine, edited by W. N. Rom, New York: Little, Brown and Company, 1992: 675-684.

5
CHAPTER
Apportionment

Charles N. Brooks, MD, and J. Mark Melhorn, MD

This chapter provides a guide to logical, defensible, and coherent apportionment that is understandable to a layperson. It does so by defining the term and describing how to apportion between contributing factors when causation is multifactorial and how to apportion for evaluation and treatment, disability. This chapter presumes the reader has a good understanding of causation analysis, including terms such as *exacerbation, aggravation, recurrence, possible,* and *probable.*

Definition

The meaning of *apportionment* depends on the context. In medicine, apportionment is most commonly relevant to causation of injury or disease. However, evaluation and treatment, disability, and impairment may also be apportioned. The American Medical Association's *Guides to the Evaluation of Permanent Impairment,* fifth edition, defines apportionment as "a distribution or allocation of causation among multiple factors that caused or significantly contributed to the injury or disease and existing impairment."[1(p599)] Its predecessor, the fourth edition, states apportionment ". . .is an estimate of the degree to which each of various occupational or non-occupational factors may have caused or contributed to a particular impairment."[2]

More generally, *medical apportionment* may be defined as an estimate of the extent to which two or more probable factors caused an injury or disease. Given this information, it is then generally possible to apportion any resulting evaluation, treatment, disability, and/or impairment.

However, if and when apportionment is indicated depends on the legal venue. Laws and rules vary significantly from one country to another and even within a country, as exemplified by the 50 states within the United States, each with its own unique workers' compensation system and differing personal injury laws. Although the principles and methods of apportionment are generally applicable, they are not specific for any particular jurisdiction. Therefore, this chapter, by necessity, will discuss apportionment in general terms with the understanding that when a physician provides an opinion, they must consider their specific jurisdictional requirements when writing their reports to comply with the applicable statutory law, case law, and departmental rules.

Apportioning Causation

When apportioning responsibility for an injury or disease, one must first consider all potential causes and then determine whether each is probable or possible. Probable causes are included in the apportionment, but possible causes are not. A compensable injury or disease may exacerbate or aggravate a preexisting condition (disease or injury), but may also be temporarily or permanently worsened by a subsequent trauma or exposure.

Apportionment often becomes an issue when a person with preexisting disease sustains a compensable injury to the same body part. For example, an occupational low-back injury prompts lumbar magnetic resonance imaging (MRI), which reveals longstanding abnormalities, including diffuse degenerative disc disease, disc bulging or protrusion at each interspace, and multilevel central and foraminal stenoses of variable severity.

A second scenario in which apportionment is often required is for two or more injuries to the same body part. A worker may have injured the right shoulder while employed by one company and reinjured the same shoulder a year later while working for a different firm. Another employee may have been exposed to the same chemical, high noise levels, or prolonged vibration while working for two or more employers. In addition, if a worker with more than one injury to the same body part was employed in the same position but the employer changed insurers, there could be uncertainty about which insurer was responsible for paying benefits.

Apportionment is a frequent issue in personal injury. For example, the vehicle of a person driving home from the chiropractor's office after receiving adjustments for neck and upper-back pain is rear-ended. Owing to increased discomfort in the neck and upper back, the person reportedly cannot work and needs more frequent treatments.

The medical literature is replete with examples of multifactorial causation of illness, e.g., pulmonary disease in coal miners who smoke or carpal tunnel syndrome (CTS) in employees whose jobs involve data entry despite studies that have shown that many factors may cause or contribute to CTS, including a variety of diseases, such as diabetes mellitus, hypothyroidism, and obesity, and physical inactivity.[3-5] In fact several studies have shown that computer keyboard use does not increase the risk of CTS and the prevalence of CTS in computer users is similar to that in the general population.[6,7] Multifactorial causation may also be applicable in injury. Tsai et al[8] found "A statistically significant association between occupational injuries and past nonoccupational injuries. . . ." In other words, employees who sustained a work-related injury were more likely to have had a prior, similar non-occupational injury than workers who did not report occupational trauma. They concluded ". . . that elements other than workplace hazards (such as lifestyle and physical and psychological factors) may predispose an individual to both occupational and non-occupational injuries."

Apportionment may be indicated when a person who is unaccustomed to heavy lifting sustains a myocardial infarction after such heavy lifting at work, but also is overweight and hypertensive and has advanced coronary artery disease.

Apportionment is frequently an issue in toxic exposures. Given the long latency period before some diseases are recognized, exposures to a given substance may have occurred over years in which the person worked for different employers with different insurers or in different states. Apportionment may be further complicated by the synergistic effect of the exposures to different toxins.

Whether a preexisting condition is apportionable usually depends on the legal venue. Epidemiologic studies often use regression analysis to assess the relative contribution of potential causes, individually and in combination. Although this method can provide information useful in apportionment, it has limitations and generally cannot provide precise percentages of contribution. Also, there are significant variations in workers' compensation statutes. In some states, a preexisting condition is not apportionable with respect to causation, disability, and/or impairment unless it was symptomatic *and* partially disabling before the occurrence of an occupational injury or disease. In other states, only preexisting symptoms are required for apportionment. Sometimes neither preexisting symptoms nor disability are required for a preexisting condition to be apportionable.

There are no hard and fast rules for apportioning causation of a condition. However, the percentages selected should be logical and defensible, i.e., consistent with the medical literature and facts of the case.

Apportionment by Duration of Exposure

Given an occupational disease with similar exposure levels over time, whether to chemicals, noise, vibration, or another factor, duration of employment with different employers may be used to apportion responsibility for the condition. For example, for a meatpacker in whom CTS developed shortly after he began working for Westside Slaughterhouse, where he worked for 2 years, and required a carpal tunnel release after 1 year of doing the same work at Quality Meats, the condition might be apportioned at 67% to Westside and 33% to Quality Meats.

Apportionment by Dose of Exposure

The dose of exposure to an injurious factor is also a basis for apportionment. For example, a 35-year-old shipyard worker had normal hearing during a preemployment physical examination, but 10 years later filed a claim for hearing loss and reported the following occupational history:

TABLE 5-1	Occupational History of Shipyard Worker	
Years	**Employer**	**Noise level exposure**
1994-1995	A	High
1996-2000	B	Low
2001-2003	C	High

Presumably being exposed to low noise levels for 5 years while working for Employer B did not contribute to the worker's hearing loss, whereas the equally high noise levels at Employers A and C did. However, because the claimant worked for Employer A for 2 years and Employer C for 3 years, two fifths, or 40%, of his hearing impairment would be apportioned to Employer A and three fifths, or 60%, to Employer C.

Apportionment by Pain Levels

Given a credible historian, one possible means of apportionment between multiple injuries involving the same body part is to inquire about pain levels on a 0 to 10 scale before and after each trauma. Although the data obtained in this manner are inherently subjective, the evaluating physician may have no better means with which to apportion effects of the various injuries.

Assume for example a 48-year-old carpenter who works through the union hall has had seven employers during the last 4 years and, during this time, sustained three low-back injuries, each involving a different firm and insurer. Physical findings were similar after each injury, including lumbar paraspinal tenderness with or without spasm and decreased lumbar motions but no neurologic deficits or signs of root tension. X-rays revealed degenerative disc disease at L4-L5 and L5-S1. Given the absence of sciatica or physical findings suggesting a need for surgery, no advanced imaging study had been obtained, and treatment had been non-operative.

CHAPTER 5

During an independent medical evaluation (IME), which was requested to apportion responsibility for the carpenter's current condition among the three occupational injuries, the carpenter denied any back pain before the first injury. Immediately thereafter, the lumbar pain was reportedly 8 on the 10-point scale but tapered to 2 during the next 2 months and remained at that level. Following the second injury the low-back pain increased to a level of 4 but reverted to 2. The third trauma caused low-back pain at a severity level of 9, although the discomfort gradually diminished to a level of 6, where it remained, as illustrated in the following:

	Preinjury	Injury 1	Injury 2	Injury 3
Low-back pain level	0	$0\rightarrow8\rightarrow2$	$2\rightarrow4\rightarrow2$	$2\rightarrow9\rightarrow6$

Responsibility for the carpenter's current condition could be apportioned in the following manner: Injury 1 resulted in a new condition or aggravated a preexisting asymptomatic condition, perhaps a tear in an already degenerated annulus fibrosis. However, even if there was a preexisting condition, the worsened condition was an aggravation, not an exacerbation, because the carpenter's status never returned to the baseline, non-painful state. Injury 2 was an exacerbation from which the carpenter fully recovered, returning to his preinjury pain level of 2 on a 10-point scale. Injury 3 constituted an aggravation because the carpenter never fully recovered; his plateau pain level was 6 after the injury versus 2 before. Therefore, his final pain level is 6 for all three injuries. Injury 1's final pain level was 2, Injury 2's final pain level was 2, and Injury 3's final pain level was 6. Apportionment is then 2 divided by 6 for Injury 1, 0 divided by 6 for Injury 2 (no change), and 4 divided by 6 for Injury 3. In summary, the carpenter's present condition is 33% attributable to injury 1, 0% to injury 2, and 67% to injury 3.

More Complex Apportionment

In some cases, physicians must rely on knowledge of pathogenesis of the condition in question, specifics of the injury or exposure, and their own judgment to estimate apportionment. A well-written report will include the rationale behind the percentages selected.

Complex scenarios may arise in which it is impossible to provide a well-reasoned apportionment, e.g., an initial athletic injury, three occupational traumas, and two motor vehicle accidents all involving the same body part. When there is no rational basis for quantitative apportionment among multiple causes, the physician should so state and defer such decision making to the adjudicator, adjuster, arbitrator, commissioner, hearing officer, judge, or jury.

Apportioning Evaluation and Treatment

Whether evaluation and treatment is apportionable also depends on the legal venue. Generally, the primary question is whether the evaluation and treatment in question would have been needed if the injury or exposure had not occurred.

When a compensable injury or exposure causes a new condition, there is no apportionment of the subsequent evaluation and treatment. Generally, apportionment is not warranted when a preexisting, asymptomatic, and untreated condition is made symptomatic and requires evaluation and treatment. The same is usually true for a preexisting symptomatic but untreated condition. Had the person's condition not worsened as a result of the compensable injury or exposure, the person would not have needed evaluation and treatment, at least not when he or she did.

Apportionment often is indicated when a claimant or plaintiff was receiving treatment for a symptomatic condition before a compensable injury or disease. Again, the question that must be answered is whether the same evaluation and treatment would have been necessary if the trauma or exposure had not occurred. If the answer is yes, the diagnostic and therapeutic endeavors are attributed 100% to the preexisting condition. If the answer is no, one must apportion subsequent evaluation and treatment between the preexisting and subsequent conditions.

Doing so may be relatively simple. For example, if a woman was receiving chiropractic adjustments and massages for neck pain twice a week before versus three times a week after being rear-ended in a motor vehicle collision, the later treatments would be apportioned two thirds (67%) to the preexisting condition and one third (33%) to effects of the rear impact.

More often, apportionment of evaluation and treatment is difficult. It requires careful analysis and skilled judgment by a physician knowledgeable about the pertinent medical literature and facts of the case and able to retroactively establish a likely prognosis for evaluation and treatment had the subject injury or exposure never occurred. As with other apportionments, the prognosis need not be stated with certainty, only as a probability. However, the percentages selected should be supported by evidence and the basis explained in a report.

CHAPTER 5

Apportioning Disability

Apportionment of disability can be difficult. It requires determination of the functional loss associated with each of two or more exposures or injuries, whether the disability was temporary or permanent, and whether it was partial or total. A prior injury that resulted in temporary total disability, followed by return to full-duty work, would probably not be considered an etiologic factor in a subsequent claim for permanent disability following a later injury. Conversely, permanent partial disability resulting from a prior injury generally would be considered apportionable in a claim for permanent total disability following a subsequent injury. In the case of a middle-aged or elderly person, apportionment must also take into account the loss of function associated with normal aging.

Apportioning Impairment

When apportioning impairment of a body part or organ system, the rating for any relevant preexisting condition is subtracted from the current percentage of impairment to obtain the net impairment due to the injury or disease in question. Aging is the most common cause of preexisting impairment. Although aging occurs in all persons, it does so at variable rates and to different extents depending on genetics and other factors. However, no one at 80 years has the same cardiopulmonary function or spinal motion that existed at 18 years. Some of the other causes of preexisting impairment include congenital or developmental anomaly, prior injury, and diseases such as degenerative arthritis.

One or more causes contributing to the impairment may also arise after the injury or disease in question. An occupational neck injury may have been aggravated (permanently worsened) by avocational activities or a later motor vehicle collision.

The *Guides,* fifth edition, retained its earlier definition of **impairment** as **"a loss, loss of use, or derangement of any body part, organ system, or organ function,"** which implies a change from a normal or 'preexisting' state. *Normal* is a range or zone representing healthy functioning and varies with age, gender, and other factors such as environmental conditions."[1(p2)] The text also states:

> Data from healthy populations, when available and widely referenced, are incorporated into chapters of the *Guides*. In some organ or body systems, such as respiratory, certain measurements of lung function have been standardized for age and gender. In other body systems, such as the musculoskeletal, age and gender differences are not reflected in most of the values. While there may be age and gender differences anticipated for some musculoskeletal values, such as range of motion in the spine and extremities, . . .the *Guides* mainly reflects average range of motion from healthy populations of mixed age and gender. . . . Evaluating physicians may use their clinical judgment, however, and comment on any significant age or gender effect for a particular individual. . . .[1(p4)]

The purpose of apportionment is an attempt to isolate effects of a compensable, usually occupational, injury or disease from other factors that may cause impairment. If an adult, particularly someone middle age or older, sustains an injury and has limited joint motion thereafter, the questions arise, "How much, if any, of the decreased motion was there before (due to aging or other causes), and how much was traumatic?" An injury involving the spine is problematic from the standpoint of apportionment because there is no corresponding uninjured body part for comparison. However, the converse is usually true in the paired extremities. Often, the contralateral joint is uninjured and can serve as a baseline for status of the involved body part before the trauma in question. Subtracting any impairments of the uninjured part from those for the injured part allows elimination of other causes of impairment and isolation of effects of the trauma.

In fact, the fifth edition of the *Guides* states, "*If a contralateral 'normal' joint has a less than average mobility*, the impairment value(s) corresponding to the uninvolved joint can serve as a baseline and are subtracted from the calculated impairment for the involved joint. The rationale for this decision should be explained in the report."[1(p453)] Corroborating this approach is the "Impairment Questions and Answers" section of a recent issue of *The Guides Newsletter*,[9] quoted in part as follows:

Question:

When rating impairment for an upper extremity disorder associated with a range of motion deficit, should I also assess the contralateral, uninjured extremity?

Answer:

. . .you should first measure range of motion of the relevant joint(s) in both upper extremities, then use the ratings specified in the *Guides*. . . .If the contralateral extremity represents normal for that examinee, any impairment of that individual's uninvolved extremity could serve as a baseline and then be subtracted from the initially calculated rating for the involved extremity.

Obviously, not everyone has a preexisting impairment. In fact, some people have better-than-average normal premorbid function. The *Guides* cites an example of a gymnast with hypermobility whose pre-injury range of motion exceeded the normal values listed. A world-class marathon runner might have above-normal pulmonary function. If, following an illness or an injury, the gymnast's range of motion and the runner's lung function are normal, both would have 0% impairment according to tables in the *Guides*. The Guides recommends that "it would be more appropriate in this instance. . .to assign an impairment rating based on the degree of change from the athlete's preinjury to postinjury state."[1(p4)]

The same principles and methods of impairment rating should be used for preexisting and current ratings. De novo estimation of the prior rating may be required. If there was a prior rating, was the impairment percentage calculated correctly? If not, it needs to be recalculated. A prior rating may have been done correctly but with a prior edition of the *Guides* that is no longer applicable, a state-specific rating method, or the *Manual for Orthopaedic Surgeons in Evaluating Permanent Physical Impairment.*[10] If so, the rating must be recalculated using current and applicable method to ensure comparison of "apples to apples."

It is often difficult to quantify preexisting impairment. In many cases, symptoms and limitations were not adequately documented, required measurements not made, and sufficiently specific diagnoses or procedures were not listed.

When Not to Apportion

Apportionment is not warranted when only one probable cause exists, even if there are other possible causes. If there is no evidence of preexisting evaluation or treatment for or disability or impairment due to the condition in question, apportionment is probably not indicated.

Apportionment may also be legally inappropriate. For example, under the Longshore and Harbor Workers' Compensation Act (LHWCA) the last responsible employer is 100% responsible for the disease or injury, even if the worker had multiple prior exposures or injuries to the same body part. Recent LHWCA case law has determined that as little as a report of an increase in preexisting and ongoing symptoms during 1 day of work is sufficient to shift responsibility from one employer to another.

Confounders in Apportionment

Causation analysis and apportionment may be confounded by a variety of factors, including the history provided, which may be incomplete due to intentionally withheld or forgotten information, false, or otherwise misleading. Health care or other pertinent records may be missing. Other confounders include degenerative disorders; aging; use of tobacco, alcohol, and illicit drugs: and lifestyle choices, such as diet and exercise or lack thereof.[11]

Causal relationships and apportionment may be misrepresented by physicians because of ignorance, financial motives, and advocacy. An erroneous conclusion may be unintentional, as in ignorance, or volitional, as with financial or advocacy motives. A known misrepresentation may be self-serving or altruistic.

An evaluating or treating physician unaware of what the current medical literature says about causes for a condition may promulgate erroneous conclusions about causation and apportionment. Similarly, a physician may blindly accept claimant history as fact without reviewing prior records or considering the plausibility of the historical information provided. Such a "parrot," so labeled because the physician repeats whatever he or she is told, may be embarrassed and impeached when subsequently confronted with information to the contrary, e.g., on cross-examination.

Although one would hope professionalism would rise above pecuniary interests, financial motives may influence physician opinion. Given a patient uninsured apart from workers' compensation, there is a tendency to ascribe the injury or illness in question to work, rather than to provide services, particularly surgery, for which no payment will be forthcoming. An analogous situation occurs with capitation. A physician who will not be paid any more for performing services unless the patient's condition is attributed to an occupational or personal injury has an inherent motive to make such an attribution. Likewise, the physician-employee of a health maintenance organization may be encouraged to ascribe to a third party the responsibility for evaluation and treatment of a patient's condition, thereby decreasing costs and/or increasing revenues for the organization.

Although less common, and perhaps not applicable in areas where managed care predominates, the converse may also be true. Given a patient with good private health insurance and a very restrictive state-imposed fee schedule for services provided under workers' compensation, a physician might, for example, be inclined to attribute need for surgery to a non-occupational cause, perhaps substantially increasing the surgical fee.

Financial motives may influence opinions expressed by evaluating and treating physicians. Apportionment conclusions drawn by a not-so-independent medical examiner may be based on what is favorable to his or her client rather than the medical literature or facts of a case. Generally, such behavior is indirectly self-serving, increasing the likelihood of a steady stream of referrals from that source.

Misrepresentations regarding causation and apportionment may also be predicated on patient advocacy. A person lacking health or disability insurance yet facing expensive diagnostic studies and treatment for, and/or prolonged disability due to a condition probably unrelated to employment may be financially and emotionally devastated. A compassionate yet not necessarily honest approach for the treating physician might be to overlook or minimize nonoccupational causes and attribute the condition primarily or exclusively to work, thereby eliminating the costs and providing an ongoing, albeit diminished, income stream for the patient.

Summary

Physicians should have a good understanding of apportionment, as defined herein and in the applicable state or federal law. Physicians should also be knowledgeable about pathogenesis of the condition in question and the facts of a case; follow a logical, rational, and, thereby, defensible thought process when drawing conclusions; and explain the basis for opinions in a coherent manner understandable to a layperson.

References

1. Cocchiarella L, Andersson GBJ, eds. *Guides to the Evaluation of Permanent Impairment.* 5th ed. Chicago, IL: American Medical Association; 2001.
2. Doege TC, Houston TP, eds. *Guides to the Evaluation of Permanent Impairment.* 4th ed. Chicago, IL: American Medical Association; 1993:315.
3. Nathan PA, Keniston RC. Carpal tunnel syndrome and its relation to general physical condition. *Hand Clin.* 1993;9:253.
4. Kerwin G, Williams CS, Seiler JG. The pathophysiology of carpal tunnel syndrome. *Hand Clin.* 1996;12:243.
5. Atcheson SG, Ward JR, Lowe W. Concurrent medical disease in work-related carpal tunnel syndrome. *Arch Intern Med.* 1998;158;1506-1512.
6. Stevens JC, Witt JC, Smith BE, Weaver AL. The frequency of carpal tunnel syndrome in computer users at a medical facility. *Neurology.* 2001;56:1568-1570.
7. Thomsen JF, Hansson GA, Mikkelsen S, Lauritzen M. Carpal tunnel syndrome in repetitive work: a follow-up study. *Am J Ind Med.* 2002;42:344-353.
8. Tsai SP, Bernacki EJ, Dowd CM. The relationship between work-related and non–work-related injuries. *J Community Health.* 1991;16:205-212.
9. Brigham CR. Impairment questions and answers. *Guides Newsletter.* March/April 1999:7.
10. American Academy of Orthopaedic Surgeons.: *Manual for Orthopaedic Surgeons in Evaluating Permanent Physical Impairment.* Chicago, IL; AAOS; 1975.
11. Brigham CR, Roth HJ. Apportionment Analysis. *Guides Newsletter.* July/August 2004:1-11.

6

The Causality Examination

Ian Blair Fries, MD

The causality evaluation of a person for causation differs from the traditional medical evaluation designed to determine the diagnosis and treatment for specific symptoms. Causation evaluation requires more insight into the events and exposures before, during, and after the onset of symptoms and understanding how reported events and exposures are related to claimed residuals. Although many of the same tools are used—history, current complaints, review of systems, physical examination, and test results—some methods and approaches are not similar to typical medical practice.

In traditional diagnosis and treatment, a physician attempts to narrow the focus, while eliciting the history, current complaints, and physical examination, to a single anatomic area and a specific diagnosis in preparation for focused treatment. Testing and additional studies may be ordered to confirm the proposed diagnosis.

Although the correct diagnosis is key to traditional and causation analysis, at the time of a causality examination, the diagnosis usually has been established, and, frequently, treatment has been provided. If the causality examination follows the same path as a traditional diagnostic or follow-up examination, important findings will be missed or misinterpreted. Therefore, the causality examination should use the current diagnosis as a springboard to an expanded examination that includes all events and exposures.

Nevertheless, the earlier the causality is identified, the less likely behavioral confounders will influence the manifestations and influence the outcome.

Standards of Causality

During the examination and analysis process, it is necessary to consider the differing standards for causality in medical and legal settings. A causality report bridges the two professions, although the bridge is tenuous. Science requires that all possibilities be explored and included in any analysis. In legal (forensic) settings, only what-is-more-likely-than-not is likely to be admissible. Conclusions that are only "possible" are typically excluded from legal consideration. (See Chapter 2 for specific jurisdictional examples.)

Elements of the Causality Examination

The causality examination consists of a review of records, interview, physical examination, test results, and conclusions. Although attempts should be made to be as complete as possible, occasionally, some elements cannot be obtained or accomplished. Complete records and test results may not be available. The person may have died. A patient may decide not to have a study, or they may be precluded from undergoing a test (e.g., metal precluding magnetic resonance imaging).

A causality examination requires more of the physician's time before, during, and after an evaluation than a traditional consultation. A physician who decides to do causality examinations must allow for the additional time requirements.

The following are goals of a causality examination:
1. Confirm that the original diagnosis was correct and due to the injury, event, or exposure
2. Verify that current symptoms and physical examination findings are consistent with the diagnosis and not indicative of a new diagnosis, which may be a complication of the original diagnosis or a result of a new event or exposure resulting in expanded or new disease
3. Confirm that the person's current complaints and findings have not been confounded by sickness behavior, whether conscious or unconscious

Record Review

It is best to review records in detail before seeing the person. Causality examinations often concern complex medical issues and lengthy treatment. Entering the examination room with little knowledge of the issues to be addressed and questions about causation may result in a muddled opinion, particularly if the patient is distracted by irrelevant issues. However, such distractions should be recorded by the examiner, which may provide clues about the person's illness perceptions.

Crucial causality information is obtained from medical records and other documents such as depositions, answers to interrogatories, accident reports, and police reports. The importance of full, complete, and legible medical records must be emphasized. The examiner should always look for primary data. Inaccurate histories and unsupported diagnoses can be inadvertently carried from report to report. Furthermore, vignetted opinions and results in later records may prove inaccurate and divergent.

It is unreasonable to expect a physician to decipher scribbled notes and weird abbreviations. The rule, "If you cannot read it, I cannot read it" applies. Occasionally, treating physicians must be compelled to transcribe illegible records.

By the finish of a record review, the examining physician should have a plan for how to approach the person during the oral history and physical examination phases. Although people may wander when recounting their history, a prepared physician can guide the interview so it will provide information about causation and other issues that must be addressed.

Interview

People often provide less accurate histories than their records, possibly owing to poor recall but sometimes purposely. However, details of injury or exposure should be obtained orally and matched to previous records, and discrepancies should be addressed in the causality report. Normally, the examining physician should attempt to clarify inconsistencies with the person examined. Treatment records may be incomplete, and the person may have valid corrections to erroneous entries. Causality often hinges on accurate dates and chronologies. Ambiguity may be a clue to lacking causal connections.

The interview may reveal consultations, tests, and courses of treatment not reflected in available records. A list of missing data should accompany a causality report, indicating the relative importance of the missing information and how it might affect the examiner's conclusions. Current complaints should be carefully elicited. Second to the history, current complaints are the most important clues to causality. A person should be asked to list current symptoms in the order of perceived seriousness. The dates of onset should be requested. Some people need guidance to focus on their current symptoms because they may expound on past inactive complaints. The person should confirm that each complaint is the result of the claimed accident or exposure.

With each complaint, the physician should elicit frequency, duration, intensity, and pattern. Ameliorating and aggravating factors should also be explored; for example, a person reported persistent ulnar hand pain following injury 2 years earlier, but during the interview, admitted the pain occurred only while delivering Karate-chops to blocks of wood.

People may claim unlikely symptoms and chronologies, e.g., ecchymoses occurring a year after trauma, double vision following an isolated ankle fracture, or swelling in the right wrist after injury to the left wrist. These are important clues of behavioral issues and unrelated diseases rather than clues to causation.

The physician should ascertain whether the symptoms have improved or worsened since onset and whether the symptoms have responded to treatment. When a person reports improvement after a procedure, it should be clarified whether the improvement was temporary or permanent. A person who has undergone surgery should be asked to specify what symptom/s is better or worse since surgery. One way to help the person clarify this is to ask, "Knowing what you know now, would you have had surgery?"

A person, who claims symptoms are continuing to worsen, denies any change in symptoms, or claims symptoms have not responded to any treatment likely has a poor prognosis. Such symptom patterns are consistent with behavioral issues.

The patient should be asked to estimate the severity of each symptom by using a scale of 0 (no symptom at all) to 10 (the worse conceivable). A person whose most serious complaint (of several) is rated 3 and is occurring twice a week differs from a person with three complaints each rated 10 and present day and night. A person reporting a constant pain rating of 10 is likely overstating the pain because with such a rating, he or she should be entirely nonfunctional. The 0 to 10 scales can be useful for complaints other than pain, e.g., numbness, swelling, and disequilibrium, because the scale is a good measure of a person's perception of many symptoms.

The way the history is elicited may offer important clues to causality. Some people may hide behind claimed or real language, speech, or hearing difficulties. It is imperative to have a disinterested interpreter so the physician can evaluate true and false veils. A family member or close friend often interjects his or her own interpretations, sometimes intentionally, and may significantly color causation and chronology.

Accurate interpretation is imperative when eliciting complaints. Feelings, sensory symptoms, and pain patterns do not cross languages easily. A facile interpreter can explain to a person the intended question and then assist the physician to understand the response. This interpretation is different from a word-for-word translation and a nuanced interpretation of a word. Strict translation of a word may not capture the essence and nuance of the word or the complaint. For example, a Chinese patient may complain that he or she has a "sour stomach." However, "sour stomach" does not exist in Western medicine. Numbness, tingling, pins and needles, and many other sensory descriptors often poorly translate across languages. Hence, word-for-word translation may be insufficient or even incorrect. A causality examination requires the clearest communication feasible.

CHAPTER 6

Symptom Diagrams

The symptom diagram is an extremely valuable tool for eliciting complaints. It is a mistake to call it a "pain diagram" because the person may then properly omit significant non-painful symptoms.

The symptom diagram clarifies laterality and location of a person's complaints. Many people describe symptom location inadequately. The words *back*, *hip*, *leg*, *arm*, and *first finger* may have differing meanings to a person and the examiner.

Right versus left confusion is common in medical records and can extend to the person. The value of a symptom diagram is illustrated in the following event.

> A patient was seen on three occasions. At first, she had left knee pain, which she claimed was due to an accident, but on the second visit, she only had pain in the right knee. On the final visit, she only had pain left knee. She ultimately claimed that the ongoing left-knee symptoms were all due to the accident before the first visit. However, the three symptom diagrams she dated and signed provided evidence that her left knee had recovered and that the current left-knee condition was not likely due to the initial event.

Symptom diagrams can be complex and sometimes communicate behavioral issues. Some people request colored pencils to complete the diagrams, or they add written notes and arrows to the diagrams. There may be insufficient room on the diagram, and symbols may spill outside the confines of the body outlines. Patients should not be discouraged from completing the diagrams as they want because the diagrams are important clues to the location and type of symptoms and behavioral issues.

A history, an admitted prior condition, or a subsequent event may cloud causality. Attaching symptoms correctly to events can be assisted by having the person complete more than one symptom diagram. For example, one diagram may show symptoms before the accident or event being considered, and a second diagram may document current symptoms.

The symptom diagrams in Figures 6-1, 6-2, and 6-3 provide insight into the person's perception of symptoms. Based on the global nature of the person's symptoms, behavior may overshadow pathophysiology as the cause. Therefore, a person with global symptoms will not likely respond to care focused on the reported neural, muscular, and skeletal symptoms. People whose behavior overshadows a pathophysiologic cause of their symptoms are poor candidates for surgery. The most effective treatment is addressing psychosocial issues.

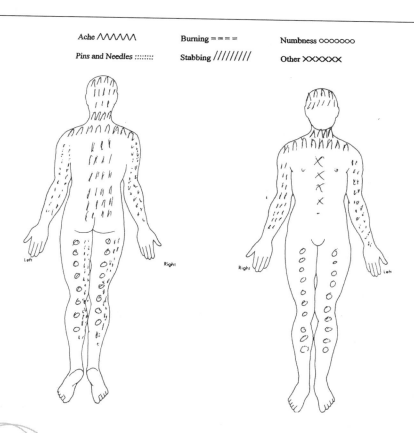

Ache /\/\/\/\/\/\   Burning = = = =   Numbness ooooooo

Pins and Needles ::::::::   Stabbing /////////   Other XXXXXX

FIGURE 6-1   Symptom Diagram 1: Symmetric Symptoms

The absolute symmetry of symptoms and locations is not physiologic. Widespread neuropathies do not spare hands and feet. There are no classic dermatomal patterns. The absence of facial symptoms and global body symptoms are characteristic of behavioral manifestations.

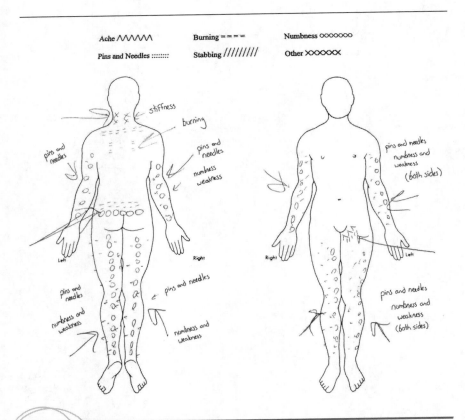

Ache ᐱᐱᐱᐱᐱᐱ   Burning = = = =   Numbness ooooooo

Pins and Needles ::::::::   Stabbing /////////   Other ✕✕✕✕✕✕

FIGURE 6-2   Symptom Diagram 2: Symmetry and additional comments.

The person who completed this diagram believes it necessary to add notes to further describe symptoms that have already been implied by the symbols within the body of the drawings. Several arrows, e.g., the left groin and low back, are not labeled but have been added to emphasize severity without imparting information about the type of symptom.

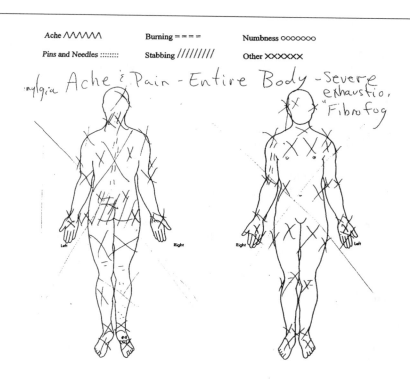

Ache ∧∧∧∧∧   Burning = = = =   Numbness ooooooo

Pins and Needles ::::::::   Stabbing //////////   Other XXXXXX

myalgia Ache & Pain - Entire Body - Severe exhaustio, "Fibro fog"

PAIN LINE - Make a mark on this line to show the amount of pain you have.

On certain days

No Pain   0 —————————— (10) Worst Possible Pain

FIGURE 6-3   Symptom Diagram 3: Overlapping symptom areas and lack of symptom description

The person who completed this diagram is expressing perceived symptoms of fibromyalgia allegedly aggravated by a motor vehicle accident. The person's inability to describe any symptoms such as aching, burning, numbness, pins and needles, or stabbing is incompatible with most organic diagnoses and even the label of fibromyalgia. The "x's" overlap, cover all surfaces, and extend beyond the body outline. This person supplements the diagram by adding "fibromyalgia ache & pain—entire body—severe exhaustion 'fibrofog,'" implying the symbols on the diagram do not provide adequate communication of her predicament.

Review of Systems

Collateral information is obtained from a careful review of systems. Previous and subsequent accidents and injuries should be explored, particularly those that may possibly affect the disorder.

Prior illnesses may explain complaints claimed due to an accident or may explain the response to injury and treatment. It is human to embrace rational explanations of an illness, and people may claim trauma as the cause of their hypertension, diabetes, rheumatoid arthritis, lupus, cancer, or other condition.

A review of systems must specifically query about mental disorders and psychiatric hospitalizations. People often do not consider psychiatric and mental health as part of their medical history. Psychiatric hospitalizations may be reported either in a form or orally by the person as admissions for somatic indications.

Hints of a mental disorder may be a general medical discharge from the military, a discontinuous work history, antisocial behavior, unemployment, or lack of social support. Psychotropic medications are often not reported because they are claimed to be for nonmental-health-related conditions, e.g., tobacco-use cessation, insomnia, weight loss, headaches, neurologic disorders, and pain. Who prescribed the medication, why, and when should be ascertained.

Physical Examination

A traditional physical examination should be performed to address all areas of claimed symptoms and concerns. Details of the traditional physical examination will not be reviewed.[1] However, specific techniques applying to causality examinations are discussed.

The causality physical examination should focus on whether physical findings support prior diagnoses, current diagnoses, and current complaints. A person occasionally has a previously undiagnosed condition, which could cause the current complaints, which then open an entirely new chain of causation. If a disparity exists among physical examination findings, history, and symptoms, causality is unlikely.

The examining physician needs to explore subjective signs and objective findings. Objective findings should carry greater weight of evidence than subjective findings in supporting a diagnosis, particularly residuals. Subjective findings are entirely dependent on the response of the person. Objective findings are readily apparent to an observer, are measurable, and do not require explanation by a person.

However, there is not a complete dichotomy between subjective and objective findings. For example, a person demonstrates active knee motion from full extension to 90° of flexion. This is an objective and measurable finding. However, why the same person did not further flex to 130° could be a lack of effort (subjective) or physical impossibility (objective). Similarly, in a weight-lifting test, a person may lift 5- and 10-pound weights with the right hand and then be unable to lift a 15-pound weight. The test has confirmed the objective ability to lift up to 10 pounds, but the inability to lift 15 pounds is a subjective claim.

Some examiners suggest that they can "objectify" subjective tests by having a person append a measurement, say a score of 8 on a 0 to 10 pain scale. However, this method does not make subjective pain any more objective.

Subjective symptoms occurring historically, at the time of examination, or on specific provocation remain subjective. However, they may be given more weight if they occur in established patterns. Thus, reported numbness restricted to right ring and little finger consistent with C7 or ulnar neuropathy may be given more weight than vague global numbness in both hands. Similarly, more value may be given to passive straight-leg lifting provoking radiating pain in an L5 or S1 distribution and even more value if radiating pain is provoked by straight-leg lifting of the opposite leg. However, these test results are still subjective.

Pain provoked during discography with negative results at a control level is considered a better indication of local disc disease than back pain alone. However, both examples carry subjective responses, depending entirely on individual perception and/or veracity. A subjective symptom or finding is always subjective and open to behavioral manipulation. People with back pain due to abdominal or pelvic disease may report that discography provokes concordant pain.

Behavioral Symptoms

The labels *non-physiologic*, *non-organic*, *functional*, *non-anatomic*, *inappropriate*, *reactive*, and *inexplicable* are pejorative. Perhaps the best label is *behavioral* because it does not imply specific causality.

Behavioral symptoms must be cautiously considered. In moderation, they may be a normal response to objective trauma, or a reasonable reaction to a medical condition. However, exaggerated behavior becomes pathologic by itself when the presentation is no longer adequately explained by an underlying physical condition. Exaggerated behavior is then the unconscious result of psychiatric pathology, or due to conscious fabrication. In either case, improvement is unlikely to follow treatment for a physical disorder. This is why all medical evaluations, not just those for causality, should include the search for behavioral signs. This is particularly indicated when a patient's course is unexpected, or inexplicable.

For example, a patient sustains a non-displaced wrist fracture that heals physically and radiologically in the expected time. However, if pain and marked dysfunction progressively increase, although there are no objective findings to support increasing symptoms, it is unlikely further treatment of the wrist will provide a cure. The patient's exaggerated behavioral symptoms may include several findings discussed later in this section.

Illness behavior may be a by-product of an injury or illness for which the person is not even undergoing a causality examination. Such a condition may be preexisting, coincidental, or subsequent.

The original disease or injury may have faded or even resolved, and the only manifestations remaining may be behavioral. Some florid presentations obscure any underlying diagnosis.

Expected illness behavior typically begins shortly after trauma and gradually fades. Exaggerated behavior either has roots well before the alleged trauma, or has a late onset when objective symptoms of trauma are fading or have resolved. It is important to obtain as many medical records as possible, spanning years before the causal event, as well as the complete records of treatment since the causal event.

A physician examining for causality must separate findings reasonably due to the causal event from those intentionally or unintentionally included manifestations that are not causally connected to the injury. Findings may also be of objective conditions completely unrelated to the specific cause.

A comprehensive causality examination must seek behavioral signs and consider their cause. There is consensus that such behavioral signs do not have pathophysiologic explanations but are how patients deport themselves in response to perceived or real disease.[2]

Although anything that follows an event could be construed as causally related, science requires a concrete connection.[3] The legal responsibility of a person or entity for the injuries of another requires more than a vicarious association. Causality by an act of God does not typically qualify for court-ordered recompense. Self-induced injury may or may not be considered in legal causality. For example, in no-fault auto or workers' compensation arenas, even an injured person at fault may have the right to recompense.

Eliciting Behavioral Signs During a Causality Physical Examination

Behavioral findings during a physical examination must be carefully considered. The presence of a sign or two may have little diagnostic value. However, a patient who exhibits multiple and/or florid signs likely has exaggerated illness behavior. The presence of these findings is usually consistent with the history and complaints.

A behavioral sign that is consistent and reproducible assumes increased weight in determining behavioral causality. Inconsistency when evoking non-behavioral signs is also a valid behavioral sign. For example, straight-leg lifting performed supine that provokes radiating lower extremity pain, which is not reproduced on straight-leg lifting while seated, is a classic discrepant sign.

Bizarre responses and complaints are clues to diagnosis and treatment. An isolated finding may be so eccentric that it stands alone as strong evidence of pathologic behavior. Obvious examples include seeing triple, complaints of urinary smoke and fire, and teeth itching. However, more often, several inexplicable findings lead the examiner to conclude that symptoms are not related to the event. Do not discard anomalous data because they do not make sense. Inexplicable findings are likely behavioral.

Some behavioral signs may be normal responses to real disease or injury. However, the more behavioral signs found, the less likely the cause is the injury and the more likely there are other causes, unconscious or conscious. People with significant chronic disease may develop a "disease personality," although they have relatively minor behavioral signs. For example, patients with reflex sympathetic dystrophy (CRPS I) present with an anxious demeanor, are passive, and not usually demanding or critical.

Florid behavioral signs are commonly seen in psychiatric disease that typically preceded the claimed causal injury. Psychiatric disease is unlikely to occur shortly after injury, although a person may want to connect the two—a more palatable alternative than conceding a preexisting mental condition. People with minor or no disease can have behavioral signs prompted by primary, secondary, or tertiary gains. Florid behavioral signs may be seen in people who are fabricating symptoms and signs without mental illness.

Behavior due to psychiatric disease may indirectly improve with successful musculoskeletal treatment, but mental health care, not orthopedic treatment, is indicated. "Desperation surgery" and even "minimally invasive surgery" typically lead to poor results in people with illness behavior. Even outcomes from indicated conservative care are atypical in the face of mental disease and behavioral manifestations.

Behavioral signs are common. For example, more than 13% of 300 consecutive people in a forensic practice consultation had several remarkable behavioral signs.[4] However, none of the people was identified by their treating physicians as having behavioral disease (0/41) and only two people (5%) of 41 were identified by a consultant. Waddell[5] described non-organic signs, which he divided into six categories. Please see box for the complete list of these signs.

CHAPTER 6

1. Tenderness
   Superficial
   Nonanatomic

2. Simulation
   Axial loading
   Simulated (pelvic) rotation

3. Distraction
   Straight-leg lifting

4. Regional
   Weakness
   Sensory disturbance

Waddell's categories have been modified into the following six categories:
   1. Inappropriate or exaggerated responses
   2. Pseudoneurologic patterns
   3. Anomalous results from muscle testing
   4. Ambiguous motion
   5. Abnormal gait
   6. Inconsistent Observations

Inappropriate or Exaggerated Responses

A person undergoing a physical examination may insist on pointing out his or her complaints on the examiner's body. The person should be encouraged to point on his or her own body. If the person says that he or she cannot reach the location of a symptom, provide a pointer (for example, a red-tipped Babinski hammer). The person may resist examination, grabbing the examining hand or wrist, may claim too much pain to allow any physical examination to proceed, may not relax to permit gentle passive joint motion, or may demur, sitting or lying on an examination table. Some people may claim they cannot step up the few inches to mount a scale to be weighed. Others cannot lift an injured foot off the ground, although they walked into the office without support. Some people may immediately lose balance when closing their eyes, without evidence of disequilibrium. Overreaction during examination may result in the person sucking air across the teeth.[6]

Other examples include inappropriate responses to sham testing. The classic is gentle vertex compression causing low back pain. If the result is positive, this test should be extended by comparing the response to bilateral superior shoulder compression and, finally, the response when the person applies pressure to his or her head with his or her own hands. Waddell pelvic rotation is a sham maneuver in which the patient's trunk is rotated by the examiner without any motion of the spine, and all motion that occurs at the hips and legs. Such motion should not cause or exacerbate spinal pain. The examiner should provide response options to a person by asking if the symptoms provoked occurred with right and/or left rotation. It is also important to document the exact symptom provoked and where it was located. The examiner should also ask whether the provoked symptom is the same as the person's complaint.

A similar principle of sham motion occurs with femoral rotation in a seated position with the examiner's hand applied to the knee. Also, torquing the ankle while performing a Steinman test for potential meniscal disease is a misdirected test because the application of force is at a distance to the expected location of a response. If these two standard tests are applied and do provoke inappropriate responses, these responses are considered as signs of behavioral symptoms.

Some behavioral responses are bizarre, such as when a person insists that severe shoulder pain is caused by passive hallux motion. Such unusual responses should be confirmed by repeating the test immediately and again later during the examination. If the response is consistently bizarre, it is strong evidence of behavioral issues. Bizarre responses can include the inability to touch a finger to nose with eyes closed, widespread sensitivity to light touch, and pain when the examiner rolls the person's skin between a thumb and index finger. Skin rolling may even cause nonphysiologic radicular symptoms.

A delayed response to a test is likely behavioral, as is the request to repeat a test before offering the provoked response. Some people revise their response several minutes later. "Doctor, do you remember when you extended my left elbow? I meant to tell you that caused my thumb to go completely dead."

A person who describes pain as 10 on a 0 to 10 pain scale should not have been able to enter the office. Such severe pain should make a person entirely nonfunctional. Even 9 out of 10 on a pain scale is suspect when a person does not appear to have more than moderate discomfort. All people should rate and mark their pain on a 10-cm pain line, which in my opinion is poorly designated as a Visual Analog Scale (VAS). People who mark scores "greater than 10" or "200" to express their pain are responding in an exaggerated manner. Similarly, people who require complex fractions or decimals to express their pain levels are displaying behavioral signs and may be responding in an exaggerated manner. Specific physical examination options or tests can be helpful to identify behavioral issues. The Mannkopf-Rumpf test, which proposes measurement of pulse increase with provoked pain to validate that pain was truly provoked,[7] has questionable reliability because pulse can increase due to any stress, including the stress of an inappropriate claim of pain.

The examiner can provoke a known-response and assesses the patient's reactions using snuffbox tenderness, forearm pain on sublimis testing, paresthesias rolling over superficial radial nerve fibers, and peroneal compartment discomfort with resisted eversion and plantar flexion are all normally expected. A person may overreact to these provocative tests. A claim that these provoked normal responses exactly reproduce symptoms due to the event or exposure is likely fabricated. Expected pain results in a normal extremity can also establish a basis for comparison.

When a person claims swelling, leg-length discrepancy, abnormal temperature, or discoloration, document the finding or lack of a finding. A tape measure, jeweler's ring-sizers, leveling blocks, a surface thermometer, and a digital camera are helpful tools (Table 6-1). They can provide strong evidence whether a patient has what is claimed.

TABLE 6-1   Examination Tools
Tape measure
Body weight scale
Goniometers, large, medium, and finger
Dual inclinometers, mechanical or electronic
Jeweler's ring sizers
Babinski hammer with red tip
Two-point discriminator (or divider or paper clip)
Four coins
Rubber gloves
Surface thermometer
Grip and pinch dynamometers
Digital camera

Pseudoneurologic Patterns

There are many behavioral sensory patterns. Stocking, glove, or total extremity numbness may have an organic cause, but in the setting of trauma, such distributions are most likely behavioral. Behavioral patterns can be non-dermatomal, non-neural, and non-myotomal. Sensory deficits may split the midline or split the coronal plane. Deficits claimed to be severe and significant may not be present on examination. The sensation from tuning-fork vibration may be lost crossing the midline or differ over parts of the same bone, e.g., tibial tubercle and medial malleolus or ulnar styloid and olecranon.

Sensory modalities may be dissociated and unassociated. The loss of pain and position perception together is unusual. The lack of coincident loss of position and vibration sensations or pain and temperature sensations suggests behavioral responses. False Tinel signs may be elicited over bony prominences and away from nerve locations.

The Bowlus and Currier test has been described.[8] The ulnar portions of the wrists are placed against each other with forearms in pronation, the fingers are then interdigitated and the hands then rotated together toward the chest. In that position, a person may inaccurately lateralize a claimed sensory loss.

Appreciation of extremity position is commonly abnormal in a behavioral setting. A person who is consistently wrong in describing the position of the hallux obviously is distinguishing position in choosing the incorrect alternative. When I examine for positional sense I provide three alternatives: "Is the big toe up or down, or are you not sure? If you are not sure, tell me. Do not guess." A person with true loss of proprioception will respond, "I don't know," whereas a behavioral response is more likely to be consistently in error.

If abnormal position sense is elicited by hallux testing, position sense should be tested sequentially at the ankles, knees, and hips until a normal level is reached. If widespread lower extremity abnormalities are elicited, position sense should also be tested at the fingers, wrists, elbows, and shoulders. A pattern may emerge that is inconsistent with a tenable neurologic diagnosis. Widespread proprioception losses are invalidated by normal gait and dexterity and normal appreciation of a vibrating tuning fork.

Psychogenic motion disorders are sometimes claimed to be caused by injury. However, true motion disorders are symptoms of central nervous system disease and not peripheral trauma. They are not caused by an accident without significant head or spinal cord injury.

Paroxysmal pseudoseizures, uncontrollable shaking, and, more commonly, posturing, may be chronic or intermittent. Psychogenic posturing commonly results in a bizarre gait disturbance, which may be a tremor, usually an intention tremor that extinguishes when attention is drawn away from the extremity. True movement disorders more typically improve with attention and use. True motion disorders have a slow onset over years, without asymptomatic intervals. However, psychogenic motion disorders have a sudden onset after trauma, followed by spontaneous remissions.

Psychogenic tremors are of variable frequency and lead to fatigue. These are not features of true neurologic motion disorders. The variable frequency of psychogenic tremor can be revealed by the entrainment test. Rhythmic motion of the normal extremity is established at a frequency different from the pathologic rhythm. True pathologic tremor rhythm will not change, but the new rhythm will likely transfer to the extremity with a psychogenic tremor. However, it is important to understand that the person may have unique skills, such as those of a drummer, and may be capable of maintaining unrelated beats with different extremities.

Electrodiagnostic testing, hypnosis, and amobarbital or benzodiazepine interviews may also help distinguish psychological from neurologic motion disorders.[9]

Two-point discrimination is a revealing test. As for proprioception, the person is given the choice of three responses: "one point," "two points" or "I cannot tell." The last answer is consistent with neuropathy. Mistaking one for two points may be physiologic as in some neuropathies and a fingertip may be hypersensitive during sensory recovery from injury. Allow the person to decide if he or she wants to look during discrimination testing. People with true sensory loss prefer not to look to ensure an accurate assessment. They want to avoid possibly influencing their responses by what they see. A patient who is consciously influencing the result is likely to watch intensely.

A finding of more than 10 mm of discrimination or of anesthesia should not be an isolated finding. Its validity is questionable in the face of normal sweat patterns, lack of pulp atrophy, no burns, no scars, and no nail changes. The results of two-point discrimination should also be compared with a person's ability to button and unbutton clothes, remove and replace jewelry to demonstrate dexterity (as illustrated in the rubber glove test example discussed subsequently).

Anomalous two-point discrimination can be supplemented by asking a person to distinguish between one and two touches of the two-point device. The ability to feel a dull point pressed against a fingertip but unable to distinguish between single and double touches is non-physiologic. A modified dexterity test based on Moberg's suggestion is called the Fries Four Coin Pickup.[4] The person sitting on the examination table is presented with a quarter, dime, nickel, and penny placed on the table top to the person's right. The person is asked to pick up the four coins with the right hand and place them on the examination table to his or her left. Then, they are to pick up the four coins with the left hand and transfer them across their body placing the coins on the table to their right. Now with coins to their right, they are asked to repeat the four-coins-pick-up with the right and then the left hand, but with their eyes closed. As a final test, the person is asked to find the dime with the eyes closed and then hand the dime to the examiner. Distinguishing the dime from the penny is the most difficult task, but can be accomplished by a hand with normal dexterity and sensation. The head, shoulder, trunk, elbow, wrist, and finger motion should be incidentally observed during the test.

Recently, I have used a rubber glove test. Watching a person don and remove a pair of rubber gloves provides a good demonstration of bimanual dexterity and sensory function. Patients may express behavioral signs by inappropriately assigning dysfunction to the hand applying and donning the glove. A patient who is fabricating symptoms will find it difficult to remain consistent during this test.

Anomalous Results from Muscle Testing

Muscle testing is an opportunity to expose many behavioral signs. A person who claims substantial chronic weakness may not have measurable atrophy. A person may be unable to move a joint through the full range of demonstrated passive motion, even with counterforce and gravity eliminated.

Feigning muscle weakness or lack of motion is often accompanied by activation of both sets of antagonistic muscles. In an attempt to prove maximal muscle activation, a person may exhibit muscle activation tremors or voluntary shaking. When resistance is applied, muscles may give way after briefly exerting normal strength. Sometimes a collapse occurs even before resistance is applied. Typically, giving way degrades rapidly with repeated testing, far faster than might be seen with normal muscle fatigue.

When a person claims complete paralysis, a joint may be held against the force of gravity. For example, a reputed flail wrist may be held extended against gravity. A knee that allegedly cannot be actively extended may drop only to 45° against gravity after being released from passive full extension. Obviously, muscle activation is required to maintain partial extension against gravity.

Strength exerted may be variable when tested by rapidly alternating right and left or when pulsed. Retesting later in the examination in another position may provide a divergent response. For example, knee extension tested seated and later prone may vary by a grade or more.

Inappropriately claimed paralyzed muscles could be activated by known synergies. The biceps and triceps muscles are activated on supination against resistance. Wrist extension reflexively occurs with firm finger flexion. The index flexor digitorum profundus is activated on strong flexor pollicis longus activation. Adjacent fingers flex and extend synchronously. Finger extensors activate with finger abduction and adduction. Toe extension accompanies ankle dorsiflexion and heel walking. People who claim they cannot close their fist may activate finger extensors to prevent passive motion of fingers into a fist. With some encouragement and gentle manipulation, fingers usually can be placed in a closed fist as the antagonistic extensors relax. After the fingers have been held passively in a fist, the person is asked to hold the position as pressure is released. Some people are able to maintain the closed fist position and then, after opening the hand, can resume the closed fist position, demonstrating what they claimed they could not do. Other people, when the fist is suddenly released, maintain the closed fist for several seconds before reverting to extensor activation and the fingers springing open. None of these responses is physiologic.

Watson[10] reported on the aforementioned tests in *The Wrist* and noted that flexor pollicis longus strength should not be exceeded in manual testing. The same principle can be applied to manual testing of hallux flexion and ankle, knee, and hip muscle strength. Overpowering a normal extremity on manual testing of these muscle groups is a sign of inconsistent effort or substantial weakness that should be matched by atrophy and other findings.

Twin hip adduction or abduction can be tested supine and seated and should not result in bilateral collapsing with a unilateral complaint. Hip abduction giving way to manual resistance, if physiologic, should be accompanied by a positive Trendelenburg test and an abductor gait. A person's claim of paralysis or severe weakness may be refuted by active deep tendon reflexes.

The Hoover test is the classic nonphysiologic finding (for full article, please see p. 99). Described 99 years ago, it confirms that problems separating objective from behavioral claims are not new.[11] A similar reverse Hoover test can be accomplished with the person prone and the examiner's hands beneath the right and left patellae. The patient is asked to lift the right or left knee, and the examiner assesses the presence or absence of downward pressure with the opposite patella.

The AMA *Guides to the Evaluation of Permanent Impairment* [12 (p.508, 16.8b)] discuss dynamometer testing at five positions as valid if the results form a bell curve. Consistent rapid alternating grip strengths are also evidence of valid muscle testing results.[12 (p508, 16.8b)]

Bilateral upper arm, forearm, thigh, and calf circumferences should be measured. Muscle bulk should be consistent with claimed muscle weakness. The pattern of muscle weakness should be neurologically consistent. Behavioral weakness usually does not match myelopathic, radicular, or peripheral nerve patterns. People with weakness in several nerve distributions or over several myotomes are more likely to have behavioral symptoms.

The mannequin sign is a rare but striking finding. The person claims that one or more digits are paralyzed and cannot be actively moved. There are no joint contractures to explain the loss of motion. The finger is typically held in semiflexion. Wide range of passive and active wrist motion occurs without any motion of the involved digit. This is an anatomic impossibility. A mannequin's joints can be moved independently. However, in a human, tendons crossing from forearm to fingers provide finger motion during passive wrist motion—the tenodesis effect. By demonstrating the lack of finger motion, the person proves activation of multiple muscles. People with the mannequin sign do not have visible skin, finger, nail, or muscle atrophy. Some claim so much pain that the finger cannot be examined, only observed.

Muscle spasms are not true late residuals of trauma. If muscle spasm is palpable or visible and then relaxes, it is likely voluntary. Extremity muscle spasms typically relax when testing antagonistic muscle strength. Spinal muscle spasm often resolves on alternating single-leg stance[12 (p382, Box 15-1)] and trunk bending right and left. Chronic peripheral muscle spasms may be indicative of neurologic disease, but in the setting of trauma are rare and, when present, are usually voluntary and behavioral.

Ambiguous Motion

Range-of-motion measurements obtained with goniometers or inclinometers are reported in degrees for documentation. Inconsistent or variable motion is commonly seen in illness behavior. Several measurements of the same joint(s) in differing positions may provide confirmation of inconsistency. A classic example is comparing straight-leg lifting when supine with that when seated. Another useful example is a discrepancy in measured passive knee flexion while supine and prone. The loss of passive knee flexion in prone position is a well-known sign of rectus femoris contracture. However, restricted prone knee flexion without muscle contracture is commonly seen in behavioral settings.

The AMA *Guides*[12(p.406)] suggest an accessory validity test for lumbosacral motion. The total range of sacral (hip) flexion and extension are measured with the person standing. This sum is compared with the measured straight-leg-lifting angle in the supine position on the most restricted side. If the straight-leg-lifting angle exceeds sacral range of motion by more than 15 degrees, lumbosacral motion measurements are considered invalid. However, for the test result to be valid, sacral flexion and extension must be less than normal, defined as less than 65° for women and 55° for men. Because hamstring and gluteal muscles are normally contracted when standing, and relaxed when supine, at sacral motion values greater than 65° and 55° this test is not valid. The test is also invalid if the person restricts passive straight lifting without signs of radiculopathy.

Observations about how motion is accomplished provide important behavioral clues. Cogwheel, stepwise, and bobbing motions are indicative of voluntary influences. People may paradoxically complain of joint pain but then demonstrate a significant "snap back" or rebound off the end of the patient's demonstrated range without apparent pain. When motion is tested in bilateral joints simultaneously, a person may restrict motion equally on the involved and uninvolved sides. For example, a person asked to abduct both shoulders simultaneously will demonstrate similar loss of motion on the claimed affected and normal sides. Simultaneous Phalen (hands held back to back) and prayer tests often reduce an exaggerated loss of wrist motion.

Abnormal Gait

Abnormalities of gait are important in assessing any person with spinal or lower extremity complaints and disease. A person who demonstrates normal gait and can tandem, tiptoe, and heel walk is unlikely to have significant spine or lower extremity disease.

Astasia-abasia is an archaic term for the inability to stand or walk in a normal manner. The gait is bizarre and does not suggest a specific organic lesion. Often the person sways wildly and nearly falls but recovers at the last moment. It is a symptom of hysteria-conversion reaction.[12]

A person may attempt to demonstrate impairment by choosing to use a cane even though it is unnecessary. However, he or she mistakenly employs it on the same side as the alleged lower extremity pathology. As the cane is not relieving any symptoms, the person does not realize his or her biomechanical error.

The person may tend to fall over a good leg, opposite the side of claimed lower extremity disease (with or without a support). There may be no observable change in gait when switching a cane to the opposite hand, or when walking while holding the cane off the floor.

Abnormal and normal gaits may alternate, sometimes depending on whether observed incidentally or during a specific gait examination. Gait may be accomplished with exaggerated effort, fatigue, groans, and sighs. Ambulation may be accompanied by convulsive tremor or violent shaking, but usually without loss of balance. A person may inappropriately adopt a cane for back pain without justifiable spinal instability or neurological pathology.[5 (p.190)]

People who exaggerate their symptoms cannot stand on one leg, although their gait is symmetrical. They cannot toe walk, yet they toe-off with each step. They cannot balance standing with legs together, but then do not demonstrate disequilibrium with ambulation. Knees may intermittently buckle, usually simultaneously. A posture of extreme trunk flexion, camptocormia, may be maintained, although it requires substantial effort and strength. Behavioral gaits include "tightrope walking" with arms extended in airplane-wing manner. Leg-dragging may be with internal or external hip rotation, but without circumduction seen with true paralysis. There may be no difference in gait in shoes or barefoot, despite claims of foot disease.

Inconsistent Observations

"You can observe a lot just by looking."

–Lawrence Peter "Yogi" Berra

Extensive normal and abnormal motion can be incidentally observed during an evaluation: how a sweater or shirt is donned over the head, buttoning and unbuttoning a blouse, taking socks off and putting them on, brassiere strap manipulation, and retrieval of a dropped object. Motion is incidentally noted when a patient demonstrates symptom location. Hairdo, makeup, and fingernail and toenail cosmesis often are inconsistent with claimed impairments. Jewelry offers many clues. Is it worn in an area of claimed pain? How is it removed and reapplied? Asking a patient to move his or her watch from one wrist to the other may provide clues to actual hand function.

During the examination, sitting and arising from a chair, mounting and dismounting the examination table, and mobility on the examination table, such as moving from a supine to a prone to a decubitus position, all provide information on a patient's disability or normality. The scoot test, asking a patient who is sitting on an examination table to move to the right or left, often provides information on range of motion and strength.

Office etiquette offers hints about a person's attitude toward his or her condition and the examining physician. People who arrive late, sometimes quite late, and do not cancel appointments they do not intend to keep often have more than medical issues. They may take a long time to complete a one-page intake form and symptom diagram, leaving all reports and films at home, and claim ignorance that a physical examination was required. They will object to disrobing, and insist previous examinations were done while they were fully clothed. The person may be inappropriately dressed with skimpy or no undergarments, and use this as an excuse to limit the physical examination. For people who forget their undergarments, the examiner can supply disposable wear.

People may claim to be doing daily exercises they cannot demonstrate. There may be no wear on the rubber tip of a cane, and no scratches on the cane handle.

CHAPTER 6

The cane is often not prescribed by a physician but was self-prescribed. The person might not bring braces and appliances he or she claims to be using daily. When an appliance is presented, it may look barely used, and the person may have difficulty fitting it or wearing it comfortably on the extremity. Skin and hair changes from alleged long-term brace wear are absent. Despite extensive use of an appliance, the person may admit to no improvement with immobilization.

Interpretation Of Behavioral Signs And Findings

So when are behavioral signs seen? They may be indications a person consciously or unconsciously wants to impress an audience—physician, spouse, family, employer, lawyer, judge, or jury—that their disorder or injury is serious. A patient may embellish if they feel their plight is not believed or if they have motives for other gains.

A person with behavioral findings may inaccurately respond to a provocative physical examination or provocative testing such as a discogram. The person may poorly respond to treatment, including physiotherapy such as work hardening and surgery, is typically out of work longer, claims greater physical impairment, and is less able to cope with pain and dysfunction.[5] Behavioral symptoms and signs may be indications of symptom magnification, augmentation, or hypervigilance; symptom, sign, or disease fabrication; or manifestations of psychiatric disease. Exaggerated behavioral symptoms are not likely to be considered evidence to support legal causation.

Diagnostic Tests

Images are the most common diagnostic test presented in a causality evaluation. However, by the time of a causality examination, additional imaging and laboratory tests are usually superfluous. It is usually easy to assign a particular time and event to fractures and dislocations. However, myriad imaging degenerative findings, particularly spinal, are difficult or impossible to date and assign causality. Further complicating attribution of causality is the poor correspondence between many imaging findings and symptoms. A large percentage of asymptomatic individuals have grossly abnormal spinal imaging—disk protrusions, facet degeneration, disk degeneration and dehydration, annular tears, spondylolyses, spinal stenosis, foraminal stenosis, and congenital deformities. As torn menisci in osteoarthritic knees are ubiquitous—regardless of symptoms—attributing a torn meniscus to a specific traumatic event is often speculative.[14] Unfortunately, the words "tear" and "herniation" suggest trauma, though that is often not the case.

Electrodiagnostic tests often provide clues to both etiology and chronology, as recent and chronic nerve injuries have differing patterns. Lack of bone scan activity shortly after trauma may be a clue that serious injury or a fracture had not occurred.

Sequential testing may provide clues to causality. Fracture healing and evolution of electrical findings, changes in bone scan all suggest chronology.

Laboratory tests may also identify diseases that explain findings, and distinguish medical from traumatic causes.

Residuals

Residuals can be divided into two types: (1) direct or indirect consequences of the claimed accident or exposure and (2) unrelated, from conditions that predated the causal event or occurred subsequently. In some jurisdictions, an evaluating physician may have to offer an opinion partitioning residuals. Apportionments may be required about preexisting conditions and subsequent accidents and occurrences. This is often the case in workers' compensation determinations.

Complications may also need consideration, although the way medicine and law approach complications differs. A treating physician considers a complication a new condition that needs proper diagnosis and then treatment, whatever the cause. Whether the complication was iatrogenic or spontaneous does not significantly influence treatment. However, legally, any complication of appropriate or inappropriate treatment is considered causally related to the primary condition. Whomever may be liable for the primary condition assumes liability for secondary conditions, and the two conditions are considered as one.

For example, a person falls, sustains a fracture that is surgically fixed, and then recovers well. However, during late removal of hardware, a major nerve is transected. Although the causes of the fracture and the nerve transection clearly differ, the defendant held responsible for the ankle fracture may be assessed responsibility for the later iatrogenic injury.

Although acute pain is expected and is causally connected to an injury, the presence of pain years later may or may not be related to the accident. Some people may only have residuals of treatment for the caused condition, like a surgical scar, or perhaps evidence of a complication of treatment. As a general guide, unexpected and inexplicable residuals are usually behavioral.

Documentation

An examining physician can expect a vigorous questioning by attorneys from both sides when causality is a legal matter. Objective documentation assists in defending opinions about causality and residuals. The results of measurements—angles, lengths, circumferences, temperatures, and weights—are often persuasive. A digital camera is an excellent adjunct. Some examiners take a portrait (photograph) as confirmation the patient was in their office. Unusual scars and other physical findings may warrant photography. When critical diagnostic films (e.g., MRI, CT scan, radiographs etc.) are presented but cannot be retained by the examining physician, digital photographs of these films may be appropriate to preserve the evidence. The particular venue may determine whether a patient can be photographed or videotaped. In some locations, judges permit the entire examination to be transcribed by a court reporter and even simultaneously videotaped.

Conclusions

The physician examining for causality should be able to answer the following questions:
1. What is the diagnosis (disease or injury)?
2. Did the accident, event, or exposure cause the disease or injury?
3. Was treatment provided required because of the accident, event, or exposure? Or did it address unrelated condition(s)
4. Did treatment modify symptoms—for better or for worse—or was care ineffective?
5. Were there preexisting conditions?
6. Was the preexisting condition permanently aggravated by the accident, event, or exposure?
7. Does the person have residuals causally related directly or indirectly to the accident, event, or exposure?
8. Did a subsequent accident, event, or exposure modify the original diagnosis or residuals?
9. What is the permanence, and how will it affect daily activities and employment (see Guides, 5th edition, Chapters 1 and 2 for more details)?
10. Did behavioral factors influence the person's course or outcome?
11. Do these behavioral factors explain claimed residuals?

This article describing the Hoover test was published 99 years ago. It has amazing clarity and remains pertinent.

A New Sign for the Detection of Malingering and Functional Paresis of the Lower Extremities

C. F. Hoover, M.D. CLEVELAND.

The sign I wish to describe is one which I have employed for the past two years. Although the cases observed number only four, I feel justified in attaching great importance to the sign because it is dependent on a normal function, which I find always exhibited in healthy persons and invariably present in the sound leg of patients suffering from hemiplegia or paresis of one leg due to some pathologic lesion.

If a normal person, lying on a couch in the dorsal position, be asked to lift the right foot off the couch with the leg extended, the left heel will be observed to dig into the couch as the right leg and thigh are elevated. If you place your hand under the tendo Achilles of the left side and sense the muscular resistance offered by the left leg you will observe that the left heel is pressed on to the couch with the same force which is exhibited in lifting the right leg off the couch. In other words, the left heel is employed to fix a point of opposition against the couch during the effort at lifting the right leg. This will always occur if the healthy person makes a free and uninhibited effort to lift the right leg. Of course the opposition offered by the other leg is not essential to a successful elevation of one leg but if a free effort of the will is made (no matter how slight the effort) the point of opposition made with the leg of the other side is invariably present unless some inhibitory impulse be sent to the opposing leg.

If the movements are carried out in the reverse order the same principle holds true; i.e., if a normal person be requested to press the right leg against the surface of the couch there will be a counter-lifting force exhibited in the left leg.

If a patient suffering from hemiplegia or monoplegia of a leg be requested to lift the extended and paretic leg off the couch it will be observed that the other leg offers the opposition above described whether there is any voluntary muscle strength exhibited or not on the affected side. I have had opportunity to observe this in a large number of hemiplegic patients and the opposition from the normal leg never failed.

If the hemiparetic patient is asked to lift the normal leg off the couch against resistance he will exhibit an opposition with paretic leg which is directly proportional to the voluntary muscular strength he is able to employ when a display of voluntary muscle power in the paretic leg is exacted.

A New Sign for the Detection of Malingering and Functional Paresis of the Lower Extremities, *continued*

When the upper extremity is involved this sign is sometimes demonstrable on the normal arm, but at other times it is wanting.

In two cases in which paresis of one leg was claimed by the plaintiffs in suits for personal injuries, they were wanting the characteristic physical signs to sustain the claim of paresis of the lower extremity as the result of injuries. Furthermore, in both of these cases, when the patient was asked to lift the normal leg off the couch, the leg which was alleged to be very paretic was opposed strongly against the surface when resistance was offered to lifting the normal leg. When the patient was requested to lift the paretic leg, there was an apparent attempt to respond to my demand, but the normal leg did not offer the least opposition. The normal leg lay perfectly limp on the couch. Had the paresis been genuine, the sound leg would have been firmly opposed against surface of the couch when an uninhibited attempt was made to lift the paretic leg.

The absolute lack of complementary opposition from the normal leg was also observed in the case of hysterical hemiplegia, when the patient was requested to lift the paralyzed leg.

In another case of hysterical para-paresis inferior, which was accompanied by abasia, the patient could bow himself into the pose of opisthotonos, but if he was requested to lift one leg off the couch there was no complemental opposition offered by the other leg and the leg which he seemingly attempted to lift would not be raised off the couch.

This sign appeals to me as being particularly valuable for the reason that it depends on the exhibition of a function from the normal leg which must always be present if the patient does not inhibit the normal impulses to the lower extremities.

In the four cases I have briefly described the complemental opposition was entirely wanting. Whether this lack of complemental opposition will always be found or not in malingerers and hysterical subjects remains for further observation to determine. But, in view of the fact that complemental opposition is always present in a normal patient and in all patients with genuine paresis and genuine paralysis, we are justified in assuming the existence of cerebral inhibition to an apparent voluntary exhibition of strength when complemental opposition is absent.

If a malingerer were familiar with the object of the examination he could, of course, satisfy the demands of the examiner. In testing for this sign the examiner should seem to fix his attention on the leg which is alleged to be paretic.

In this manner I believe that one will always be able to trick a malingerer or hysterical subject into betraying the falsity of his claim.

I demonstrated the character and significance of this sign to one of the patients described. He promptly abandoned a crutch and cane, an orthopedic corset and blue spectacles and returned to work for the company against whom he had brought suit. The same course was adopted with the hysterical abasic patient. His gait became quite normal after a half hour's persuasion. Whether he later relapsed or not I do not know.

The sign in genuine hemiplegia, which Babinski describes for differentiating between genuine and functional hemiplegias depends on the affected side for its exhibition. I have found Babinski's sign unsatisfactory. The fact that this sign of complemental opposition is always present in normal subjects and in genuine paresis of the lower extremity, and the fact that it depends on invariable function of the normal side gives it a very broad application.

JAMA. AUG. 29, 1908; 51; pp: 746-747. © 1908 American Medical Association. All Rights Reserved.

References

1. Grace TG, ed. Independent Medical Evaluations. Rosemont, IL: American Academy of Orthopaedic Surgeons; 2001.
2. Melhorn, JM. Chapter 7 Upper Extremity: RTW by Consensus Documents. In: 8th Annual Occupational Orthopaedics and Workers' Compensation: A Multidisciplinary Perspective, Rosemont, IL: American Academy of Orthopaedic Surgeons; 2006.
3. Melhorn, JM. Chapter 10 Arm Pain: Prevention and Return to Work. In: Occupational Orthopaedics and Workers' Compensation: A Multidisciplinary Perspective. J. M. Melhorn and J. S. Barr Jr, eds. Rosemont, IL: American Academy of Orthopaedic Surgeons; 2001.
4. Melhorn, JM and Ian BF. 7th Annual Occupational Orthopaedics and Workers' Compensation: A Multidisciplinary Perspective. Rosemont, IL: American Academy of Orthopaedic Surgeons; 2005.
5. Waddell G. *The Back Pain Revolution.* 2nd ed. Edinburgh, Scotland: Churchill Livingstone; 2004.
6. Melhorn, JM. Return to Work - Workplace Guides. In: Workers' compensation case management: a multidisciplinary perspective, edited by J. M. Melhorn and J. P. Zeppieri, Rosemont, IL: American Academy of Orthopaedic Surgeons, 1999: 451-458.
7. Guilick WG. *Mental Diseases: A Handbook Dealing With Diagnosis and Classification.* St Louis, MO: CV Mosby; 1918:133.
8. Bowlus WE, Currier RD. A test for hysterical hemianalgesia. *N Engl J Med.* 1963;269:1253.
9. Hallett M, Fahn S, Jankovic J, et al. *Psychogenic Movement Disorders.* Philadelphia, PA: Lippincott Williams & Williams; 2006.

CHAPTER 6

10. Watson HK. Examination of the wrist. In: Watson HK, Weinzweig J, eds. *The Wrist.* Philadelphia, PA: Lippincott Williams & Wilkins; 2001:47-59.

11. Hoover CF. A new sign for the detection of malingering and functional paresis of the lower extremities. *JAMA.* 1908;51:746-747.

12. American Medical Association. *Guides to the Evaluation of Permanent Impairment.* 5th ed. Chicago, IL: AMA; 2000:508, 16.8b.

13. Spraycar M, Randolph E, eds. *Stedman's Medical Dictionary.* 26th ed. Baltimore, MD: Williams & Wilkins; 1995:158.

14. Bhattacharyya T, et al. The Clinical Importance of Meniscal Tears Demonstrated by Magnetic Resonance Imaging in Osteoarthritis of the Knee. *JBJS* 2003; 85:4-9.

Bibliography

Block A, Gatchel R, Deardoff W, Gyer R. *The Psychology of Spine Surgery.* Washington, DC: American Psychological Association; 2003.

Blom A, Taylor A, Whithouse S, Orr B, Smith E. A new sign of inappropriate lower back pain. *Ann R Coll Surg Engl.* 2000;84:342-343. [heel-tap test]

Centeno C.Waddell's signs revisited [editorial]? *Spine.* 2004;29:13:1392.

Deyo R. Pain and public policy. *N Engl J Med.* 2000;342:1211-1213. ["Treatments are sometimes imposed as if desperation were a legitimate indication, circumventing the need for objective evidence . . . "]

Ferrari R. *The Whiplash Encyclopedia.* Gaithersburg, MD: Aspen Publications; 1999.

Gaines W, Hegmann K. Effectiveness of Waddell's non-organic signs in predicting a delayed return to regular work in patients experiencing acute occupational low back pain. *Spine.* 1999;24:396-401.

Hadler N. *Occupational Musculoskeletal Disease.* 3rd ed. Philadelphia, PA: Lippincott Williams & Wilkins; 2004.

Menard M, et al. Pattern of performance in workers with low back pain during comprehensive motor performance evaluation. *Spine.* 1994;19:132:1359-1366.

Pearl J. *Causality: The Art and Science of Cause and Effect.* Cambridge, MA: Cambridge University Press; 2000:331-357 [epilogue].

Politan P, Cox B, Gatchel R, Mayer T. A prospective study of Waddell signs in patients with chronic low back pain. *Spine.* 1997;22:14:1618-1621.

Rainville J, Jouve C, Finno M, Limke J. Comparison of four tests of quadriceps strength in L3 or L4 radiculopathies. *Spine.* 2003;28:21:2466-2471.

Scaer R. *The Body Bears the Burden: Trauma, Dissociation, and Disease.* New York, NY: Haworth Medical Press; 2001.

Waddell G. Non-organic signs [editorial:]. *Spine.* 2004;29:13:1393.

Werneke M, Harris D, Lichter R. Clinical effectiveness of behavioral signs for screening chronic low-back pain patients in a work-oriented physical rehabilitation program. *Spine.* 1993;18:16:2412-2418.

7

Report Writing

Paul F. Waldner, JD, and Gary Freeman, MD, JD

Wayne was a very precise person. From the way he lined up his shoes in his closet, to his arrangement of ties by color, to his job as an electrical engineer, everything he did, he did with precision. Every morning he had a bowl of oatmeal with two spoonfuls of raisins, one spoonful of sugar, and a half cup of skim milk. He had two pieces of whole-wheat toast, orange marmalade, and one banana. He drank a small glass of orange juice and a cup of coffee. One cup. After breakfast he brushed his teeth, put the dog outside, and left for work precisely at 7:15 AM.

On the morning of his death, Wayne did something totally out of character; he had a second cup of coffee. Engrossed in the article about the construction of a cogeneration plant that was on the front page of the business section of the morning paper, Wayne poured himself another cup, finished his breakfast, brushed his teeth, let the dog out, and left for work at 7:25 AM.

The intersection of his street and the railroad track was framed by tall weeds on both sides. There had been no mowing for months. The stop sign was on the other side of the tracks. Wayne never saw the train approaching because his field of vision from his sports car was blocked by the weeds. The impact was horrific. Wayne was ejected from the vehicle and killed instantly.

If he had just stuck to his routine, if he had just had one cup of coffee, Wayne would have made it to work that morning.

The cause of Wayne's death? The second cup of coffee.

The concept of "causation" in a legal context can be baffling for health care professionals: Baffling because it seems to never be the same. Baffling because whether there's causation in any particular case depends on the circumstances, the definition, and the principles that might be applicable. Given the exact facts, there may be sufficient causation in a workers' compensation case but insufficient causation in an automobile accident case. Given the exact facts, there may be insufficient causation in a construction accident case but sufficient causation in a case involving a defective product. When asked about the sufficiency of causation by a layperson, lawyers frequently give the answer that clients hate the most: It *depends.*

The purpose of this chapter is to acquaint health care professionals with the general definitions, principles, and concepts that all must be considered when the question of causation is being answered.

In Wayne's case, the weeds were arguably a proximate cause of the accident. The second cup of coffee was a producing cause of the accident. The distinction between these concepts will be discussed in greater detail. Hopefully, this discussion will assist in writing reports and in giving depositions and trial testimony.

Causation: The Link in the Chain

Most claims that arise out of an injury involve three basic elements that must be proven: liability, damages, and causation. First, *liability* must be proven. It must be established that the person or entity against whom the claim is being made is in some way legally responsible for the injury. *Damages,* or the nature and extent of the injury, must be proven. Damages include economic losses, e.g., lost wages, medical bills, and property damage, and non-economic losses, e.g., pain, mental anguish, and disfigurement. *Causation* is the element that links liability and damages. If someone was negligent and someone was injured, it must be proven that the negligence caused the injury.

> Mary had been worried about the lump in her right breast. She showed it to her physician. He laughed and told her to forget about it, it was nothing. Two days later, she sought and obtained a second opinion from another physician. A needle aspiration was done. A malignancy was discovered. Mary had a uni-lateral mastectomy.

Was Mary's first physician negligent? Of course. Was she injured? Of course she was; she lost her breast. Is there causation linking the two? No. Had Mary's cancer been diagnosed 48 hours earlier, the result would have been the same. Does Mary have a malpractice claim? No; she has only two of the three necessary elements. Her first physician ran the stop sign but did not hit anyone. Just negligence and injury mean nothing legally without the two being linked by causation.

Proximate Cause

Here is the textbook definition of *proximate cause*:

> The proximate cause of an injury is the primary or moving cause that produces the injury and without which the accident could not have happened, if the injury is one which might be reasonably anticipated or foreseen as a natural conse-quence of the wrongful act.[1]

The phrase "which might be reasonably anticipated or foreseen" is the part of the definition that seems to get the most attention. Back to Wayne's accident. Was the second cup of coffee a proximate cause of his death? It could hardly have been anticipated or foreseen that drinking a second cup would result in being hit by a train and killed. Were the weeds a proximate cause of the accident? Sure looks like it. If the approaching train cannot be seen, it can be anticipated or foreseen that a person will drive across the tracks and, if a train's coming, might be hit and killed. Same facts, but when you focus on one event or condition (the second cup of coffee) there is insufficient causation; and when you focus on another (the unmowed intersection) there is causation—all because of the reasonably anticipated or foreseen part of the definition.

Producing Cause

This category of causation is sometimes referred to as *cause in fact*. Here is the definition:

> A producing cause of an injury for which compensation is sought is that [said] cause which, in a natural and continuous sequence, produces the injury, and without which the injury would not have occurred.[1]

Gone from the definition is the "anticipated or foreseen" requirement. *Producing cause* lacks the element of foreseeability, which is the cornerstone of proximate cause. Did one event produce another? If the first event is taken out of the picture, does the second one happen? Was Wayne's second cup of coffee a producing cause of his death? Sure was. Take it away, and he leaves his house 10 minutes earlier. And if he is at the railroad tracks 10 minutes earlier, he and the train never collide.

Producing cause is much less a burden on the claimant than proximate cause. Producing cause is usually the standard applied in workers' compensation claims, admiralty claims (Jones Act), and railroad claims (Federal Employers Liability Act).

Medical-Legal Standard

Every jurisdiction has a threshold standard for the admissibility of medical opinions. In many jurisdictions, the standard is reasonable medical probability. In others, it is a reasonable degree of medical certainty. In a few, it is simply more likely than not.

What the standards all have in common is that compliance with the standard is an absolute requirement for the admission into evidence of an opinion in a medical case. The question, "Doctor, is it possible . . . " is usually cut off in mid-sentence by an objection. Courts want to know what is probable, not what is possible. The courts recognize that medicine is an inexact science. For that reason, the standard is never one of certainty. The standard is virtually always some variant of what is probable or likely, something that if converted to percentages would indicate something more than 50%.

It is important to know the applicable standard before writing a report or giving a deposition or trial testimony. The standard for any medical witness and the requirements for the testimony to be considered evidentiary is clearly conveyed in statements such as, "In my opinion and based on reasonable medical probability, I . . . ." Therefore, the standard should be known, memorized, and used. Furthermore, knowing and using the standard appropriately in reports and testimony will prevent many avoidable problems.

Daubert v Merrell Dow Pharmaceuticals, Inc[2]

At one time, all an expert witness had to do to express an opinion in a legal case was prove to the judge that he or she was smart. A person who went to college and medical school, completed a residency, and practiced orthopedic surgery could give an opinion, for example, that the automobile accident caused the ruptured disc at L5-S1.

Then, in 1993, the US Supreme Court changed all of that.

Anyone who might ever be asked to give an opinion in a legal claim should know about this decision. Unfortunately, it has a name that causes considerable head scratching about its pronunciation. It is pronounced "daw-burt," not "daw-bear." *Daubert* was a pharmaceutical case. Like most drug cases, the principal issue is causation. Someone took a drug, something bad happened, and the central question was whether the drug caused it. In pre-Daubert cases, all the claimant needed was a "really smart person" on the witness stand to point the finger of guilt at the drug. The opinion was admissible because a really smart person said it. *Daubert* changed all of that. Now, four criteria must be met for an opinion to be admissible:

1. The methods on which the testimony is based are centered on a testable hypothesis.
2. There is a known or potential rate of error associated with the method.
3. The method has been subject to peer review.
4. The method is generally accepted in the relevant scientific community.

Any health care provider who is asked to give causation testimony—in a workers' compensation claim, an automobile accident case, or a product liability

CHAPTER 7

lawsuit—must measure his or her opinions regarding causation against these criteria. These criteria should be reviewed before any testimony is given at deposition or trial because it should be anticipated that each of these four areas will be challenged by someone.

The Report

Most claims for compensation of any kind, e.g., workers' compensation, social security, maritime, negligence, and malpractice, will require the health care provider to write a report. Meticulous attention must be given to this task because the report will later become the questioning attorney's road map for deposition or trial testimony. The report is not office dictation. It is not clinical notes or correspondence with a colleague. It is the document that will be referred to in order to determine the nature and extent of the injury, the extent of any disability or impairment, and, in many cases, the critical element of causation.

A suggested outline for the report is as follows:
1. A brief summary of the case
2. A list of all records reviewed
3. The history given and the source(s) of the history
4. Qualifications of the report writer
5. The results of the physical examination
6. The results of any tests
7. The diagnosis
8. A description of the treatment given or expected to be given
9. The prognosis, including, when appropriate, disability and impairment ratings
10. An opinion about the cause of the injury

Obviously, there would be variations on this outline depending on the kind of claim involved. But the previous 10 criteria are fairly standard for most claims that involve an injury.

One cannot overstate the importance of a thorough and complete history because that is usually the foundation on which the causation testimony is structured.

The most common objection to expert reports is that they are conclusionary. An opinion cannot be given without stating a conclusion, can it? An opinion *is* a conclusion. But the courts require that a complete explanation be given before the conclusion is stated. In causation opinions, for example, the explanation could be a discussion of the mechanism of injury, the temporal relationship between the event and the symptoms, or the nature of the symptoms themselves.

The report should be written with the following in mind: This is the document that will be the framework of your testimony in a deposition or a trial. This is the document that people who will be questioning you will be referring to most frequently during your examination. Your report can be your best friend or your worst enemy.

The Type of Claim Is Important

As mentioned earlier, there are different species of causation. Knowing which one applies to the case at hand is helpful.

In most negligence cases, proximate cause must be proven. Automobile accidents, slip-and-falls, construction site accidents, and similar events, all usually require proof that the resulting injury was foreseeable. In most product liability, maritime, railroad, and workers' compensation cases, it has to be proven simply that an event or condition caused an injury or the producing cause standard applies.

A medical witness, when giving causation opinions, usually is not asked to comment on whether the injury was foreseeable. The important issue for medical witnesses is whether the event or condition caused the injury, not whether the injury was foreseeable. An important exception to this would be medical negligence cases.

It would be a good practice for medical witnesses to inquire about the type of claim and the exact nature of causation testimony that will be required in a report before writing the report.

Defending the Causation Opinion

A medical witness who has thoroughly reviewed the chart, done a MEDLINE search on the most recent relevant articles, re-read the applicable chapter in Campbell's *Operative Orthopaedics*, gone through all four *Daubert* criteria, and is ready for giving a deposition or trial testimony should be ready for questions like these:

CHAPTER 7

Doctor, did you notice that he had injured the same level of his back 2 years before this injury?

Your response: Yes, but he went back to work in 3 weeks and worked continuously as an ironworker up to the date of this injury.

But don't you think that the first injury caused his ruptured disc?

Your response: To restate my opinion, the first injury healed and was over with. The overwhelming probability is that the injury we're here to talk about ruptured his disc. Let me put it this way: the first injury was like a road rock putting a little chip in your windshield. *This* injury was like someone throwing a brick through it.

Doctor, what's the basis for your opinion that my client's disc wasn't ruptured in the car wreck?

Your response: My opinion is based on my education and my experience in treating back injuries of every description for the last 20 years. It's also based on the medical literature and on the history I was given. It's also based on the alleged mechanism of injury. It is my opinion that a rear-end collision at less than 15 mph will not rupture a lumbar disc in a seat-belted driver.

Doctor, is it *possible* that the accident at work caused the symptoms he reported to you during the independent medical examination (IME)?

Your response: The number of possibilities for any event is infinite. But, if you're after what's *likely,* I can assure you that what's likely is the work injury had nothing to do with those symptoms.

Doctor, do you know *for sure* that the prior back injuries we've discussed didn't combine to make his surgery necessary?

Your response: No. Very little in medicine is known with absolute certainty. But, I do know that they *probably* didn't.

Frequently, the most accurate answer that should be given in response to a question about causation would be one of the following:

- I don't know.
- I don't have enough information to answer your question.
- I'm not qualified to answer your question.
- I don't have an opinion about what caused the injury.
- There are many *possible* causes but, in my opinion,
  not one *probable* cause.

Determining the cause of an accident, an injury, a disability or an impairment within the guidelines of the rules may be a daunting or even impossible task. At some point, making an honest assessment to determine the probable cause becomes little more than an educated guess. The witness is not required to know everything or even have an opinion on everything. When the issue of causation is simply too close to call, the witness should remember that an opinion is not required.

Summary

When a physician is treating an injury, the exact cause of that injury can be way down on the list of the things that are important to consider. There are just so many ways to treat a fractured tibia, and just how the tibia was fractured probably does not enter into the equation. But in treating injuries, a physician should also consider that injuries frequently result in a claim of some kind. It might be a legal claim against another person, a claim for disability insurance against the patient's carrier, or a claim for disability benefits under Medicare or workers' compensation, but all of these species of claims have at least one thing in common: what caused the injury or resulting disability or impairment is of great importance to the claim. If the condition was not caused by the work, there is no basis for a workers' compensation claim. If the automobile accident did not cause the back problems, there is no basis for the lawsuit. The extent to which a causation determination by a physician is important and even may be outcome determinative should never be underappreciated.

Knowing the medical-legal standard, being familiar with the various forms of causation, and being able to defend the causation opinion are all of high importance to any physician who ever treats an injured patient.

References

1. *Black's Law Dictionary, Revised.* 4th ed. St. Paul, Minnesota: West Publishing Co; 1968.
2. *Daubert v Merrell Dow Pharmaceuticals,* 509 US 579 (1993).

CHAPTER 7

CHAPTER

Spinal Disorders Causation

Donald Krawciw, MD, CCFP, Dip Sports Med

The causation of spinal disorders, particularly traumatic causation, is one of the most commonly encountered questions in general medicolegal occupational medicine or independent medical examination (IME) practice. This chapter discusses the basic similarities and differences between legal and scientific causation arguments as they apply to spinal disorders, epidemiologic or scientific causation arguments in more detail, and the scientific data relevant to some of the more commonly encountered disorders of the cervical, thoracic, and lumbar spine, beginning with mechanical neck and low back pain. This chapter does not address systemic spinal disorders such as malignancy, inflammatory disease, and radiation of pain from non-spinal structures.

Differential Diagnosis

The differential diagnosis for low back pain includes mechanical and nonmechanical causes and referred pain from visceral disease. Mechanical low back pain can include spondylosis (facet pain), spondylolysis, spondylolisthesis, disc herniation, spinal stenosis, and fractures.[1-19]

Non-mechanical low back pain can be caused by neoplasia, infection, abscesses, metabolic bone disease (e.g., Paget), and different forms of inflammatory arthritis.[20-23] Low back pain related to visceral disease may be referred from pelvic organs, kidney disease, vascular disease, and gastrointestinal disease.[24-27] The specific pathologic picture of mechanical low back pain is difficult to ascertain. Despite the sophistication of modern medicine, the pain-generating structure can usually not be determined. A diagnosis of pain related to non-mechanical low back pain is easier to discern because in many cases, objective pathologic findings can be defined.

Scientific vs. Legal Cause

What is *cause*? As Aristotle taught in his metaphysics,[28] it depends on the context of the question. Some causes are necessary, others are sufficient. Some are general, others specific. Much of the fundamental thinking and wording of modern IME reports has changed little in essence, only in translation from the Attic Greek of 300 BC.

"Does the flap of a butterfly's wings in Brazil set off a tornado in Texas?"[29,30]

"Does twisting on stairs at work result in an artificial knee replacement 20 years later?"

With the first statement in 1972, sometimes called the "Butterfly effect," Edward Lorenz, Massachusetts Institute of Technology, popularized chaos theory, adding yet another chapter to Aristotle, Hume, and others in the human debate about the cause of things.

Scientific and legal analyses of causation approach evidence differently. This topic is further developed elsewhere in this text. Scientific causation considers population-based, randomized studies of large groups as the strongest evidence. Legal causation accords much weight to specific anecdotal details of the case. Scientific cause follows an inductive logic and looks at the reproducibility of hypotheses by different observers. Legal cause follows deductive logic and looks at the weight of expert opinion and may choose to select one opinion over all the others if it is thought to be most credible. The Daubert Rules of Evidence in the United States and Civil Procedure Rules in the United Kingdom seek to minimize the effect of biased expert opinion. Scientific cause and legal cause are, therefore, cousins, not twins.[31-33]

TABLE 8-1   Scientific vs. Legal Cause

Scientific Cause	Legal Cause
Predominant, underlying, cause in fact	Proximate
Inductive argument	Deductive logic
Populations	Individual case
Stochastic, chaos theory	Deterministic
Randomized trials	Weighing of expert opinion
Multifactorial	Unifactorial
Etiology	Responsibility, liability

Scientific Cause (Etiology) of Spinal Disorders

Epidemiologists seek first to identify a disease using a case definition. This definition should be robust, with good interrater reliability. The case definition should be demonstrably distinct from the background "normal" population, with a reasonably well-defined cutoff. The moniker "disorder" or "disease" is attached to the case definition if it can be demonstrated to increase the risk of morbidity or mortality in the population. A *tautological or circular case definition* is one in which the disease is defined by its alleged cause or treatment. A *radiologic diagnosis* is a condition described on X-ray or other imaging that may or may not have a clear clinical correlate. A *symptomatic or subjective diagnosis* is a collection of subjective symptoms. A *diagnosis of exclusion* is the inverse of a diagnostic entity—it is the absence of diagnoses.[34] Steurer and others[35] developed these taxonomic issues further.

Epidemiology aims to direct us to a cause but generally gets us no closer than an association, which is a bidirectional relationship between one variable and another.

The strength of association is measured by different study designs that maximize power and minimize bias and confounding. Generally, prospective studies are preferred over retrospective studies for assessing cause.[36,37]

In the case of low back pain, epidemiologic studies have been hampered by the lack of a consistent case definition for low back pain and the lack of validated outcome measures to reliably assess the extent of low back pain and disability in the population.[38] There is a great need to reduce interrater variation and minimize sources of bias in this field of research. Hopefully, progress will be made by the work of evidenced-based diagnostic methods groups.

Because of the high prevalence and variability of back pain in the general population, statistical methods for determining clinically important differences in outcomes are still being developed.[39,40] Ultimately, we are left with a list of risk factors with varying levels of association with the condition of interest.

Different philosophical heuristics are then used to argue causation by applying deductive logic to statistical data.[37,41] The most common heuristic is referred to as the Hill principles of causation[41], which is somewhat akin to the Koch postulates of infection. In general terms, the Hill principles of causation are embodied and supported by different study designs:

- Mechanistic or biomechanical studies on animal or cadaveric models (biologic plausibility)
- Cohort studies that demonstrate an association (strength of association)
- Interventional or crossover studies that demonstrate a reversal of causation

Another commonly used heuristic is the attributable-fraction method. If a risk factor has a relative risk of 2 or more, it can be argued that the causal risk for a person is 50% or more, or "within reasonable medical certainty/probability."[42] An alternative heuristic might assign relative weights to the relative risk measurement and its statistical significance (confidence intervals) before concluding that the risk to a person is more than 50%.

Often spinal changes present at multiple levels are argued to be degenerative, whereas a single-level change can be more suggestive of traumatic injury. However, one should be cautious when applying deterministic logic in individual cases in the absence of good population data. Great care should be taken to avoid causal fallacies such as *post hoc ergo propter hoc* (covered in Chapter 3) .[43]

Experimental Sources of Data

Anatomic, Biomechanical, and Cadaveric studies

The studies can be termed *preclinical* because they often involve animal or cadaveric subjects in the absence of clinical manifestations. This type research gained momentum in the 1930s when Mixter and Barr[44] postulated that disorders of the intervertebral disc might be the cause of most back pain. More modern progression of this line of basic research takes us to the use of high-tesla magnetic resonance imaging (MRI) and functional MRI to further delineate anatomic variants and biochemical correlates of structure.

Although these studies represent the key first step toward the anatomic diagnosis of disease, the reader is cautioned that studies demonstrating a correlation with clinical findings in a population are the next step. In other words, the prevalence of these findings in symptomatic and asymptomatic people needs to be studied before an anatomic finding can be classified as a normal variant or pathologic.

Biomechanical research studies the spine using mechanical engineering principles of strain and fatigue. The development of mechanical wear can be correlated to extremes of loading and repetitive movement. However, such studies demonstrating damage at high mechanical load may or may not necessarily extrapolate in a linear manner to produce damage at physiologic loads. (See the "Repetitive Injury (Overuse or Toxicologic) Paradigm.")

CHAPTER 8

Injection Studies

This research seeks to identify pain-generating structures by documenting symptom improvement after injection of anesthetic near various structures. This research is helpful in cases in which there is an independent "gold standard" case definition of the condition being treated, such as disc herniation. The research is ambiguous when the clinical entity is itself defined by the outcome of the injection in the absence of any gold standard (a tautology).

Ergonomic Studies

Similar to biomechanical studies, this research looks for association between biomechanical work functions and clinical outcomes, typically pain.

Genetic Studies

These studies are only now coming to the forefront of spinal research. The use of registries of twins allows for the genetic correlation of symptomatic and anatomic or radiologic outcomes. In some cases, molecular biologic markers can then be sought in the search for a putative gene. With the revolution in molecular genetics, this avenue holds much promise for progress in our understanding of spinal disorders.

Environmental Causation: Degeneration vs. Trauma

It has been difficult to study the effect of acute trauma in a scientific manner because trauma can generally only be identified retrospectively. Furthermore, traumatic explanations of injury lend themselves easily to the legal tort process, and so tautological "tort" language can easily be adopted to diagnose medical conditions. The terms *posttraumatic, cumulative trauma disorder, whiplash,* and *strain* are not necessarily clinical diagnoses per se, but they reflect causal assumptions. Attempts to support this theory are hampered by the lack of a clear case definition for "back strain." As described by Deyo et al[45]: "strain and sprain have never been anatomically or histologically characterized."

Recently, Caragee et al[46,47] described a cohort that was followed up prospectively and asked to keep a record of episodes of injury. Although still subject to recall bias, this method holds some promise for studying the temporal link of trauma and outcome in spine pain.

Clinical Syndromes

Neck and Low Back Pain

Although records of cases of low back pain are first documented among the Egyptians, spinal pain first commonly came to be attributed to injury or trauma in the Victorian era, with the rise of Ehrichsen's "railway spine" as a diagnosis. The theory was that back pain in people who rode on railroads was due to the excessive speed achieved by steam engine trains, speeds not previously attainable. Not coincidentally, this occurred alongside the rise of the workers' compensation system in England, where it was adopted from Bismarck's German model.[48(pp 47-69)]

Low back pain affects more than 70% of the population in developed countries and poses a major socioeconomic burden, accounting for 13% of sickness absences in the United Kingdom. The annual incidence in adults is up to 45%, with people aged 35 to 55 years affected most often. Although 90% of episodes of acute low back pain resolve within 6 weeks, chronic pain develops in up to 7% of patients.[49]

Approximately 80% of Americans experience at least one episode of back pain during their lifetime, with 15% to 20% reporting back pain at some time during a 1-year period. In Australians, the lifetime incidence is 80%; 1-year prevalence is 68%.[50,51]

A systematic literature review of acute low back pain by Pengel et al[52] concluded that rapid improvements in pain (58% reduction of initial scores), disability (58%), and return to work (82%) occurred within 1 month. There was further improvement until about 3 months. Thereafter, levels for pain, disability, and return to work remained almost constant to 12 months of follow up; 73% of patients had at least one recurrence within 12 months.

Some reviewers of low back pain describe a subcategory known as *sacroiliac joint pain*. This term is often used interchangeably with *sacroiliac dysfunction,* which typically implies a dynamic instability of the sacroiliac joint. Although much has been written on this condition, particularly by Bogduk,[53] other reviewers conclude that sacroiliac dysfunction (or mechanical, non-inflammatory sacroiliac pain) is controversial and overdiagnosed—there is little scientific evidence to correlate history and examination findings with this diagnosis.[54-59] However, this conclusion should not preclude careful examination and imaging to rule out potential pathology in the joint.

Scientific Paradigms for Low Back Pain

We are still in the "preantibiotic" era of understanding the cause of back pain. Low back pain is like a sandbox in which theorists build castles. A historic overview on the diagnosis of back pain in the 20th century notes how neural, muscular, and osseous causes have been postulated, with an increase in emphasis in "discogenic" pain since the Mixter and Barr article of 1938.[44] As with many taxonomic controversies, "lumpers" and "splitters" have emerged. For an introduction to the essential issues in low back pain diagnosis, the reader is urged to read the historical development of the topic by Lutz et al[60] and the 2002 debate between Deyo[59] and Abraham and Killackey-Jones[61] in the *Archives of Internal Medicine.* Both genetic and environmental themes play a role in the following paradigms:

Idiopathic Paradigm: The Null Hypothesis of Causation   This view takes the perspective that we simply do not know with any satisfactory level of probability what causes most cases of low back pain. The term *nonspecific low back pain* is often used in this context. Back pain is, thus, a symptom without explanation and a diagnosis of exclusion. "About 90% of all patients with low back pain will have non-specific low back pain, which, in essence, is a diagnosis based on exclusion of specific pathology."[62]

"Nonspecific terms, such as strain, sprain, or degenerative processes, are commonly used. Strain and sprain have never been anatomically or histologically characterized, and patients given these diagnoses might accurately be said to have idiopathic low back pain."[45] "The underlying cause of low back pain is unknown."[59]

Acute Injury Paradigm   This is the standard paradigm in Western medicine for acute low back pain. A person lifts a heavy box, feels a pop or a crack, and is thought to have a back strain. The strain gradually resolves over time as the soft tissue injury heals.

The problem with this model is that no histologic evidence of *acute strain* has ever been found. In a cohort of 200 patients followed up for back pain for 5 years, there was no significant association between pain and episodes of minor trauma. There were also no new MRI findings in the group that experienced minor trauma.[46,47] Also, back pain tends to recur,[63] which is not in keeping with an acute injury.

Finally, trauma has been difficult to study in a controlled setting. Biomechanical studies of automobile injury have evaluated the impact of sudden axial loads on cadaveric specimens.[64] Whether the anatomic changes seen in cadavers are ecologically valid representations of the changes seen in living tissues has not been well established. On this basis, some have concluded that there is little prospective scientific evidence to suggest that such episodes of chronic recurrent low back pain are related to musculoskeletal injury.[65]

Neck pain seems to be analogous to back pain, albeit less well studied. Joslin et al[66] followed up a "whiplash" cohort for 3.5 years and concluded that functional recovery after neck injury was unrelated to the physical insult. The authors concluded that increased morbidity in patients with whiplash is likely to be psychological and is associated with litigation.[66]

Repetitive Injury (Overuse or Toxicologic) Paradigm Kuiper et al[67, 68] considered back injury to be due to repetitive loading. A consensus meeting supported the causal relationship. The concept is a toxicologic approach to loading: a certain dose of repetitive loading or mechanical trauma over time causes damage, akin to fatigue fractures that occur in inorganic materials.

Decades of ergonomic research, including a literature review by the National Institute of Occupational Safety and Health (NIOSH) in 1997,[69] have identified activities thought to be harmful to the back. A summary by Waddell lists lifting and vibration as two physical risk factors with "strong evidence" of "moderate effect."[48(p109)] An attempt has been made to encapsulate the level of harm in lifting equations.[70-72]

According to NIOSH, the recommended weight that should not be exceeded assuming *ideal* lifting conditions and techniques is 51 lb. Ideal conditions are not realistic when calculating a recommended weight limit for most tasks; thus, 51 lb will invariably be reduced to a lower weight. A small cohort of 10 young military trainees was shown to vastly and repetitively exceed NIOSH loading limits during 14 weeks, without MRI evidence of spinal injury.[73]

Degeneration (Gompertzian) Paradigm This is another traditional view of the back that is common among physicians. The idea is that degeneration of the supporting structures of the spine (discs and facet joints) leads to pain that gradually worsens with aging. Degeneration would, therefore, represent a parametric bound on the daily fluctuations of back pain—"unpredictable in the short term, but broadly predictable in the long term."[74] (Gompertz was a mathematician whose equations are frequently used to model mortality and other outcomes in aging populations.)

One problem with the degenerative model is that X-ray changes of degeneration cannot consistently predict low back pain.[75-78] Furthermore, back pain tends to improve, rather than worsen, as people enter their senior years, except for the small cohort in whom recognizable spinal stenosis, a specific cause of back pain, develops.

Furthermore, there is good evidence to suggest that lumbar disc degeneration noted on MRI is not significantly associated with occupational exposure but is more likely due to genetic influences and possibly smoking.[79-85] Disc herniation may also have a genetic basis.[86]

Chronic Disease Paradigm This paradigm is perhaps best summarized by considering back pain as a condition "of a relapsing-remitting nature, with peaks and valleys of pain."[48(p75)] This definition is based on the South Manchester natural history studies by Croft's group.[87] Symptoms recur periodically, somewhat akin to the symptoms of diabetes and asthma.

A 1998 study by Croft et al[88] indicated that 90% of patients with back pain stopped consulting with their physician after 3 months. However, only 20% to 25% had fully recovered from pain and disability at 1 year.

In a 2004 Canadian study, neck pain was present in 13.6% of men and 22.7% of women. Approximately one third experienced persistence or recurrence of symptoms at 1 year. Neck pain seems to be a chronic episodic condition characterized by episodes of persistent, recurrent, or fluctuating pain and disability.[89]

In some sense, the difference between acute and recurrent injury and chronic disease is merely a matter of perspective between viewing the trees or the forest.

Variation of Normal Paradigm Hadler,[90] a rheumatologist, espouses the principle of a wider acceptance of normalcy. Back pain, he argues, is a normal part of the human condition, like headache, abdominal pain, and fatigue. We have too narrowly defined wellness and misclassify many healthy people who experience common symptoms as diseased, causing iatrogenic disability.[90-92]

Some authors argue that there is little prospective scientific evidence to suggest that episodes of chronic recurrent low back pain are related to occupational musculoskeletal injury.[63,65]

Underuse or Sports Medicine Paradigm Some suggest that the current epidemic of back pain is due to inactivity and lack of physical conditioning. Many occupational physicians believe that participation in work activities has a salubrious effect, not only on the back, but also on general well-being and morbidity.[93] Recent work by Videman et al[94] on disc degeneration may support this hypothesis as well.

Hormesis, Threshold, or Nonlinear J-Curve Paradigm This concept is taken from the toxicology dose-response literature, in which many toxins do not manifest harm below a threshold exposure level or may even be beneficial at low or midrange doses. Extremes of underuse and overuse are harmful.[95] The attraction of this model is the synthesis of perspectives that loading and activity are beneficial,[93,94] neutral,[46,47] or harmful.[70-72]

Biopsychosocial and Other Models Traditionally, a biomechanical or anatomic explanation for low back pain has been pursued by researchers.[96] However, psychological factors, such as somatization and fear avoidance, as well as behavioral economics, have a critical role in the development of chronic back pain.[97-101] For example, increased morbidity in patients with whiplash is associated with psychological factors and litigation.[66]

Hearkening to Lorenz' butterfly, some theorists look beyond a unidirectional cause-effect model of low back pain to complexity science, which incorporates recursive or circular feedback interactions of multiple causes into a system modeled on chaos theory.[74,102,103]

Legal Cause of Low Back Pain

> The important question for the law is not how judges can best do justice to science, but rather how courts can better render justice under conditions of uncertainty and ignorance.
>
> S. Jasanoff.[104]

Occupational liability for low back pain generally falls into the domain of workers' compensation in North American jurisdictions. The basic premise of workers' compensation is the great compromise of Bismarck—a worker receives wage indemnity and treatment benefits from an employer-funded pool in exchange for relinquishing the right to a civil tort suit against the employer. In most US and Canadian jurisdictions, a workers' compensation system is the "sole remedy" for an injured worker, unless criminal charges are involved. In the United Kingdom and some Australian states, a hybrid system still allows access to tort redress.

Workers' compensation is generally a state or provincial service, governed by administrative statutes. Each jurisdiction, therefore, adopts a slightly different set of statutory laws and policies regarding compensability of low back injury. In general, however, the language of tort is best aligned with the injury model of back pain, which presupposes a traumatic event to the spine and consequent physical damages.

Hallowed among most British common law traditions is the "thin-skull" (or fragile-spine) principle, which directs the court to find liability with the proximate cause of injury. In the case of an elderly woman with osteoporosis who falls down the stairs in a private home and sustains a compression fracture, the homeowner is found liable, not the osteoporotic condition.[105]

A legal decision about cause takes a scientific opinion into account as one of many opinions that must be weighed. A legal inquiry into cause necessitates consideration whether there was an injury (usually traumatic) and where liability for that injury should be directed. Assignment of cause in civil injury cases is closely intertwined with the assignment of liability for damages and compensation. It therefore invokes nonscientific principles of fairness and justice to the injured party. Consider these Canadian civil law opinions:

> Causation in law is not identical to scientific causation.
>
> Causation in law must be established on the balance of probabilities, taking into account all the evidence: factual, statistical and that which the judge is entitled to presume.
>
> In some cases, where a fault presents a clear danger and where such a danger materializes, it may be reasonable to presume a causal link, unless there is a demonstration or indication to the contrary.
>
> Statistical evidence may be helpful as indicative but is not determinative. In particular, where statistical evidence does not indicate causation on the balance of probabilities, causation in law may nonetheless exist where evidence in the case supports such a finding.
>
> Even where statistical and factual evidence do not support a finding of causation on the balance of probabilities with respect to particular damage (e.g. death or sickness), such evidence may still justify a finding of causation with respect to lesser damage (e.g. slightly shorter life, greater pain).[106]

> It is not now necessary, nor has it ever been, for the plaintiff to establish that the defendant's negligence was the *sole cause* of the injury [emphasis added]. There will frequently be a myriad of other background events which were necessary preconditions to the injury occurring. To borrow an example from Professor Fleming (The Law of Torts [8th ed. 1992] at p. 193), a "fire ignited in a wastepaper basket is. . . caused not only by the dropping of a lighted match, but also by the presence of combustible material and oxygen, a failure of the cleaner to empty the basket and so forth." As long as a defendant is *part* of the cause of an injury, the defendant is liable, even though his act alone was not enough to create the injury. There is no basis for a reduction of liability because of the existence of other preconditions: defendants remain liable for all injuries caused or contributed to by their negligence.[107]

In low back pain, tort law and the injury model of low back pain have had a sym-biotic relationship since Victorian times. Our medical and societal understanding of low back pain tends, therefore, to be somewhat biased toward an injury paradigm, perhaps because much of the low back pain in the physician's office involves third-party liability and insurance coverage issues.

In many workers' compensation and civil jurisdictions, an occupational trauma to the back is looked at from the perspective of a proximate cause, as the straw that broke the camel's back (thin-skull principle). Preexisting degenerative or idiopathic low back pain is considered the predominant or underlying cause but does not absolve the proximate cause of liability.

If, however, the occupational exposure is thought to be minimal, within the range of normal activities, the argument for proximate cause is weakened. The precise threshold of proximity will relate to local differences in statutory and case law definitions of causation.

Many jurisdictions use the concept of apportionment of damages to weigh the contributions of a predominant and proximate cause. Under Canadian common law, for example, liability cannot be apportioned, but damages can.[105]

Oregon Example

In Oregon, the state passed a law stipulating that work injuries be considered from the perspective of predominant or "major contributing cause" only. This law was appealed to the Supreme Court of Oregon, which upheld the right of the plaintiff to seek damages for proximate cause. Workers were thereby restored the right to file suit against their employers on the basis of proximate cause.[108]

Medicolegal Causal "Analysis":
The Interface Between Scientific and Legal Proof

> The laws of probability, so true in general, so fallacious in particular.
>
> Edward Gibbon (1737-1794)[109]

Translation of a general causation argument into a specific one requires a blend of inductive and deductive logic. This cannot follow any formula, but generally one attempts to establish the purported causative agent ("mechanism of injury") with more than 50% likelihood and the purported effect ("diagnosis") with more than 50% likelihood and then address whether the cause-effect relationship is biologically plausible. Bradford Hill[41] suggested some guidelines on forming such an opinion—temporal relationship, dose response, mechanistic plausibility, and others. Ultimately, this becomes a deductive judgment about how reliably the specific facts of the case can be predicted or inferred from general principles. As Harber and Schusterman[41] mention in their article on causation heuristics, such approaches incorporate scientific and social elements to reach a conclusion.

Causation analysis travels along a mental continuum from speculation to possibility to probability to certainty. One tends to move forward along the path with arguments that support biologic plausibility, perhaps also with social judgments and risk perceptions that invoke a precautionary principle. One tends to move in the other direction by *reductio ad nihilem*, an appeal to the null hypothesis of causation—"we cannot know what is not known."

A commonly used heuristic blend of inductive and deductive logic occurs when using attributable fraction calculations for a population to conclude that an exposure is greater than 50% likely to cause an effect **in** a person.[42] As mentioned earlier, an alternative perspective is that a smaller relative risk with tight confidence intervals may well translate into a probability of cause in a specific person. The mean and variation need to somehow be weighed in any causal argument that looks to statistical data for support.

Radiculopathy with Disc Herniation

This refers to the finding of peripheral neurologic deficits in a dermatomal or myotomal distribution without upper motor neuron findings to suggest involvement of the spinal cord itself (myelopathy) or the brain. Generally there is also radicular pain, aggravated in the neck by the Spurling maneuver or in the low back by straight-leg-lifting maneuvers. This is commonly associated with a herniated disc, most commonly at the L4-L5 and L5-S1 levels in the low back or at the C5-C6 and C6-C7 levels in the neck. Sciatic pain is most prevalent between the ages of 45 and 64 years.[110-112]

Most case definitions use radiculopathy and disc herniation somewhat interchangeably, which is problematic to causation arguments because there is a significant prevalence of asymptomatic cervical and lumbar disc herniation in the general population. In the neck, posterior disc protrusion and foraminal stenosis with demonstrable compression of the spinal cord was observed in 7.6% of asymptomatic subjects, mostly older than 50 years[113]; 20% younger than 60 years and 36% older than 60 years were found to have asymptomatic lumbar disc herniation on MRI.[114]

Furthermore, the differential diagnosis of radiculopathy goes beyond disc herniation to encompass any intrinsic or extrinsic (compressive) insult to the nerve root anywhere along its path. For example, an osteophyte or a facet joint ganglion cyst could lead to compression at the foramen. Uterine fibroids and other pelvic lesions could compress the lumbosacral nerve roots.

However, disc herniations are likely the most common cause of radiculopathy, so the discussion will focus disc herniations. The prevalence of disc herniations requiring surgical intervention in the United States has been estimated as 1% to 3%.[115]

Etiology (Scientific Causation)

Disc herniations are hypothesized to be a consequence of degenerative change of the annulus fibrosus. Genetic factors, age-related disc degeneration, ischemic degeneration, and trauma have all been put forward as factors in causation. Biomechanical studies have looked at the effects of trauma. Epidemiologic studies provide some insight into the relationship with age. Studies in twins of disc degeneration on MRI allow some inference about a genetic relationship.

It is generally believed that intradiscal fragmentation precedes and is the driving force behind annular rupture. Cadaveric studies describe a progression of degenerative changes in the annulus fibrosus starting in early adult life. Fissuring of the annulus progresses outward from the inner annular layer, leading eventually to a complete annular tear. The herniation of nucleus pulposus occurs through the annular tear.[116] The extruded disc material seems to have inflammatory potential. A mechanical compression of a nerve root and a chemical cytokine irritation of the nerve root have been proposed to explain the connection between a disc herniation and the clinical finding of radiculopathy.[117]

Methodological challenges exist in establishing the causative factors because of the difficulty, as in all research of back diseases, of identifying clinically relevant case definitions. Radiologists disagree on the definition of "disc bulge" vs "disc herniation." Can studies on causes of "disc degeneration" be said to generalize to disc herniation? Is the finding of disc herniation on MRI correlated in any significant way to the clinical picture of radiculopathy or sciatica? How do we define radiculopathy?

Much of the basic research in this area focuses on the biomechanical cadaver studies. Research by Adams et al[118] in the United Kingdom used fatigue principles of mechanical engineering to study the effect of loading a spinal segment. Single-load studies suggest that normal intervertebral discs can prolapse in vitro if loaded with supraphysiologic forces in bending and compression. However, such forces are difficult to quantify because the distribution of spinal forces generated from a 40-lb lift depend a great deal on intrinsic muscular and

CHAPTER 8

ligamentous tone and biomechanics. Repetitive loading studies suggest that intervertebral discs can prolapse in vitro if loaded within normal physiologic limits.[118] A review of automotive injury literature failed to support the hypothesis of acute herniation due to traumatic loading,[64] raising the possibility that disc herniation may be partially caused by repetitive trauma, as opposed to a single lifting event.

However, if we consider disc herniation to be a feature of disc degeneration, there is now substantial evidence to link disc degeneration on MRI with genetic influences, age, and smoking. Occupational factors do not seem to be strongly correlated.[79-82]

One possible conclusion from the cited literature is that disc herniations are caused primarily by genetic, age-related, and/or ischemic degeneration (atherosclerosis). Trauma, most likely repetitive loading fatigue, seems to be of secondary importance.

Other conclusions are also possible. For example, repetitive loading may be a confounding component of age-related degeneration. The recent study by Videman et al[94] argues against this, suggesting that loading may be neutral or beneficial. However, it appears unlikely that a single heavy lift is the primary "scientific" cause of a disc herniation.

A common medicolegal question relates to recurrent disc herniations. Does a recurrent herniation at the same level as a prior episode relate to new trauma or to the prior episode? Following lumbar discectomy, there is a recurrence rate of 5% to 8%.[116] Whether this could be generalized to all recurrences of disc herniation is unclear. Various medicolegal arguments can be made, depending on the choice of paradigm. A chronic disease or degenerative paradigm could argue that recurrent herniations are a manifestation of ongoing disc degeneration.

Legal Causation

The Thin-Skull Principle In English common law, the thin-skull principle means one takes the victim as one finds him or her. A defendant is liable for a plaintiff's injuries even if the injuries are unusually severe owing to preexisting conditions. The thin-skull rule or eggshell plaintiff is recognized in American civil law decisions as well.[117]

The application of the thin-skull principle by the courts is thought to bring "better social cost accounting."[105]

"it premises, as it were, a norm of vulnerability of the average person and makes the wrongdoer rather than the victim bear the damage suffered by those falling short of the norm."[120]

The Crumbling-Skull Principle This principle does not relate to liability, but to assessment of damages. Damages may be reduced in cases in which it is established that a preexisting condition would have deteriorated over time even in the absence of injury. The American analogy is called substantial factor analysis.[121] This principle is not applied uniformly in all American or Canadian jurisdictions. In French Canada and jurisdictions under the Napoleonic civil code, a "loss of chance rule" is used.[105]

A Disc Herniation on Trial, 1996 In the Canadian Supreme Court case of *Athey v Leonati,* 1996, the question was raised whether the defendant should be liable for a disc herniation after a motor vehicle accident because the plaintiff (injured party) had a "predisposition" to disc herniation.

The Judicial Committee ruled:

> In the present case, the suggested apportionment is between tortious and non-tortious causes. Apportionment between tortious and non-tortious causes is contrary to the principles of tort law, because the defendant would escape full liability even though he or she caused or contributed to the plaintiff's entire injuries. The plaintiff would not be adequately compensated, since the plaintiff would not be placed in the position he or she would have been in absent the defendant's negligence.

The "crumbling skull" argument is the respondents' strongest submission, but in my view it does not succeed on the facts as found by the trial judge. There was no finding of any measurable risk that the disc herniation would have occurred without the accident, and there was therefore no basis to reduce the award to take into account any such risk.[107]

Lumbar Spinal Stenosis

Although neurogenic claudication was described by Charcot in 1858, this syndrome has been described and treated for only 30 years or so.[122] Anatomic compression of the spinal canal results in compressive neuropathy of the spinal nerve roots below the level of the conus, most commonly at the L3-L4 and L4-L5 levels. The typical occurrence is in patients in their 60s through 90s.

The differential diagnosis of compressive lesions in the canal is long. Although congenital stenosis is less common than acquired stenosis, an element of congenital narrowing of the canal is not uncommon. Acquired stenosis is typically a manifestation of degenerative change in the ligaments (calcification and hypertrophy), facets (spondylosis), and discs (central bulging). Spondylolisthesis may also contribute.[122] Posttraumatic stenosis is possible in cases of fractures into the canal or other traumatic causes of altered spinal canal anatomy.

Cervical Myelopathy

Myelopathy refers to a disease process that disrupts the intrinsic function of the spinal cord. The differential diagnosis is extensive, grouped into many categories, including infectious, metabolic, inflammatory, and other systemic causes. In the setting of neck pain, however, degenerative cervical stenosis is a common scenario. This stenosis is most common in elderly people. As with lumbar stenosis, posttraumatic stenosis is possible in cases of anatomic encroachment on the spinal canal (e.g., fracture).[123]

Radiologic Diagnoses

Most radiologic diagnoses are not well correlated clinically with low back pain.[78,124] The 2005 study by Jarvik et al[125] followed up on 123 patients for 3 years and concluded: "We did not find an association between new LBP [low back pain] and type 1 endplate changes, disc degeneration, annular tears, or facet degeneration". . . . "New imaging findings have a low incidence; disc extrusions and nerve root contact may be the most important of these findings."[125]

Spondylosis (Facet Arthritis) The term *spondylosis* refers to arthritis of the bony spinal elements. Spondylosis is an exceedingly common radiologic finding, and prevalence increases with age. Although spondylosis is commonly invoked as a pain generator, outcome studies have been unable to reliably correlate this finding with pain.[78]

Degenerative Discs The radiologic finding of degenerative discs (ie, loss of disc height, and water content) is common in both sexes after 40 years of age. The most common site of cervical degenerative change is C5-C6. However, radiologic findings of cervical degenerative discs or arthritis are not predictive of pain or disability.[114,126]

Spondylolisthesis Beutler et al[127] did not show a link between spondylolisthesis and low back pain. Large studies of blue-collar workers and military personnel have not identified spondylolisthesis as a condition that predisposes the person to greater risk of disability from low back pain than that of the general population.[128] The lack of correlation observed by some authors between patient outcomes and the presence of solid arthrodesis or pseudarthrosis after fusion surgery does not support a strict etiologic association between segmental motion and low back pain. Also, in a study of the natural history of radiographic instability in the lumbar spine, "restabilization" was found to occur in up to 20% of patients over time.[129]

Spondylolysis Some sources suggest there is little correlation between a finding of spondylolysis and back pain or disability.[130] People with backache have no greater incidence of isthmic spondylolysis and spondylolisthesis than do people without backache. The presence of the lesion may not necessarily be the cause of the patient's back pain.[131] However, one study of isthmic spondylolisthesis in 111 patients undergoing fusion or aggressive exercise noted an improvement in low back pain and function in the fused group at 2 years.[132] Another study showed a modest improvement at 1 year in a fusion group over improvement in an exercise group.[133] Ranson et al[134] showed an increased incidence of pars interarticularis stress fractures in cricket bowlers but concluded that the relationship between the radiologic findings and pain and dysfunction remains unclear.

Scoliosis The large study by Weinstein et al[135] did not show a significant link between scoliosis and disability from low back pain. Another study found no link between pain and mild scoliosis; a more severe scoliosis (>4 cm of coronal displacement) was correlated with pain.[136] In fact, the US Preventive Services Task Force has recommended against routine screening in asymptomatic adolescents for idiopathic scoliosis and cites fair evidence that screening is ineffective or that harm outweighs benefit.[137]

Transitional Vertebrae Having a lumbosacral transitional vertebra increases the risk of early degeneration in the disc above this anomaly. This effect seems to be obscured by age-related changes in middle age. The degenerative process is slowed in the lower disc. For these effects, the presence of a transitional vertebra should be noticed when morphologic methods are used in research on the lumbosacral spine. A transitional vertebra is not associated with any type of low back pain.[138]

Annular Tears (High-Intensity Zones) The text edited by Bogduk[52] postulates that most cases of chronic low back pain may be due to annular tears. A cadaveric study reported an association between annular tears and low back pain.[134] However, from the radiologic in vivo perspective, high-intensity zones do not change or improve spontaneously in a large proportion of cases during a period of time. Furthermore, there is no statistical correlation between high-intensity zones changes and change in a patient's symptoms.[125,140]

Tarlov Cysts The majority of Tarlov cysts are incidental findings on MRI.[141]

Schmorl Nodes Schmorl nodes are common in middle-aged women and are strongly genetically determined. They are associated with lumbar degenerative change, but are not themselves an independent risk factor for back pain.[142]

Summary

It has been suggested by some that we need to move away from an injury model for managing spinal disorders, perhaps "demedicalize" these conditions altogether. Some of these choices involve societal values and policy and statutory decisions, which transcend purely scientific perspectives.

I would suggest that the role of the medicolegal consultant in this setting is to provide a clear and unbiased illumination of the science, cognizant that the legal perspective may lead to legal conclusions about causation that differ from the scientific conclusions.

Disclosure

My background is in engineering, family medicine, and sports medicine. I am an occupational physician and employee of WorkSafeBC, the Workers Compensation Board of British Columbia, Canada. Although the material in this review represents my opinion alone and not necessarily that of the Workers Compensation Board, this is a disclosed source of potential bias.

References

1. Lurie JD. What diagnostic tests are useful for low back pain? *Best Pract Res Clin Rheumatol.* 2005; 19:557-575.
2. Takahashi I, Kikuchi S, Sato K, Iwabuchi M. Effects of the mechanical load on forward bending motion of the trunk: Comparison between patients with motion-induced intermittent low back pain and healthy subjects. *Spine.* 2007;32:E73-8.
3. Wang JP, Zhong ZC, Cheng CK, et al. Finite element analysis of the spondylolysis in lumbar spine. *Biomed Mater Eng.* 2006; 16:301-308.
4. McIntosh G, Hall H, Boyle C. Contribution of nonspinal comorbidity to low back pain outcomes. *Clin J Pain.* 2006;22:765-769.
5. Langevin HM, Sherman KJ. Pathophysiological model for chronic low back pain integrating connective tissue and nervous system mechanisms. *Med Hypotheses.* 2007;68:74-80.
6. Chan D, Song Y, Sham P, Cheung KM. Genetics of disc degeneration. *Eur Spine J.* 2006;15(suppl 3):S317-S325.
7. Bakker EW, Verhagen AP, Lucas C, et al. Daily spinal mechanical loading as a risk factor for acute non-specific low back pain: a case-control study using the 24-hour schedule. *Eur Spine J.* 2007;16:107-113.
8. Cavanaugh JM, Lu Y, Chen C, Kallakuri S. Pain generation in lumbar and cervical facet joints. *J Bone Joint Surg Am.* 2006;88(suppl 2):63-67.
9. Van der Wall H, Magee M, Reiter L, et al. Degenerative spondylolysis: a concise report of scintigraphic observations. *Rheumatology (Oxford).* 2006;45:209-211.
10. O'Sullivan P. Diagnosis and classification of chronic low back pain disorders: maladaptive movement and motor control impairments as underlying mechanism. *Man Ther.* 2005;10:242-255.
11. Panjabi MM. A hypothesis of chronic back pain: ligament subfailure injuries lead to muscle control dysfunction. *Eur Spine J.* 2006;15:668-676.
12. Mulleman D, Mammou S, Griffoul I, et al. Pathophysiology of disk-related low back pain and sciatica, II: evidence supporting treatment with TNF-alpha antagonists. *Joint Bone Spine.* 2006;73:270-277.
13. Flamme CH. Obesity and low back pain—biology, biomechanics and epidemiology [in German]. *Orthopade.* 2005;34:652-657.
14. Valat JP. Factors involved in progression to chronicity of mechanical low back pain. *Joint Bone Spine.* 2005;72:193-195.
15. Kawakami M. Pathophysiology of radicular pain [in Japanese]. *Clin Calcium.* 2005;15:57-62.
16. Adams MA. Biomechanics of back pain. *Acupunct Med.* 2004;22:178-188.
17. Bejia I, Younes M, Zrour S, et al. Factors predicting outcomes of mechanical sciatica: a review of 1092 cases. *Joint Bone Spine.* 2004;71:567-571.
18. Park P, Garton HJ, Gala VC, et al. Adjacent segment disease after lumbar or lumbosacral fusion: review of the literature. *Spine.* 2004; 29:1938-1944.
19. Colloca CJ, Keller TS. Active trunk extensor contributions to dynamic posteroanterior lumbar spinal stiffness. *J Manipulative Physiol Ther.* 2004; 27:229-237.
20. Grabois M. Management of chronic low back pain. *Am J Phys Med Rehabil.* 2005;(suppl 84):S29-S41.

CHAPTER 8

21. Kuritzky L. Steps in the management of low back pain. *Hosp Pract (Minneap)*. 1996; 31:109-24; discussion 124, 130.

22. Borenstein DG. Chronic low back pain. *Rheum Dis Clin North Am.* 1996; 22:439-456.

23. McCowin PR, Borenstein D, Wiesel SW. The current approach to the medical diagnosis of low back pain. *Orthop Clin North Am.* 1991; 22:315-325.

24. Troyer MR. Differential diagnosis of endometriosis in a young adult woman with nonspecific low back pain. *Phys Ther.* 2007; 87:801-810.

25. Sparkes V, Prevost AT, Hunter JO. Derivation and identification of questions that act as predictors of abdominal pain of musculoskeletal origin. *Eur J Gastroenterol Hepatol.* 2003; 15:1021-1027.

26. Mazanec DJ. Evaluating back pain in older patients. *Cleve Clin J Med.* 1999; 66:89-91, 95-99.

27. Diehl AK. Symptoms of gallstone disease. *Baillieres Clin Gastroenterol.* 1992; 6:635-637.

28. Aristotle. The Metaphysics. Available at: http://etext.library.adelaide.edu.au/a/aristotle/metaphysics/. Accessed Sept 10, 2007.

29. Lorenz E. *Predictability: does the flap of a butterfly's wings in Brazil set off a tornado in Texas?* Presented at the meeting of the American Association for the Advancement of Science; December 1972. Washington D.C.

30. Gleick J. *Chaos: Making a New Science.* London, England: Abacus; 1987.

31. Ozonoff D. Legal causation and responsibility for causing harm. *Am J Public Health.* 2005; 95(suppl 1):S35-8.

32. Coggon D, Martyn C. Time and chance: the stochastic nature of disease causation. *Lancet.* 2005;365:1434-1437.

33. Freckleton I, Mendelson D, eds, *Causation in Law and Medicine.* Burlington, VT: Ashgate / Dartmouth Publishing; 2002.

34. Sackett D, et al. *Clinical Epidemiology: A Basic Science for Clinical Medicine.* 2nd ed. Boston: Little Brown; 1991: chap 1-5.

35. Steurer J, Bachman L, Miettinen O. Etiology in a taxonomy of illnesses. *Eur J Epidemiol.* 2006; 21:85-89.

36. Gordis L. *Epidemiology.* 3rd ed. Philadelphia, PA: Saunders; 2004.

37. Shrier I. Understanding causal inference: the future direction in sports injury prevention. *Clin J Sport Med.* 2007; 17:220-224.

38. Herkowitz HN, et al, eds. *The Lumbar Spine.* 3rd ed. Philadelphia, PA: Lippincott Williams & Wilkins; 2004:chap. 12 & 13.

39. Jordan K, Dunn KM, Lewis M, Croft P. A minimal clinically important difference was derived for the Roland-Morris Disability Questionnaire for low back pain. *J Clin Epidemiol.* 2006; 59:45-52.

40. van der Roer N, Ostelo RW, Bekkering GE, van Tulder MW, de Vet HC. Minimal clinically important change for pain intensity, functional status, and general health status in patients with nonspecific low back pain. *Spine.* 2006; 31:578-582.

41. Harber P, Shusterman D. Medical causation analysis heuristics. *J Occup Environ Med.* 1996;38:577-586.

42. Taylor AN. The Prescription of Disease. Presented at: the Industrial Injuries Advisory Council of the UK, Belfast N Ireland, Mar 2007. Available at: http://www.iiac.org.uk/pdf/reports/PrescriptionOfDisease.pdf. Accessed Sept. 10, 2007.

43. Lacerte M, Forcier P. Medicolegal causal analysis *Phys Med Rehabil Clin N Am.* 2002; 13:371-408.

44. Mixter WJ, Barr JS. Ruptures of the intervertebral disc with involvement of the spinal canal. N Engl J Med. 1934;211:210-211.

45. Deyo RA, Weinstein JN. Primary care: low back pain. *N Engl J Med.* 2001;344:363-370.

46. Carragee E, Alamin T, Cheng I, Franklin T, van den Haak E, Hurwitz E. Are first-time episodes of serious LBP associated with new MRI findings? *Spine J.* 2006;6:624-635.

47. Carragee E, Alamin T, Cheng I, Franklin T, Hurwitz E. Does minor trauma cause serious low back illness? *Spine.* 2006; 31:2942-2949.

48. Waddell G. *Low Back Pain Revolution.* 2nd ed. New York, NY: Churchill Livingstone; 2004.

49. Speed C. Low back pain. *BMJ.* 2004;328:1119-1121.

50. Andersson GJ. Epidemiology of Spinal Disorders. In: Frymoyer JW Ducker TB Hadler NM et al. *The Adult Spine: Principles and Practice,* 2nd ed. New York: Raven Press; 1997:93-141.

51. Walker BF, Muller R, Grant WD. Low back pain in Australian adults: Prevalence and associated disability. *J Manipulative Physiological Therapeutics.* 2004; 27:238-244.

52. Pengel LH, Herbert RD, Maher CG, Refshauge KM. Acute low back pain: Systematic review of its prognosis. *BMJ.* 2003; 327:323.

53. Bogduk N, ed. *Medical Management of Acute and Chronic Low Back Pain.* New York, NY: Elsevier; 2002. Pain Research and Clinical Management Series; Vol. 13.

54. Bamji AN. Low back pain: Sacroiliac joint pain may be myth. *BMJ.* 2004; 329:232.

55. Dreyfuss P, Michaelsen M, Pauza K, McLarty J, Bogduk N. The value of medical history and physical examination in diagnosing sacroiliac joint pain. *Spine.* 1996; 21:2594-2602.

56. Dreyfuss P, Dreyer SJ, Cole A, Mayo K. Sacroiliac joint pain. *J Am Acad Orthop Surg.* 2004; 12:255-265.

57. Sturesson B, Uden A, Vleeming A. A radiostereometric analysis of movements of the sacroiliac joints during the standing hip flexion test. *Spine.* 2000; 25:364-368.

58. Sturesson B, Uden A, Vleeming A. A radiostereometric analysis of the movements of the sacroiliac joints in the reciprocal straddle position. *Spine.* 2000; 25:214-217.

59. Deyo R. Diagnostic evaluation of LBP: Reaching a specific diagnosis is often impossible. *Arch Intern Med.* 2002; 162:1444-1447.

60. Lutz GK, Butzlaff M, Schultz-Venrath U. Looking back on back pain: Trial and error of diagnoses in the 20th century. *Spine.* 2003;28:1899-1905.

61. Abraham I, Killackey-Jones B. Lack of evidence-based research for idiopathic low back pain: the importance of a specific diagnosis. *Arch Intern Med.* 2002;162:1442-1444.

62. Koes BW, van Tulder MW, Thomas S. Diagnosis and treatment of low back pain. *BMJ.* 2006;332:1430-1434.

63. Maul I, Laubli T, Klipstein A, Krueger H. Course of low back pain among nurses: A longitudinal study across eight years. *Occup Environ Med.* 2003;60:497-503.

64. King A, Cavanaugh JM, Levine RS. Does acute disc rupture really exist? a review. Poster presented at: 33rd meeting of the International Society for the Study of the Lumbar Spine; Bergen, Norway June 2006. Poster 39.

65. Harkness EF, Macfarlane GJ, Nahit ES, Silman AJ, McBeth J. Risk factors for new-onset low back pain amongst cohorts of newly employed workers. *Rheumatology (Oxford)*. 2003;42:959-968.

66. Joslin CC, Khan SN, Bannister GC. Long-term disability after neck injury. A comparative study. *J Bone Joint Surg Br*. 2004;86:1032-1034.

67. Kuiper JI, Burdorf A, Frings-Dresen MH, et al. Assessing the work-relatedness of nonspecific low-back pain. *Scand J Work Environ Health*. 2005;31:237-243.

68. Coggon D. Does it help to know the work-relatedness of back pain in individual cases? Scand J Work Environ Health. 2003 Dec; 29(6):441-2.

69. Bernard B, ed. *Musculoskeletal Disorders and Workplace Factors. Washington, DC:* US Dept of Health and Human Services, National Institute for Occupational Safety and Health (NIOSH); 1997. Publication 97-141.

70. Waters T, et al. Revised NIOSH Lifting Equation for the Design and Evaluation of Manual Lifting Tasks. *Ergonomics*. 1993;36:749-776.

71. NIOSH. Lifting equation. http://0-www.cdc.gov.mill1.sjlibrary.org/niosh/pot_lift. html. Accessed Sept 10, 2007.

72. Waters T. *State of the Science in Ergonomics*. Presented at: 4th Annual Safe Patient Handling and Movement Conference. Orlando, FL April 2005. http://www. nursingworld.org/OJIN. Accessed Sept 10, 2007.

73. Aharony S, Milgrom C, Wolf T, et al. Magnetic resonance imaging showed no signs of overuse or permanent injury to the lumbar sacral spine during a special forces training course. *Spine J*. Mar 2, 2007 [Epub ahead of print]. doi:10.1016/ j.spinee.2007.01.001. Accessed September 10, 2007.

74. Ridley M. *Genome*. New York: Harper Collins; 1999:312.

75. Jarvik JG, Hollingworth W, Martin B, et al. Rapid magnetic resonance imaging vs. radiographs for patients with low back pain: A randomized controlled trial. *JAMA*. 2003; 289:2810-2818.

76. Borenstein DG, O'Mara JW,Jr, Boden SD, et al. The value of magnetic resonance imaging of the lumbar spine to predict low-back pain in asymptomatic subjects: A seven-year follow-up study. *J Bone Joint Surg Am*. 2001; 83-A: 1306-1311.

77. Videman T, Battie MC, Gibbons LE, Maravilla K, Manninen H, Kaprio J. Associations between back pain history and lumbar MRI findings. *Spine*. 2003; 28:582-588.

78. Carragee EJ, Alamin TF, Miller JL, Carragee JM. Discographic, MRI and psychosocial determinants of low back pain disability and remission: A prospective study in subjects with benign persistent back pain. *Spine J*. 2005; 5:24-35.

79. Battie MC, Videman T, Gill K, et al. 1991 Volvo award in clinical sciences. Smoking and lumbar intervertebral disc degeneration: An MRI study of identical twins. *Spine*. 1991;16:1015-1021.

80. Battie MC, Videman T, Gibbons LE, Fisher LD, Manninen H, Gill K. 1995 Volvo award in clinical sciences. Determinants of lumbar disc degeneration. A study relating lifetime exposures and magnetic resonance imaging findings in identical twins. *Spine*. 1995; 20:2601-2612.

81. Videman T, Battie MC, Ripatti S, Gill K, Manninen H, Kaprio J. Determinants of the progression in lumbar degeneration: A 5-year follow-up study of adult male monozygotic twins. *Spine.* 2006; 31:671-678.
82. Battie MC, Videman T, Gibbons LE, et al. Occupational driving and lumbar disc degeneration: A case-control study. *Lancet.* 2002;360:1369-1374.
83. Sambrook PN, MacGregor AJ, Spector TD. Genetic influences on cervical and lumbar disc degeneration: A magnetic resonance imaging study in twins. *Arthritis Rheum.* 1999;42:366-372.
84. MacGregor AJ, Andrew T, Sambrook PN, Spector TD. Structural, psychological, and genetic influences on low back and neck pain: A study of adult female twins. *Arthritis Rheum.* 2004; 51:160-167.
85. Seki S, Kawaguchi Y, Chiba K, et al. A functional SNP in CILP, encoding cartilage intermediate layer protein, is associated with susceptibility to lumbar disc disease. *Nat Genet.* 2005; 37:607-612.
86. Bhardwaj R, Midha R. Synchronous lumbar disc herniation in adult twins. Case report. *Can J Neurol Sci.* 2004; 31:554-557.
87. Papageorgiou AC, Croft PR, Thomas E, Ferry S, Jayson MI, Silman AJ. Influence of previous pain experience on the episode incidence of low back pain: Results from the south Manchester back pain study. *Pain.* 1996; 66:181-185.
88. Croft PR, Macfarlane GJ, Papageorgiou AC, Thomas E, Silman AJ. Outcome of low back pain in general practice: A prospective study. *BMJ.* 1998; 316:1356-1359.
89. Cote P, Cassidy JD, Carroll LJ, Kristman V. The annual incidence and course of neck pain in the general population: A population-based cohort study. *Pain.* 2004; 112:267-273.
90. Hadler NM. *Occupational Musculoskeletal Disorders.* 3rd ed. Philadelphia, PA: Lippincott Williams & Wilkins; 2004.
91. Hadler NM. *The Last Well Person: How to Stay Well Despite the Health-Care System.* Toronto, Canada: McGill-Queen's University Press; 2004.
92. Hadler N. Cumulative trauma disorders. *J Occup Environ Med.* 1990; 32:38-41.
93. Stovitz SD, Johnson RJ. "Underuse" as a cause for musculoskeletal injuries: Is it time that we started reframing our message? *Br J Sports Med.* 2006;40:738-739.
94. Videman T, Levalahti E, Battie MC. The effects of anthropometrics, lifting strength, and physical activities in disc degeneration. *Spine.* 2007;32:1406-1413.
95. Rosenberg J, Israel L. Chapter 13 Clinical Toxicology. In: LaDou J, ed. *Current Occupational and Environmental Medicine.* 4th ed. New York, NY: McGraw-Hill; 2007:181.
96. Weiner BK. Difficult medical problems: on explanatory models and a pragmatic alternative. *Med Hypotheses.* 2007;68:474-479.
97. Gatchel RJ, Gardea MA. Psychosocial issues: their importance in predicting disability, response to treatment, and search for compensation. *Neurol Clin.* 1996;17:149-166.
98. Hoogendoorn WE, van Poppel MNM, Bongers PM, Koes BW, Bouter LM. Systematic review of psychosocial factors at work and private life as risk factors for back pain. *Spine.* 2000;25:2114-2125.
99. Krause N, Dasinger LK, Deegan LJ, Rudolph L, Brand RJ. Psychosocial job factors and return-to-work after compensated low back injury: a disability phase-specific analysis. *Am J Ind Med.* 2001;40:374-392.

CHAPTER 8

100. DeBerard MS, Masters KS, Colledge AL, Holmes EB. Presurgical biopsychosocial variables predict medical and compensation costs of lumbar fusion in Utah workers' compensation patients. *Spine J.* 2003; 3:420-429.

101 Schultz IZ, Crook J, Meloche GR, et al. Psychosocial factors predictive of occupational low back disability: towards development of a return-to-work model. *Pain.* 2004;107:77-85.

102. Borrell-Carrio F, Suchman AL, Epstein RM. The biopsychosocial model 25 years later: Principles, practice, and scientific inquiry. *Ann Fam Med.* 2004;2:576-582.

103 Reis S, Griffiths F, et al. Complexity and low back pain. Presented at: 8th International Forum on Low Back Pain in Primary Care; June 2006; Amsterdam, the Netherlands.

104. Jasanoff S. Law's knowledge: Science for justice in legal settings. *Am J Public Health.* 2005;95(suppl 1):S49-58.

105. Linden AM. *Canadian Tort Law.* 7th ed. Toronto: Butterworth; 2001.

106. *Laferrière v Lawson.* 1 S.C.R. 541 (1991). http://scc.lexum.umontreal.ca/en/1991/1991rcs1-541/1991rcs1-541.html. Accessed Sept 10, 2007.

107. *Athey v Leonati.* 3 S.C.R. 458 (1996). http://scc.lexum.umontreal.ca/en/1996/1996rcs3-458/1996rcs3-458.html. Accessed Sept 10, 2007.

108. *Smothers v Gresham Transfer, Inc.* 332 Or 83, 23 P3d 333 (2001). http://www.publications.ojd.state.or.us/S44512.htm. Accessed Sept 10, 2007. See also Welch EM. Oregon Major Contributing Cause Study. 2000. http://www.cbs.state.or.us/wcd/administration/finalmcc.pdf. Accessed Sept 10, 2007.

109. Gibbon E. *Memoirs of My Life and Writings.* London, England; New York, NY: Penguin Classics; 1984.

110. Praemer A., et al. *Musculoskeletal Conditions in the United States.* Rosemont, IL: AAOS Press; 1999.

111. Carrette S Fehlings MG. Clinical practice: cervical radiculopathy. *N Engl J Med.* 2005;353:392-399.

112. Koes BW, van Tulder MW, Peul WC. Diagnosis and treatment of sciatica. *BMJ.* 2007;334:1313-1317.

113. Matsumoto M, Fujimura Y, Suzuki N, et al. MRI of cervical intervertebral discs in asymptomatic subjects. *J Bone Joint Surg Br.* 1998;80-B:19-24.

114. Boden SD, Davis DO, Dina TS, Patronas NJ, Wiesel SW. Abnormal magnetic-resonance scans of the lumbar spine in asymptomatic subjects. A prospective investigation. *J Bone Joint Surg Am.* 1990;72:403-408.

115. Bendo JA, Awad JN. Chapter 31 Lumbar Disk Herniation. In: Spivak J, Connolly P, eds. *Orthopedic Knowledge Update: Spine 3.* Rosemont, IL: AAOS Press; 2006.

116. Johnson MG, Errico TJ. Chapter 34 Lumbar Disc Herniation. In: Fardon D, Garfin S, eds. *Orthopedic Knowledge Update: Spine 2.* Rosemont, IL: AAOS Press; 2002.

117. Rhee J, Schaufele M, Abdu W. Chapter 28 Radiculopathy and the Herniated Disk. In: Marsh J, ed. *Instructional Course Lectures 2007.* Rosemont, IL: American Academy of Orthopedic Surgeons; 2007:287-299.

118. Adams M, Bogduk N, Burton K, Dolan P. *The Biomechanics of Back Pain,* New York, NY: Churchill Livingstone; 2002: chapter 12.

119. Restatement of the law, Second, torts 2d. St. Paul, MN: American Law Institute Publishers; 1965: Section 435 (1).

120. *Cotic v Gray.* 17 C.C.L.T. 138 (Ont. C.A.), aff'd (1984), 26 C.C.L.T. 163 (S.C.C.) (1981).

121. Restatement of the law, second, torts 2d. St. Paul, MN: American Law Institute Publishers; 1965: Sections 431, 433.

122. Truumees E. Chapter 29 Spinal Stenosis. In: Pellegrini V, ed. *Instructional Course Lectures 2005.* Rosemont, IL: American Academy of Orthopedic Surgeons; 2005:87-302.

123. Lapsiwala S, et al. Chapter 15 Myelopathy. In: Clark C, ed. *The Cervical Spine.* 4th ed. Philadelphia, PA: Lippincott; 2005:199.

124. Kleinstuck F, Dvorak J, Mannion AF. Are "structural abnormalities" on magnetic resonance imaging a contraindication to the successful conservative treatment of chronic nonspecific low back pain? *Spine.* 2006; 31:2250-2257.

125. Jarvik JG, Hollingworth W, Heagerty PJ, Haynor DR, Boyko EJ, Deyo RA. Three-year incidence of low back pain in an initially asymptomatic cohort: Clinical and imaging risk factors. *Spine.* 2005; 30:1541-8; discussion 1549.

126. Peterson C, Bolton J, Wood AR, Humphreys BK. A cross-sectional study correlating degeneration of the cervical spine with disability and pain in United Kingdom patients. *Spine.* 2003; 28:129-133.

127. Beutler WJ, Fredrickson BE, Murtland A, Sweeney CA, Grant WD, Baker D. The natural history of spondylolysis and spondylolisthesis: 45-year follow-up evaluation. *Spine.* 2003;28:1027-35; discussion 1035.

128. Connolly PJ, Fredrickson BE. Chapter 37 Surgical Management of Isthmic and Dysplastic Spondylolisthesis and Spondylolysis. In: Fardon D, Garfin S, eds. *Orthopedic Knowledge Update Spine.* 2nd ed. Rosemont, IL: American Academy of Orthopedic Surgeons; 2002:354.

129. Kwon BK, et al. Indications, techniques, and outcomes of posterior surgery for chronic low back pain. *Orthop Clin North Am.* 2003;34:297-308.

130. Kuri J, et al. *The Spine at Trial: Practical Medicolegal Concepts About the Spine.* Chicago, IL: American Bar Association Press; 2002.

131. Hoaglund F. Chapter 6 Musculoskeletal Injuries. In: Ladou J, ed. *Current Occupational and Environmental Medicine.* 4th ed. New York, NY: McGraw-Hill; 2007:63.

132. Moller H, Hedlund R. Surgery versus conservative management in adult isthmic spondylolisthesis—a prospective randomized study: Part 1. *Spine.* 2000; 25:1711-1715.

133. Ekman P, Moller H, Hedlund R. The long-term effect of posterolateral fusion in adult isthmic spondylolisthesis: A randomized controlled study. *Spine J.* 2005;5:36-44.

134. Ranson CA, Kerslake RW, Burnett AF, Batt ME, Abdi S. Magnetic resonance imaging of the lumbar spine in asymptomatic professional fast bowlers in cricket. *J Bone Joint Surg Br.* 2005;87:1111-1116.

135. Weinstein SL, Dolan LA, Spratt KF, Peterson KK, Spoonamore MJ, Ponseti IV. Health and function of patients with untreated idiopathic scoliosis: A 50-year natural history study. *JAMA.* 2003;289:559-567.

136. Glassman SD, Berven S, Bridwell K, Horton W, Dimar JR. Correlation of radiographic parameters and clinical symptoms in adult scoliosis. *Spine.* 2005;30:682-688.

137. US Preventive Services Task Force (USPSTF) Recommendation: Idiopathic Scoliosis in Adolescents (2004). http://www.ahrq.gov/clinic/3rduspstf/scoliosis/scoliors.htm Aug/04. Accessed Sept 10, 2007.

138. Luoma K, Vehmas T, Raininko R, Luukkonen R, Riihimaki H. Lumbosacral transitional vertebra: Relation to disc degeneration and low back pain. *Spine*. 2004;29:200-205.

139. Videman T, Nurminen M. The occurrence of annular tears and their relation to lifetime back pain history: A cadaveric study using barium sulfate discography. *Spine*. 2004;29:2668-2676.

140. Mitra D, Cassar-Pullicino VN, McCall IW. Longitudinal study of high intensity zones on MR of lumbar intervertebral discs. *Clin Radiol*. 2004;59:1002-1008.

141. Langdown AJ, Grundy JR, Birch NC. The clinical relevance of tarlov cysts. *J Spinal Disord Tech*. 2005;18:29-33.

142. Williams FM, Manek NJ, Sambrook PN, Spector TD, Macgregor AJ. Schmorl's nodes: Common, highly heritable, and related to lumbar disc disease. *Arthritis Rheum*. 2007; 57:855-860.

CHAPTER

Upper Limb

J. Mark Melhorn, MD, Douglas Martin, MD,
Charles N. Brooks, MD, and Shirley Seaman, PA-C

The most common upper limb conditions about which physicians are asked to opine regarding causation are masses, including ganglions of thumb and finger tendon sheaths and about the wrist; Dupuytren disease (contracture); osteoarthritis of the thumb carpometacarpal joint; trigger digits; de Quervain disease; painful elbow (lateral and medial epicondylitis); peripheral nerve entrapments, including carpal and cubital tunnel syndrome; and shoulder tendinopathy, including impingement syndrome and rotator cuff tear. Each diagnosis is reviewed for epidemiologic risk factors as outlined in Chapter 4, Methodology (step 1, literature review; step 2, quality score from review by three-member panel; step 3, determination of study design; step 4, multiplying the quality score by the weighting factor; and step 5 determine the strength of evidence).

Ganglions of Tendon Sheaths in Hand and Digits

Ganglions (ganglia) are the most common soft tissue tumor of the hand and digits, accounting for 50% to 70% of such masses. Also known as ganglion cysts, these benign lesions arise from an adjacent joint capsule or tendon sheath and consist of a sac filled with thick, clear liquid identical to synovial fluid. They usually occur singly and in specific locations. The exact cause of ganglions, which may develop and resolve spontaneously, remains uncertain. The most popular theory suggests they form after trauma to or degeneration of the tissue layer responsible for producing synovial fluid. The cyst arises from accumulation of this fluid outside the joint or tendon sheath. Alternatively, fluid may leak out through a torn or degenerated joint capsule or tendon sheath and continue to accumulate ectopically if a one-way valve is created.

Occupational Risk Factors for Ganglions of Tendon Sheaths

Several occupational risk factors have been proposed for ganglions of tendon sheaths. These proposed risk factors include the following:

- Combination of risk factors (e.g., force and repetition, force and posture)
- Vibration
- Highly repetitive work alone or in combination with other factors
- Forceful work
- Awkward postures
- Keyboard activities
- Cold environment

- Length of employment
- Dominant hand

The *evidence* for each of these risk factors is *insufficient.*

Nonoccupational Risk Factors for Ganglions of Tendon Sheaths

Several nonoccupational risk factors have also been proposed:
- Age
- Body mass index (BMI)
- Sex
- Biopsychosocial factors
- Diabetes

As with the proposed occupational risk factors, there is *insufficient evidence.*

Table 9-1 shows the results for the literature searches for ganglions of tendon sheaths, and Table 9-2 shows representative references and comments.

TABLE 9-1	Results of Literature Search for Ganglions of Tendon Sheaths
Step	**Result**
Step 1: search all fields for combination of	
Search 1: mass & finger & causation	31 articles; none addressed causation
Search 2: ganglion & finger & causation	82 articles; three addressed causation
Search 3: mass & finger & etiology	453 articles; 64 non-English, 30 duplicates, none that addressed causation
Search 4: ganglion & finger & etiology	82 articles; all duplicates and none that addressed causation
Search 5: digital & myxoid & cysts	9 articles; none that addressed causation
Steps 2, 3 and 4	Completed; representative references provided

CHAPTER 9

TABLE 9-2   Representative References and Comments for Ganglions of Tendon Sheaths

Risk Factor	References and Comments
Combination of risk factors (e.g., force and repetition, force and posture)	None
Vibration	None
Highly repetitive work alone or in combination with other factors	None
Forceful work	None
Awkward postures	None
Keyboard activities	None
Cold environment	None
Length of employment	None
Dominant hand	No correlation with hand dominance[1]
Age	Population study completed during 30 years reviewed 128 patients with flexor tendon sheath ganglions; majority of patients, female with sex ratio of 2.6 to 1; most in third to fifth decade of life; no correlation between hand dominance, previous trauma, or illnesses involving the hand and formation of ganglions; middle finger the most commonly affected digit; 69% of the ganglions located on A1 and A2 pulleys; recurrence rate, high (89%) after multiple percutaneous punctures; none recurred after surgical excision[1]
BMI	None
Sex	Females, with sex ratio of 2.6 to 1[1]
Biopsychosocial factors	None
Diabetes	None
Confounders	None

Ganglions of Hand and Wrist

Ganglions (ganglia) are the most common soft tissue tumor of the wrist and hand, accounting for 50% to 70% of such masses. Also known as ganglion cysts, these benign lesions arise from an adjacent joint capsule or tendon sheath and consist of a sac filled with thick, clear liquid identical to synovial fluid. They usually occur singly and in specific locations. The exact cause of ganglions, which may develop and resolve spontaneously, remains uncertain. The most popular theory suggests they form after trauma to or degeneration of the tissue layer responsible for producing synovial fluid. The cyst arises from accumulation of this fluid outside the joint or tendon sheath. Alternatively, fluid may leak out through a torn or degenerated joint capsule or tendon sheath and continue to accumulate ectopically if a one-way valve is created.

Occupational Risk Factors for Ganglions of Hand and Wrist

As with ganglions of tendon sheaths, several occupational risk factors have also been proposed for ganglions of hand and wrist. These proposed risk factors include the following:

- Combination of risk factors (e.g., force and repetition, force and posture)
- Vibration
- Highly repetitive work alone or in combination with other factors
- Forceful work
- Awkward postures
- Keyboard activities
- Cold environment
- Length of employment
- Dominant hand

The *evidence* for each of these risk factors is *insufficient.*

Nonoccupational Risk Factors for Ganglions of Hand and Wrist

Nonoccupational risk factors have also been proposed:

- Age
- BMI
- Sex
- Biopsychosocial factors
- Diabetes

As with the proposed occupational risk factors, there is *insufficient evidence.*

Table 9-3 shows the results for the literature searches for ganglions of hand and wrist, and Table 9-4 shows representative references and comments.

TABLE 9-3 Results of Literature Search for Ganglions of Hand and Wrist

Step	Result
Step 1: search all fields for combination of	
Search 1: mass & hand & causation	359 articles; 1 addressing causation
Search 2: ganglion & hand & causation	372 articles; no additional articles addressing causation
Search 3: ganglion & wrist & causation	3 articles; all duplicates
Search 4: ganglion & wrist & etiology	118 articles; all duplicates
Search 5: ganglion & etiology & work	273 articles; none addressing causation
Steps 2, 3 and 4	Completed; representative references provided

TABLE 9-4 Representative References and Comments for Ganglions of Hand and Wrist

Risk Factor	References and Comments
Combination of risk factors (eg, force and repetition, force and posture)	None
Vibration	None
Highly repetitive work alone or in combination with other factors	None
Forceful work	None
Awkward postures	None
Keyboard activities	None
Cold environment	None
Length of employment	None
Dominant hand	None

TABLE 9-4 Representative References and Comments for Ganglions of Hand and Wrist (continued)

Risk Factor	References and Comments
Age	Retrospective review of the results of operation on 71 volar wrist ganglions demonstrated a recurrence rate of 28%, occurring between 1 and 144 mo (median, 5 mo); highest risk of recurrence was in males younger than 30 years, in a manual occupation, operated on by a junior surgeon[2]
BMI	None
Sex	Retrospective review showed the highest risk of recurrence after excision was in males[2]
Biopsychosocial factors	None
Diabetes	None
Confounders	None

Dupuytren Disease (Contracture)

Dupuytren disease (DD; palmar fibromatosis) is a nonmalignant fibroproliferative disease that causes progressive, permanent nodular thickening and contracture of the palmar fascia with eventual flexion contracture of the digits. Although the exact cause of DD is unknown; familial, racial, and physiologic factors have been suggested.

Occupational Risk Factors for Dupuytren's Disease(DD)

The proposed occupational risk factors and their level of evidence for DD are as follows:
- Combination of risk factors (e.g., force and repetition, force and posture): insufficient evidence
- Vibration: strong evidence
- Highly repetitive work alone or in combination with other factors: insufficient evidence

- Forceful work: insufficient evidence
- Awkward postures: insufficient evidence
- Keyboard activities: insufficient evidence
- Cold environment: insufficient evidence
- Length of employment: insufficient evidence
- Dominant hand: insufficient evidence

Nonoccupational Risk Factors for DD

The proposed nonoccupational risk factors and their level of evidence for DD are as follows:
- Age: some evidence
- BMI: insufficient evidence
- Sex: insufficient evidence
- Biopsychosocial factors: insufficient evidence
- Diabetes: strong evidence
- Genetic factors: strong evidence

Table 9-5 shows the results of the literature searches for DD.

TABLE 9-5   Results of Literature Search for DD

Step	Result
Step 1	
Search 1: All fields for the combination Dupuytren & causation	46 articles; 17 discussed causation relative to risk factors
Steps 2, 3 and 4	Completed; representative references provided

Representative References With Comments for DD

Combination of Risk Factors

For a combination of risk factors (e.g., force and repetition, force and posture), there was *insufficient evidence*. A retrospective study found that occupational activities (not specifically defined) showed no statistical significance with familial analysis for the development of DD.[3] A retrospective survey study of 1100 men revealed that 19.5% of male climbers had developed DD. There was a significantly higher lifetime intensity of climbing activity in people with the disease, and an earlier age of onset of the disease was found in climbers compared with the general population. The authors of this study concluded that their results strengthened the hypothesis that repetitive trauma to the palmar fascia predisposes to the development of DD in men.[4] A retrospective population study in Germany found 1.9 million with DD. The population had a higher use of alcohol, tobacco, and heavy manual labor workers.[5]

Vibration

For vibration, there was *strong evidence.* A population study[6] found the prevalence of Dupuytren contracture (DC) at a British PVC bagging and packing plant in which workers were exposed to repetitive manual work to be 5.5 times that at a local plant without packing and twice the expected prevalence in a United Kingdom working population previously studied.[7] A retrospective study[8] found that DD was observed more frequently among claimants with vibration white finger than control subjects (odds ratio [OR], 2.1; 95% confidence interval [CI], 1.1-3.9).[7] Two population studies, one by Bovenzi[9] with an OR of 2.6 (95% CI, 1.2-5.5) and another by Cocco et al[10] found DD to be more frequent among vibration-exposed workers than control subjects, whereas a third study[7] found some evidence of a dose-response relationship. A population study of 66 jackhammer drillers and 35 blasters involved clinical screening for hand-arm vibration syndrome. Examination revealed soft tissue wasting in the hands (26 cases), ulnar nerve impairment (23 cases), median nerve impairment (16 cases), and DC (4 cases).[11]

Highly Repetitive Work Alone or in Combination With Other Factors

Highly repetitive work alone or in combination with other factors had *insufficient evidence.*

Forceful Work

For forceful work, there was *insufficient evidence.* A meta-analysis of DD investigated whether there was evidence that DC is associated with frequent or repetitive manual work or hand vibration. For the meta-analysis, the published literature was searched for studies meeting the following criteria: (1) in English or having an English abstract; (2) controlled studies; (3) DC was an identified health outcome; and (4) the study group was exposed to repetitive or frequent manual work, vibration, or acute traumatic injury. Relevant non-English articles identified through English abstracts were translated. The validity of studies meeting the selection criteria was assessed using a series of questions adapted from those of Stock.[12] Of

10 studies that met the initial selection criteria, 4 met the criteria for methodologic quality, 1 addressing the relationship between manual work and DC and 3 of vibration and DC. No controlled studies of acute trauma and DC were identified.[7] A population survey study of 5206 ironworkers found that 196 were affected, and a work history (specific work not provided) showed a correlation between hard manual work for many years and DD, especially in the younger age group.[13]

Posture, Keyboarding, Cold, Employment Duration, and Hand Dominance

There was *insufficient evidence* for awkward postures, keyboard activities, cold environment, length of employment, and dominant hand.

Age

For age, there was some evidence. A retrospective review found that DD was linked to ethnicity (white), age (increases after age 50 years), and positive family history.[14]

Body Mass Index

For the BMI, there was *insufficient evidence.* A retrospective follow-up study of people with diabetes found a prevalence of DD of 4% at baseline. Dupuytren disease was significantly associated with the age of the patient and the duration of diabetes but not with the age at the onset of diabetes, BMI, or the control of diabetes.[15]

Sex

For sex, there was *insufficient evidence.* A population study found that DD is more common in men than women.[16]

Biopsychosocial Factors

Biopsychosocial factors were supported by insufficient *evidence.* A retrospective population study in Germany found 1.9 million people with DD. People with DD had a higher incidence of alcohol use and tobacco and were more likely to perform heavy manual labor.[5]

Diabetes

For diabetes, there was *strong evidence*. A case-control study of DD that indi-vidually matched subjects by age, sex, and general health included 821 cases and 1642 controls with 588 men (71.6%), with a mean age at diagnosis of 62 years (range, 24-97 years). Diabetes was a significant risk factor for DD (OR, 1.75), and there was an increased risk for medically treated diabetes (OR, 3.56) and insulin-controlled (OR, 4.38) rather than diet-controlled diabetes.[17] A retrospec-tive population study in Germany found that people with diabetes have a less severe form of DD.[5] A retrospective population study found DD associated with other medical conditions, such as alcoholism, smoking, and diabetes.[18]

Genetic Factors

For genetic factors, there was strong evidence. A retrospective review found that DD was linked to ethnicity (white), age (increases after age 50 years), and posi-tive family history.[14] A retrospective study found that familial occurrence of DD and its presence in identical twins suggests a genetic basis for the condition. The sibling recurrence-risk ratio (λ) equaled 2.9 and ranged from 2.6 to 3.3 based on the 95% CIs for the population prevalence, suggesting a high genetic basis for DD. A younger age of onset and greater severity of DD were associated significantly with a positive family history of DD.[3] A retrospective study found that DD is common in southern Europe (although usually considered a northern European disease), and the prevalence of DD was highly age-dependent, rang-ing from 17% for men between 50 and 59 years to 60% in the oldest men. The prevalence among women was lower.[19] A retrospective study found endocrine disorders such as diabetes, hyperthyroidism, hypothyroidism, hyperparathyroid-ism, hypoparathyroidism, hyperadrenocorticism, and acromegaly to be more common in people with DD.[20] The racial distribution in a retrospective popula-tion study of 9938 patients was as follows: black, 412 (estimated prevalence of 130 per 100,000 population); white, 9071 (734 per 100,000); Hispanic white, 234 (237 per 100,000); Native American, 11 (144 per 100,000); Asian, 8 (67 per 100,000); and unknown race, 202. The characteristics of the disease in blacks are similar to those in whites. In both groups, the disease has a late onset, affects predominantly the ulnar digits, and is associated with other medical conditions, such as alcoholism, smoking, and diabetes. Unlike DD in whites, however, the disease is rarely bilateral in blacks. The differential prevalence among racial groups suggests a genetic component to the pathogenesis of the disease.[18]

Confounders

A retrospective study found palmar fascial proliferations sometimes present as a different entity without the typical DD characteristics, usually with unilateral involvement and without a family history or ectopic manifestations.

Environmental factors, especially trauma, surgery, and diabetes, were important in the pathogenesis of non-Dupuytren palmar fascial disease, but the patients did not seem to be genetically predisposed to DD. Typical DD and non-Dupuytren palmar fascial disease are different clinical entities that run different courses with dissimilar prognoses. This should be taken into account in future epidemiologic and outcome studies.[21]

Epilepsy (OR, 1.12) and antiepileptic medications were not associated with DD. Ascertainment bias in previous studies may explain the reported association with epilepsy.[17]

No association could be detected between DD and smoking, alcohol consumption, or living in rural or urban areas.[19] A case-control study of 222 subjects matched for age, operation date, and sex used patients having other orthopedic operations as control subjects. Dupuytren contracture needing operation was strongly associated with current cigarette smoking (adjusted OR, 2.8; 95% CI, 1.5-5.2). The mean lifetime cigarette consumption was 16.7 pack-years for subjects with DD vs 12.0 pack-years for control subjects ($P = .016$). Dupuytren contracture was also associated with an Alcohol Use Disorders Test score greater than 7 (adjusted OR, 1.9; 95% CI,1.02-3.57). Mean weekly alcohol consumption was 7.3 units for cases vs 5.4 units for control subjects ($P = .016$). The excess risk associated with alcohol did not seem to be due to a confounding effect of smoking or vice versa. Smoking increases the risk of developing DC and may contribute to its prevalence in people with alcoholism, who tend to smoke heavily.[19] A population study revealed that DD was present in 13.75% of elderly ex-servicemen living at the Royal Hospital Chelsea, (The Royal Hospital Chelsea, London SW3 4SR Tel: 020 7881 5200 Fax: 020 7881 5463). Five men (9.1%) reported the condition in a parent or sibling, but none was aware of an affected child. The prevalence of heavy drinking, type 2 diabetes mellitus, or manual occupation was statistically the same in people with and without the condition. Overall, both hands were equally affected, but they differed in severity in 29 men. In milder cases, the left hand was the more severely affected (grades 1 and 2); the reverse was true when the difference in severity was greater (grade 3).[16]

Osteoarthritis of the Thumb Carpometacarpal Joint

Degenerative arthritis (also called osteoarthritis, degenerative joint disease, and degenerative arthrosis) of the carpometacarpal joint (CMCJ) of the thumb is the most common type and location of arthritis in the hand. It is more prevalent in women between 40 and 70 years (up to one third of women older than 40 years will have radiographic changes). The actual degenerative process is not completely understood. Although it involves "wear and tear," other factors have a role, including previous trauma, repetitive stress for long periods, joint configuration, and ligamentous laxity secondary to hormonal influences or normal aging. Hypermobility of the first metacarpophalangeal joint is a contributing factor owing to force concentration on the palmar trapeziometacarpal joint. However, rheumatoid arthritis or gout may also involve the CMCJ.

Occupational Risk Factors for Osteoarthritis of the CMCJ of the Thumb

Occupational risk factors for osteoarthritis of the CMCJ of the thumb include the following:

- Combination of risk factors (e.g., force and repetition, force and posture)
- Vibration
- Highly repetitive work alone or in combination with other factors
- Forceful work
- Awkward postures
- Keyboard activities
- Cold environment
- Length of employment
- Dominant hand

There is *insufficient evidence* for all of these factors.

Nonoccupational Risk Factors for Osteoarthritis of the CMCJ of the Thumb

There are also several proposed non-occupational risk factors for osteoarthritis of the CMCJ of the thumb:

- Age: strong evidence
- BMI: some evidence
- Sex: some evidence

- Biopsychosocial factors: insufficient evidence
- Diabetes: insufficient evidence

Table 9-6 shows the results of the literature searches for osteoarthritis of the CMCJ of the thumb, and Table 9-7 gives the representative references and comments.

TABLE 9-6   Results of Literature Search for Osteoarthritis of the CMCJ of the Thumb

Step	Result
Step 1: Search all fields for the combination of	
Search 1: osteoarthritis thumb CMCJ & causation	3 articles
Osteoarthritis Thumb & causation	14 articles; 2 duplicates; only 2 addressing causation
Osteoarthritis CMCJ Thumb & causation	3 articles; 2 duplicates; none addressing causation
Arthritis thumb CMCJ Joint & causation	3 articles; being duplicates.
Arthritis thumb	16 articles
Arthritis CMCJ thumb & causation	3 articles; all duplicates
Search 2: arthritis thumb & etiology	230 articles; 52 non-English; only 7 addressing causation or etiology associated with risk factors
Steps 2, 3 and 4	Completed; representative references provided

TABLE 9-7 Representative References and Comments for
Osteoarthritis of the CMCJ of the Thumb

Risk Factor	References and Comments
Combination of risk factors (eg, force and repetition, force and posture)	None
Vibration	None
Highly repetitive work alone or in combination with other factors	One-to-one matched case control study for sex, age, and occupational strain found women at increased risk of CMCJ arthritis for typists (OR, 5.0; CI, 1.27-19.59) and for work involving dexterity (OR, 2.0; CI, 0.77-5.23); in both sexes, an elevated OR for osteoarthritis in the finger joints for repetitive work (OR, 3.8; CI, 1.52-9.49) but not for the CMCJ of the thumb[22]; retrospective population review between 1978 and 1980 of a representative population sample of 8000 Finns found no significant association between the physical workload history and CMCJ osteoarthritis of the thumb[23]
Forceful work	None
Awkward postures	None
Keyboard activities	None
Cold environment	None
Length of employment	Case report study reviewed job-related (ironing activity for laundry) static-dynamic stress and CMCJ arthritis of the thumb; concluded that occupational conditions may contribute to arthritis of the CMCJ in dominant thumb in people older than 50 years of age and employed >10 y[24]
Dominant hand	None

TABLE 9-7   Representative References and Comments for
Osteoarthritis of the CMCJ of the Thumb (continued)

Risk Factor	References and Comments
Age	Prevalence of degenerative arthritis in all thumb and finger joints, including CMCJ, increases with age[25]; case report study reviewed job-related (ironing laundry) static-dynamic stress and arthritis of the thumb CMCJ; concluded occupational conditions may contribute to arthritis of the CMCJ in dominant thumb in people older than 50 years and employed >10 y[24]
BMI	Retrospective population review between 1978 and 1980 of a representative population sample of 8000 Finns: adjusted OR, 1.29 (95% CI, 1.15-1.43) per 5 kg/m^2 increment in BMI[23]
Sex	Sex-specific analyses of hand dominance demonstrated the majority of people with unilateral osteoarthritis of the second distal or third proximal interphalangeal joint had disease in dominant hand; among subjects with unilateral first CMCJ osteoarthritis, both sexes had a tendency for disease in nondominant hand[25]
Biopsychosocial factors	None
Diabetes	None
Genetic factors	Population study in Iceland found CMCJ arthritis in 1% of people; average pairwise kinship coefficient (KC) for patients and relative risk (RR) of arthritis in relatives of patients were matched to 1,000 control sets of similar composition in number, age, and sex, generated from genealogy database; KC for patients significantly higher than for control sets and proportional to the degree of thumb CMCJ involvement; RR in sisters of women in the study was 2.0 ($P < .001$); RR in spouses not significantly different from control subjects; RR increased with the severity of disease; for sisters of women with severe CMCJ involvement: RR, 6.9; increased risk extended beyond the nuclear family, with significantly increased risk in cousins[26]

Additional information was found about joint-specific disease, age, sex, and hand dominance. In a longitudinal study the joint-specific prevalence of radiographic osteoarthritis of the hand among a group of community-dwelling people aged 40 years or older was quantified and reported by age, sex, and dominant hand. The distal interphalangeal joint (DIPJ) had the highest osteoarthritis prevalence, whereas the proximal interphalangeal joint (PIPJ) showed the lowest. Joint-specific osteoarthritis prevalence rates for second DIPJ, third PIPJ, and first CMCJ were 35%, 18%, and 21%, respectively. As expected, hand osteoarthritis prevalence for all joints increased with age. With exceptions, women had higher osteoarthritis prevalence rates for the three sites examined. However, among men aged 40 to 49 years, the rate of osteoarthritis in the second DIPJ rate was higher (13%) than in women (8%). In addition, men in that age group had an elevated rate of osteoarthritis in the first CMCJ (9%) compared with that in women (5%). Sex-specific analyses of hand dominance demonstrated that the majority of people with unilateral osteoarthritis of the second DIPJ or third PIPJ had disease in the dominant hand. However, among people with unilateral osteoarthritis of the first CMCJ, both sexes had a tendency to have disease in the nondominant hand.[25]

Genetic and environmental factors might also be implicated in the risk for osteoarthritis. A population-based, cross-sectional study reviewed radiographs of the hands of 157 women in Japan and 655 women in the United States aged 71 years or older and knee radiographs of 358 women in Japan and 815 women in the United States aged 63 years or older. Logistic regression with the US group as referent to determine the prevalence OR of osteoarthritis among Japanese women showed the age-adjusted prevalence of osteoarthritis of the knee in Japanese women was higher than in white women (OR, 1.96; 95% CI, 1.50-2.56), whereas the prevalence of osteoarthritis of the hand, other than DIPJ in Japanese women, was lower than in white women (OR for PIPJ, 0.66; 95% CI, 0.46-0.93; OR for metacarpophalangeal joint, 0.62; 95% CI, 0.42-0.90), especially osteoarthritis of the base of thumb (OR, 0.15; 95% CI, 0.11-0.22). The authors concluded that site-specific differences in the prevalence of osteoarthritis may be attributed to genetic and/or environmental factors.[27]

Confounders

Among people with unilateral osteoarthritis of the first CMCJ, both sexes had a tendency to have disease in the nondominant hand.[25] A prospective study investigated the effect of mechanical stress on the development of osteoarthritis of the finger by comparing women from two occupations with different hand load but the same socioeconomic grade. The prevalence of osteoarthritis in any digit joint and in any DIPJ was higher among teachers compared with dentists (59%

vs 48%; $P = .020$ and 58% vs 47%; $P < .010$, respectively). Osteoarthritis of the finger showed more clustering in the ring and little fingers and more row clustering and symmetry in the teachers than in the dentists (age-adjusted OR, 1.57; 95% CI, 1.10-2.23; OR, 1.84; 95% CI, 1.28-2.64; and OR, 1.98; 95% CI, 1.38-2.86, respectively). The OR of more severe osteoarthritis (grade 3 or more) in the right thumb and index and middle fingers was significantly elevated among dentists compared with teachers (OR, 2.61; 95% CI, 1.03-6.59). The authors concluded that finger osteoarthritis in middle-aged women is highly prevalent and often polyarticular. Hand use may have a protective effect on osteoarthritis of the finger joint, whereas continuing joint overload may lead to joint impairment or arthritis.[28]

A retrospective population review between 1978 and 1980 selected a representative sample of 8000 Finns 30 years old or older. Subjects were invited to have a comprehensive health examination for review of arthritis of the CMCJ. Age-adjusted prevalence of osteoarthritis of the CMCJ of the thumb was 7% for men and 15% for women. After adjustment for age, sex, and other alleged risk factors, BMI was found to be directly proportional to the prevalence of osteoarthritis of the CMCJ of the thumb in both sexes. The adjusted OR was 1.29 (95% CI, 1.15-1.43) per 5-kg/m^2 increment in BMI. No significant association was found between the physical workload history and osteoarthritis of the CMCJ of the thumb. Restricted mobility of the thumb, local tenderness, and swelling were frequently found in conjunction with radiographic evidence of osteoarthritis of the CMCJ of the thumb. Advanced (grade 3 or 4) thumb CMCJ osteoarthritis predicted the total mortality rate in men (adjusted RR, 1.32; 95% CI, 1.03-1.69). Radiographic signs of osteoarthritis of the CMCJ of the thumb did not predict work disability. The authors concluded that obesity is a strong determinant of osteoarthritis of the CMCJ of the thumb in both sexes. The effect of osteoarthritis of the CMCJ of the thumb on disability and mortality in the general population is modest.[23]

A population study to investigate the prevalence and pattern of radiographically evident osteoarthritis of the hand joints and its association with self-reported hand pain and disability in 3906 people aged 55 years or older showed that 67% of women and 54.8% of men had osteoarthritis in at least one hand joint. The DIPJs were affected in 47.3% of participants, the CMCJ of the thumb in 35.8%, the PIPJs in 18.2%, and metacarpophalangeal joints in 8.2% (right or left hand). The authors concluded that radiographically evident osteoarthritis of the hand is common in elderly people, especially women. Co-occurrence of arthritis in different joint groups of the hand is more common than single-joint disease. There is a modest to weak association between arthritis of the hand and hand pain and disability, varying with the site of involvement.[29]

Trigger Digits

Triggering of upper limb digits may occur when the flexor tendon is enlarged, the A1 pulley is narrowed, or there is some combination of these factors. Inflammatory swelling of the tendon sheath and resultant stenosing tenosynovitis may be the most common cause of triggering. The edema results in "pinching" of the flexor tendon at the A1 pulley, which in turn causes a nodule to form within the tendon when fibers bunch up and lose their normal spiral arrangement. The inflammation of the tenosynovium may be primary, eg, with rheumatoid arthritis or gout. However, metabolic disorders such as diabetes mellitus and amyloidosis can cause connective tissue changes with similar synovial enlargement. The inflammation can also be secondary due to irritation of the tenosynovium as an enlarged tendon passes through the pulley. Possible causes of tendon enlargement include scarring from a partial tendon laceration and idiopathic nodule formation. Less commonly, occupational or avocational activities can cause inflammation and triggering. Blunt trauma is another possible but unusual cause. Many cases of trigger digit are idiopathic (of unknown cause).[30]

Occupational Risk Factors for Trigger Digits

The occupational risk factors for trigger digits are as follows:
- Combination of risk factors (e.g., force and repetition, force and posture): some evidence
- Vibration: some evidence
- Highly repetitive work alone or in combination with other factors: some evidence
- Forceful work: some evidence
- Awkward postures: some evidence
- Keyboard activities: insufficient evidence
- Cold environment: insufficient evidence
- Length of employment: insufficient evidence
- Dominant hand: insufficient evidence

Nonoccupational Risk Factors for Trigger Digits

Nonoccupational risk factors are as follows:
- Age: insufficient evidence (some reports of inverse relationship with age)
- BMI: insufficient evidence (obesity increases risk of multiple trigger digits)
- Sex: insufficient evidence (risk increased for females)
- Biopsychosocial factors: insufficient evidence
- Diabetes: strong evidence

Table 9-8 shows the results of the literature searches for trigger digits, and Table 9-9 gives the representative references and comments.

TABLE 9-8	Results of Literature Search for Trigger Digits
Step	**Result**
Step 1: search all fields for the combination of *	
Search 1: trigger finger & cause	18 articles
Search 2: trigger finger & epidemiology	4 articles
Search 3: trigger finger & etiology	8 articles
Search 4: trigger finger & work	6 articles
Search 5: trigger finger & age	23 articles
Search 6: trigger finger & vibration	2 articles
Search 7: trigger finger & biopsychosocial factors	2 articles
Search 8: trigger finger & diabetes	19 articles
Search 9: trigger finger & tool use	2 articles[†]
Steps 2, 3 and 4	Completed; representative references provided

* Multiple search combinations were used to identify relevant articles. There was considerable overlap of articles between search criteria.

† To this, 8 articles from the July 1997 "Musculoskeletal Disorders and Workplace Factors: A Critical Review of Epidemiological Evidence for Work-related Musculoskeletal Disorders of the Neck, Upper Extremity, and Low Back" were added with specific data extrapolated from the "hand wrist tendonitis" section dealing with trigger digit alone.

TABLE 9-9   Representative References and Comments for Trigger Digits

Risk Factor	References and Comments
Combination of risk factors (e.g., force and repetition, force and posture)	Higher order references[31-33] indicate strong evidence of combination of risk factors increasing risk over any individual single factor, but number of studies inadequate to garner a "strong evidence" recommendation
Vibration	Use of vibrating hand tools increases risk[32]
Highly repetitive work alone or in combination with other factors	Repetitive bending and twisting of hand and wrist increase risk[31-33]
Forceful work	Only one good study addressed forceful grip[31]; forceful grip in meatpacking worker increased risk[34]
Awkward postures	Video analysis of assembly line work with unusual postures showed increased risk[31]; awkward postures of factory workers[35]; unusual job mechanics of self-reported job description[36]
Keyboard activities	None
Cold environment	Case series reviewing trigger finger in frozen food workers did not list this diagnosis as a common injury[37]
Length of employment	One study implied inverse relationship, indicating increased incidence rate if employed <3 y in a repetitive job[32]
Dominant hand	None
Age	None
BMI	Obese and morbidly obese persons have increased risk of more than two trigger digits on one hand and more than four trigger digits on both hands[38]
Sex	Females report increased incidence of all hand and wrist tendinitis[32]; not confirmed by other studies and selection bias of study populations questioned by other studies

TABLE 9-9 Representative References and Comments for Trigger Digits
(continued)

Risk Factor	References and Comments
Biopsychosocial factors	Relationship of depression with self-reported upper extremity health status addressed by only one study that indicated an association with trigger digit and depression plus pain anxiety[39]
Diabetes	Relationship of diabetes as an independent risk factor for trigger digit development studied more than any other risk factor in the literature[40-42]

Confounders

Multiple studies discuss a variety of anatomic variants as risk factors for trigger finger development[43-46]; congenital anomaly[47,48]; other confounders include increased incidence with use of aromatase inhibitors used in breast cancer treatment[49]; increased incidence of trigger digit with comorbid carpal tunnel syndrome[50-52]; increased incidence reported with prior partial flexor tendon laceration injury[53]; relationship with certain tumors, including giant cell tumor, osteochondroma, and cavernous hemangioma[54,55]; relationship with thyroid disease[56]; increased incidence after motor vehicle accident[57]; and association with systemic rheumatologic conditions.[58]

de Quervain Disease

de Quervain disease is generally defined as stenosing tenosynovitis of the abductor pollicis longus and extensor pollicis brevis tendons at the first extensor (dorsal) compartment of the wrist. However, the original description by de Quervain was of tenovaginitis, a thickening of the extensor retinaculum, not tenosynovitis. There has also been controversy concerning the implication of inflammation in the disorder. Hence, for these reasons, use of the eponym, de Quervain disease, may be preferable.

Occupational Risk Factors for de Quervain Disease

The following are proposed occupational risk factors for de Quervain disease:
- Combination of risk factors (e.g., force and repetition, force and posture): some evidence
- Vibration: insufficient evidence
- Highly repetitive work alone or in combination with other factors: some evidence
- Forceful work: some evidence
- Awkward postures: some evidence
- Keyboard activities: insufficient evidence
- Cold environment: insufficient evidence
- Length of employment: insufficient evidence (trend of increased incidence if on job less than 3 years)
- Dominant hand: insufficient evidence

Nonoccupational Risk Factors for de Quervain Disease

The following are proposed nonoccupational risk factors for de Quervain disease:
- Age: insufficient evidence (de Quervain disease peaks in the younger-than-40-years age group)
- BMI: insufficient evidence
- Sex: insufficient evidence (conflicting reports in the literature as to sex prevalence, which some have postulated to occur as a result of height differences between men and women at stationary workstations leading to differences in postures)
- Biopsychosocial factors: insufficient evidence
- Diabetes: insufficient evidence

Table 9-10 shows the results of the literature searches for de Quervain disease, and Table 9-11 gives the representative references and comments.

TABLE 9-10   Results of Literature Search for de Quervain Disease

Step	Result
Step 1: Search all fields for the combination of*	
Search 1: de Quervain & radial styloid tenosynovitis causation	2 articles
Search 2: de Quervain & radial styloid tenosynovitis and epidemiology	5 articles
Search 3: de Quervain & radial styloid tenosynovitis and age	1 article
Search 4: de Quervain & radial styloid tenosynovitis and etiology	11 articles[†]
Steps 2, 3 and 4	Completed; representative references provided

* Multiple searches were performed owing to the small number of articles found concerning de Quervain and radial styloid tenosynovitis in general. Several articles overlapped the search criteria.

†To this, 8 articles from the July 1997 "Musculoskeletal Disorders and Workplace Factors: A Critical Review of Epidemiological Evidence for Work-related Musculoskeletal Disorders of the Neck, Upper Extremity, and Low Back"[162] were added with specific data extrapolated from the "hand wrist tendonitis" section dealing with de Quervain disease alone.

TABLE 9-11   Representative References and Comments for de Quervain Disease

Risk Factor	References and Comments
Combination of risk factors (e.g., force and repetition, force and posture)	Higher order references[33,35] indicated strong evidence of a combination of risk factors increasing risk over any individual single factor, but number of studies inadequate to garner a "strong evidence" recommendation; increased incidence in volleyball players overall with a higher incidence in professional than in amateur players argues for combination of repeated trauma, force, and posture as a strong risk factor[59]; increased incidence in certain video game players argues for increased risk due to combination of repetition and awkward posture[60]
Vibration	None

TABLE 9-11   Representative References and Comments
for de Quervain Disease (continued)

Risk Factor	References and Comments
Highly repetitive work alone or in combination with other factors	Repetitive bending and twisting of hand and wrist increases risk[33,35,36,61-63]; See comment with "Forceful work" about combination of repetition and force
Forceful work	Certain jobs requiring high force in grip have increased risk: jobs studied included meat processors,[64] auto assemblers,[61] textile workers,[63] and meat cutters[36]; higher order reference comparing force and repetition across seven manufacturing plants indicated a dramatic risk increase in high force–high repetition jobs compared with high force–low repetition and low force–low repetition[33]
Awkward postures	Deviated wrist postures increase risk[35,61,62]
Keyboard activities	None
Cold environment	None
Length of employment	Possibly an inverse relationship between years on the job as predictor of de Quervain disease[63]; may be a complex interplay among years on the job, age, and sex, indicating that the longer on the job, the less likely the disorder will develop, but effect is statistically small[33]
Dominant hand	None
Age	Peak incidence rate in younger-than-40-years age group[61] See discussion for "Length of employment"
BMI	None
Sex	Conflicting information; increased report rate in men thought perhaps due to more frequent tool use than women[61]; differences in posture owing to height differences between men and women postulated to account for differences in reporting rates at stationary workstations[63]; studies of sex differences hampered by large number of women vs men in certain manufacturing groups of workers[63]
Biopsychosocial factors	Only one study addressed relationship of depression with self-reported upper extremity health status; indicated an association with depression plus pain anxiety[39]
Diabetes	None

Confounders

Some articles discuss the significance (or lack thereof) of anatomic morphology of the first dorsal compartment in relation to the presence of a septum or other anatomic variant of the tendon sheath. There seems to be a small statistical argument favoring these anatomic variants as predictors of the development of de Quervain disease in relation to the presence of septation of the first dorsal compartment. However, not all studies reached the same conclusions. It seems that this factor has a more significant role in surgical management of the disorder because failure to recognize these variants may lead to incomplete surgical release of one or both tendons, resulting in unrelieved or recurrent disease.[65-67] A radial styloid abnormality such as cortical erosion, sclerosis, or periosteal bone apposition may be a manifestation of de Quervain disease, but questions remain as to the significance of radial styloid abnormalities as risk factors for the development of de Quervain disease.[68,69] Most studies exclude subjects with a history of trauma, arthritis, and other disease; there are no studies that directly compare de Quervain disease with systemic conditions or prior trauma.[35]

Painful Elbow
(Lateral and Medial Epicondylitis)

Tennis elbow is a painful disorder that originates at the common extensor origin on the lateral humeral epicondyle. Traditionally, it has been described as *lateral epicondylitis,* despite the fact that repeated studies of pathologic findings do not show inflammation. Rather, histologic studies show an angiofibroblastic dysplasia from microtears of the tendon. Hence, *lateral epicondylopathy* may be semantically more correct. Similar disease in the common flexor origin at the medial elbow has been labeled *golfer's elbow, medial epicondylitis,* and *medial epicondylopathy.*

Occupational Risk Factors for Tennis Elbow

The following are the occupational risk factors for tennis elbow:
- Combination of risk factors (e.g., force and repetition, force and posture): very strong evidence
- Vibration: insufficient evidence
- Highly repetitive work alone or in combination with other factors: insufficient evidence

- Forceful work: some evidence
- Awkward postures: some evidence
- Keyboard activities: insufficient evidence
- Cold environment: insufficient evidence
- Length of employment: insufficient evidence
- Dominant hand: insufficient evidence

Nonoccupational Risk Factors for Tennis Elbow

The following are the nonoccupational risk factors for tennis elbow:
- Age: insufficient evidence; increased risk in fourth and fifth decades
- BMI: insufficient evidence
- Sex: insufficient evidence
- Biopsychosocial factors: insufficient evidence
- Diabetes: insufficient evidence

Table 9-12 shows the results of the literature searches for tennis elbow, and Table 9-13 gives the representative references and comments.

TABLE 9-12	Results of Literature Search for Tennis Elbow
Step	**Result**
Step 1: Search all fields for the combination of	
Search 1: tennis elbow & causation	21 articles
Search 2: tennis elbow & cause	31 articles
Search 3: tennis elbow & etiology	199 articles
Search 4: tennis elbow & work	65 articles
Search 5: tennis elbow & occupation	8 articles*
Steps 2, 3 and 4	Completed; representative references provided

*To this, articles from the July 1997 "Musculoskeletal Disorders and Workplace Factors: A Critical Review of Epidemiological Evidence for Work-related Musculoskeletal Disorders of the Neck, Upper Extremity, and Low Back" were added.

Risk Factor	References and Comments
TABLE 9-13 Representative References and Comments for Tennis Elbow	
Combination of risk factors (e.g., force and repetition, force and posture)	Strong evidence. Good-quality studies consistently show strong relationship between combination of risk factors and tennis elbow, especially at higher exposure levels; relationship demonstrated in certain working populations (construction workers, meatpackers)[35,70-76]; strong support in sports medicine literature; incidence of tennis elbow strongly correlates with combination of force of grip, position, and frequency of playing racquet sports[77-79]
Vibration	Insufficient evidence. One high-quality study shows vibration as independent risk factor[80]; vibratory transmission to elbow also postulated as risk factor in amateur racquet sport players[81,82]
Highly repetitive work alone or in combination with other factors	Insufficient evidence. A few studies show high repetition as small independent risk factor, but in most, another risk factor is combined with repetition (force, posture)[70-72]
Forceful work	Some evidence. Association with forceful work as an independent risk factor and tennis elbow, but number of studies is small[35,74,83,84]
Awkward postures	Some evidence. A few high-quality studies show posture as a clear independent risk factor[84-87]; sports medicine studies of racquet players show the difference in grip mechanics between beginning and advanced players has a correlation[79]
Keyboard activities	Insufficient evidence. There seems to be an association of longer duration of symptoms in keyboard workers who have previously developed tennis elbow from some other cause[88]
Cold environment	Insufficient evidence
Length of employment	Insufficient evidence. Increased risk with length of employment in public works department workers[89]; peak incidence in fourth and fifth decades, with decreasing risk in later life[90]
Dominant hand	Insufficient evidence

TABLE 9-13 Representative References and Comments for Tennis Elbow
(continued)

Risk Factor	References and Comments
Age	Some studies show increased incidence in older workers; when confounders eliminated, age alone not a legitimate independent risk factor[89,90]
BMI	Insufficient evidence
Sex	Insufficient evidence
Biopsychosocial factors	Insufficient evidence. Low social support and low decision-making authority in workplace increase risk[76,81]
Diabetes	Insufficient evidence

Confounders

Lack of normal shoulder internal rotation is a risk factor.[86] A study of twins showed that genetic factors have a role, with a twofold to threefold increase in incidence above chance and when controlling for other risk factors.[91] The presence of posterolateral elbow plica was seen in surgically treated patients.[92] Carpal tunnel syndrome is frequently associated with tennis elbow.[93,94] Alcoholism was associated with tennis elbow in one study.[95] Decreased upper extremity reaction times were linked to an increase in tennis elbow.[96] People with tennis elbow have an increase in vascularity shown by Doppler studies.[97] Litigation is associated with increased incidence and longer duration of tennis elbow.[98] In many studies looking at quantifiable risk factors, the number and/or intensity of repetitions and forceful contractions are not identified. It is difficult to control for common nonoccupational activities, and many people with symptomatic tennis elbow continue to work, which leads to bias.

Carpal Tunnel Syndrome

Carpal tunnel syndrome (CTS) is a constellation of symptoms and signs resulting from compression of the median nerve in the carpal tunnel. Symptoms typically include numbness, paresthesias, dysesthesias, and/or pain in the radial palm and palmar aspect of the thumb, index, middle, and perhaps ring fingers. The sensory complaints sometimes also extend proximally in the limb and often occur or worsen at night.

No one physical examination test absolutely confirms this diagnosis. Because electrodiagnostic testing is considered the "gold standard" for diagnosis, the best studies on CTS risk factors include nerve conduction testing (NCT) as a requirement for inclusion. Electromyography may also be helpful.

According to the World Health Organization, CTS is a multifactorial disease, which may be work-related, but also occurs in the general population. Hence, occupational exposures are not necessarily risk factors in every case of CTS. Anatomic abnormalities, other personal characteristics, fluid abnormalities, inflammatory and neuropathic diseases, and other environmental factors may also have an etiologic role. However, CTS may be caused, in part or in whole, by adverse working conditions. Preexisting CTS may be aggravated, accelerated, or exacerbated by workplace exposures. Carpal tunnel syndrome may also impair working capacity.[99]

Many studies used the following definitions for workplace risk factors:

High repetitions: cycle time of less than 30 seconds or more than 50% of the cycle time involved in performing fundamentally the same activity

High force: jobs in which the estimated average hand force requirements are more than 4 kg; no effective way to measure actual grip force used on most jobs

Awkward wrist posture: posturing in more than 45° of wrist flexion or extension, without excessive radial or ulnar deviation

Vibrating power tools: not clearly defined

Most CTS incidence studies use the surveillance definition from the National Institute for Occupational Safety and Health (NIOSH) for this condition, which requires two symptoms and one examination finding. However, in an occupation with a 10% prevalence of CTS, using the NIOSH definition, 85% of the people who meet the NIOSH requirements would not have true (NCT-confirmed) CTS.[100,101]

One perspective is as follows:

Even if a patient experiences symptoms only at work, an honest clinician is still unable to describe the extent to which the patient's CTS is related to the job. It is unfortunate that workers' compensation determinations must be made in individual cases, where it is impossible to quantify the contribution of the job to the clinical problem.[102(pp421-434)]

Occupational Risk Factors for CTS

The occupational risk factors for CTS are as follows:

- Combination of risk factors (e.g., force and repetition, force and posture): strong evidence; national and international epidemiologic surveillance data consistently demonstrated that highest rates of CTS occur in occupations with high physical demands that include intensive manual exertion, such as meatpacking, poultry processing, and automobile assembly work
- Vibration: some evidence
- Highly repetitive work alone or in combination with other factors: some evidence; widely varied definitions for repetitive work, making association difficult
- Forceful work: some evidence
- Carpal tunnel or wrist size: some evidence
- Awkward postures: insufficient evidence; lack of evidence possibly associated with individual variability in work methods among workers in similar jobs and influence of differing body posture while measuring postural characteristics of jobs; some evidence of postural factors in laboratory-based studies of extreme postures
- Keyboard activities: insufficient evidence
- Cold environment: insufficient evidence
- Length of employment: insufficient evidence
- Dominant hand: insufficient evidence

Nonoccupational Risk Factors for CTS

The nonoccupational risk factors for CTS include the following:

- Age: very strong evidence; risk increases with increasing age
- BMI: very strong evidence; high BMI increases risk
- Sex: strong evidence; female
- Biopsychosocial factors: strong evidence (The biopsychosocial approach looks at the mind and body of an individual as two important and interrelated systems.[103] Pain and other neuromusculoskeletal symptoms that may be related to conditions such as CTS are reported differently by each individual.[104] Examining physicians must broaden their evaluation to consider how developmental, psychological, cognitive, family, occupational, and economic factors affect the expression of pain and disability.[105] If the three components of the word are reviewed, a more complete understanding of pain must include biological, psychological, and social factors.[106] Biological refers to the medical or physical aspects of pain. Psychological[107] refers to the mental, emotional, and behavioral[108] aspects of pain. Social refers to the individual's interactions with other people. According to the biopsychosocial model, it is impossible to fully

understand the problem of pain or symptoms using physical or medical concepts alone. In contrast with the biomedical model, which separates body and mind, the biopsychosocial model is holistic in that mind and body are seen as inextricably intertwined. Unfortunately, cultural biases against psychological and psychiatric diagnoses can result in disincentives for biobehavioral treatment and have been noted to increase the tendency for patients to somaticize and for physicians to inappropriately medically treat.108 This biopsychosocial concept has been expressed by Halder as "insights that will lead to restructuring of health care, so that patients with musculoskeletal disorders, particularly those with the illness of work incapacity, will be treated with concern and compassion." (Halder NM: Point of View. Spine 19:1116-1994)

- Diabetes: strong evidence
- Smoking: insufficient evidence

Table 9-14 shows the results of the literature searches for CTS, and Table 9-15 gives the representative references and comments.

TABLE 9-14 Results of Literature Search for CTS

Step	Results
Step 1: Search all fields for the combination of	
Search 1: carpal tunnel & causation	301 articles with 199 after 1996
Search 2: carpal tunnel & epidemiology & etiology & cross-sectional studies	39 articles with 16 after 1996; of these, 5 unavailable in English, and 5 did not address carpal tunnel leaving only 6
Search 3: keyboards & carpal tunnel	39 articles, with 21 after 1996; of these, 5 not available in English, 4 did not address carpal tunnel, 2 duplicates, leaving only 10*
Steps 2, 3 and 4	were completed. Representative references are provided.

* The available studies were added to the 30 epidemiologic studies used in the July 1997 Musculoskeletal Disorders and Workplace Factors: A Critical Review of Epidemiologic Evidence for Work-related Musculoskeletal Disorders of the Neck, Upper Extremity, and Low Back.[109]

TABLE 9-14 References and Comments for CTS

Risk Factor	References and Comments
Combination of risk factors (eg, force and repetition, force and posture)	Repetitive hyperflexion and twisting of wrists[110] and regular and prolonged use of handheld vibratory tools increases the risk of CTS >twofold[111]; stressful manual work,[112] type of grasp, and repetitiveness not significantly different and not statistically significant[84]; RR, 8.3 for forceful and repetitive wrist motion (95% CI, 2.6-26.4) for a history of CTS-like symptoms[113]; high-force and repetition, no relationship found[114]; repetitive tasks,[115] predisposing factors were stressful manual work,[112] manual handling, and repetitive work[116]; combination of factors, high-velocity and high-force manual work is a risk factor[118]; repetitiveness a contributing factor,[119] sustained forceful movement and repetitive motion,[83] force and duration of wrist flexion,[120] and combinations of above listed factors[117,121]
Vibration	Exposure to vibration, OR, 1.9[122]; vibrations associated with job tasks[123]; prospective longitudinal study found risk associated with vibration[124]; increased prevalence statistically significant[125]
Highly repetitive work alone or in combination with other factors	Some evidence for combinations of factors[83]; high-velocity and high-force manual work a risk factor[118]; stressful manual work a risk factor[112]; type of grasp and repetitiveness not significantly different and not statistically significant[84]; repetitive jobs,[115] failed to detect a relationship for highly-repetitive tasks,[114] motion repetitiveness a risk factor (OR, 8.8)[121]; repetitiveness a contributing factor[119]. Conflicting information was reported in the study; showing no consistent association found between type and the level of occupational hand activity[126]; longitudinal study showed age and hand dominance more important than any job-related factor[127]; three studies concluded there was conflicting information[123,128,129]

CHAPTER 9

TABLE 9-14 References and Comments for CTS (continued)

Risk Factor	References and Comments
Forceful work	Type of grasp and repetitiveness not significantly different and not statistically significant[84]; RR, 8.3 for forceful and repetitive wrist motion (95% CI, 2.6-26.4) with a history of CTS-like symptoms[113]; no relationship found for high force[114]; sustained forceful movement [83]; exertion of force >1 kg (OR, 9.0)[121]; pinch grasp, no effect[130.] Sustained forceful movement is a label for activities that require a forceful grip or hold to be applied for more than two minutes.
Carpal tunnel size or wrist size	Wrist index,[131] wrist depth-width ratio,[132-127] hand and wrist anthropometrics found to be independent risk factors for CTS in females but not males[137]; square wrists[138] and square wrist dimensions were risk factors[139]
Awkward postures	Insufficient evidence. Repetitive hyperflexion and twisting of wrists,[110] differences in wrist posture not statistically significant[84]; non-neutral wrist and elbow postures,[140] exposure to wrist bend and twist, OR, 5.5[122] prolonged and highly repetitious flexion and extension of the wrist, especially when allied with a forceful grip,[141] awkward positions,[117] activities involving flexing or extending the wrist,[130] computer workers who kept their wrists extended by more than 20° at greater risk,[142] awkward positions,[83] no association with posture[121]
Keyboard activities	Insufficient evidence for keyboard risk[143,144]; keyboard not risk factor[145]; no trend for risk to increase with more time spent keyboarding[146]; no evidence on keyboard and computer work[141]; keyboard not factor[148]; keyboard not factor[123,145, 147]; no effect of typing[130]; no effect from keyboard redesign[149]
Cold environment	Local exposure to cold contributing factors[119]
Length of employment	No association between the length of employment (OR, 1.13; 95% CI, 0.77-1.66; $P = .591$)[110]; prevalence not associated with length of employment[126]; total frequency of symptoms displayed a positive linear correlation with employment duration ($r = 0.618$; $P = .004$)[117]

TABLE 9-14 References and Comments for CTS (continued)

Risk Factor	References and Comments
Dominant hand	Each hand seems to be at independent risk depending on that hand's activity[150]; hand dominance, no effect[132]; dominant hand, no effect[123]; prevalence of bilateral slowing of conduction of median nerve not associated with bimanual occupational hand activity[126]; hand dominance, no effect[151]; longitudinal study showed age and hand dominance more important than any job-related factor[127]
Age	Risk increases with increasing age: older than 40 years[152,153]; age[131]; increased BMI a significant independent risk factor for CTS in patients younger than 63 years but less important in older patients[154]; age[132]; older than 39 years, OR, 1.2[122]; age[139,151,154,155,156,158,159]; greater age[123]; older[157]; longitudinal study showed age and hand dominance more important than any job-related factor[127]; aging[160]*
BMI	Higher BMI increases risk: BMI >30[152]; obesity (OR, 4.4; 95% CI,: 1.1-17.1)[161]; BMI risk,[162] BMI risk,[109] BMI[131]; increased BMI a significant independent risk factor for CTS in patients younger than 63 years but less important in older patients[154]; BMI,[132] BMI,[137] obesity (BMI > 29),[112] BMI >5, OR, 2.0[122]; obesity,[138,155,163]; relative overweight[123]; increasing weight[139]; higher BMI[139]; obese (BMI > 29) people 2.5 times more likely than slender people (BMI < 20) to be diagnosed with CTS[164]; BMI[165]; being overweight[157]; BMI[158]*†
Sex	Strong evidence. Female sex, OR, 2.3[122]; female[123,137,139,155,163]; higher risk in women with diabetes[167]

TABLE 9-14 References and Comments for CTS (continued)

Risk Factor	References and Comments
Biopsychosocial factors	Ergonomic stressors and physical factors independent risk factors for CTS[168]; history of CTS[152]; lower self-reported social support[140]; psychological distress at baseline (OR, 4.3; 95% CI, 1.0-18.6)[161]; ergonomic stressors[162]; ergonomic factors[109]; results emphasize complexity of the determinants of CTS, role of psychosocial factors at work, and potentially negative effects of some practices of companies aimed at enhancing their competitiveness[169]; results indicate that three sets of risk factors independently affect the incidence of upper-limb disorders: biomechanical constraints, psychosocial factors, and personal factors[170]; role of psychological distress in workers exposed to a high level of physical exposure and psychological demand highlighted[161]‡
Diabetes	History of diabetes[140]; diabetes mellitus[172]; Type 1 diabetes related to age and duration of diabetes[173]; diabetes mellitus[112]; diabetes may be a weak risk factor, especially among women[155]; higher risk in women with diabetes[167]
Smoking	History of cigarette smoking, OR, 1.6[122]
Genetic factors	Case report of familial CTS occurring in seven members of three generations of a black family: 20 members of four generations had NCTs; age of subjects affected by CTS ranged from 29 to 67 years; familial CTS seems to have an autosomal dominant pattern of CTS inheritance with high penetrance[174]

* Retrospective review of 900 people randomly selected from a group of 2500 railroad workers with a diagnosis of CTS confirmed by NCT. The authors concluded that in this population claiming CTS caused by railroad occupations, there was a significant association between CTS and BMI, age, and wrist index but not job classification. More than half of the study group and one third of the surgical subset had normal nerve study data.[131]

† Prospective study for BMI and square wrist pattern (wrist depth-width ratio) demonstrated increased risk with increasing BMI and increasing square wrist pattern.[166]

‡ Considering psychosocial and biomechanical factors as separate exposures is a somewhat artificial distinction because the two classes of stressors are strongly linked. Both result from core aspects of the organization: its technology, culture, and work organization. Biomechanical and psychosocial risk factors both result from the way work is organized, the technology and sector of the company, and the organizational policies and culture that drive work organization. Thus, the two classes of stressors are generally highly correlated in a workplace.[133] Therefore, to the extent that the quality of the evidence is poor, any subsequent inference will be weakened.[171]

Confounders

One confounder was a history of tendinitis of the wrist, hand, or finger.[140] In addition, CTS occurred twice as often in both hands as in the dominant hand alone, suggesting that nonoccupational factors could be more important than occupational in the development of CTS.[120] Rheumatoid arthritis[172] and pregnancy[172] were confounders. There was no correlation for job classification.[131] A lower exercise level resulted in higher risk,[132] as did oophorectomy.[175] No relationship was found with employment duration or with work produced per year,[176] but dissatisfaction with work, lack of job control, short cycle time, and having to press repeatedly with the hand were associated with CTS.[169] An OR of 2.24 was found for "just in time" production.[169] White race had an OR of 16.7[122] and a history of cigarette smoking an OR of 1.6.[122,123] Education of more than 12 years had an OR of 1.2.[122] An annual family income more than $20,000 had an OR of 1.5.[122] Workplace demands seem to bear an uncertain relationship.[163] The mechanism whereby a weight gain of about 6 lb increases the risk of disease 8% requires explanation.[145] The presence of an endocrine disorder is marginally related to risk.[123] No relationship was found between specific job categories or job tasks.[123] A lower exercise level[139,151] and oral contraceptive use increased risk for tendinitis.[139]

People who ingest caffeine alone or in combination with tobacco were at the highest risk.[177] No consistent association was found between the type and level of occupational hand activity and the prevalence or the severity of slowing.[126] Age and dominance were more important than any job-related factor in the prediction of slowing after 5 years.[127] Occupational hand use,[151] duration of employment,[151] and industry type were not predictive of CTS.[151] Individual factors, such as BMI, age, wrist dimensions, and physical activity are far more important for determining who develops clinical CTS than are job-related factors, such as specific job, force or repetitions, duration of employment, or industry.[157] Physical inactivity increased risk for tendinitis.[157] Oral contraceptive use had a 2.0 times higher OR.[83] Employment experience had no effect.[160] Occupational risk factors have a substantial role in the development of CTS symptoms.[178] A lack of change in tasks or lack of breaks for at least 15% of the daily work time had an OR of 6.0,[121] workstation design an OR of 5.0,[121] and lack of job rotation an OR of 6.3.[121] Hysterectomy without oophorectomy demonstrated an increased risk for tendinitis.[130] Last menstrual period occurring 6 to 12 months previously also had an increased risk for tendinitis.[130] Widely varying incidence rates in geographically different locations with almost identical workplace conditions were found, and it was concluded that job and personal satisfaction should be considered as confounders for CTS in the workplace.[148] A prospective study for BMI and square wrist pattern (wrist depth-width ratio) demonstrated increased risk with increasing BMI and increasing square wrist pattern.[166]

Carpal Tunnel Update

CTS Causation Meta-analysis

Research presented in February 2007, at the 74th annual meeting of the American Academy of Orthopaedic Surgeons corroborates earlier studies indicating there may be a genetic predisposition to CTS.[179] A review of 117 studies on CTS published in the medical literature using a quantitative scale based on the Hill Criteria of Causation, which included temporal relationship, strength, dose-response relationship, consistency, plausibility, consideration of alternate explanations, experiment, specificity, and coherence was completed. Average scores for biological factors (e.g., genetics, race, and age) were double those of occupational factors (e.g., job type, repetitive hand use, and vibration), and the average strength of causal association (OR) was about three times as strong for biological factors as it was for occupational factors. David Ring, MD, stated "the quality and strength of evidence supporting genetic or inherent risk factors was felt to be moderate while the quality and strength of evidence supporting occupational risk factors was felt to be poor." Ring confirmed that the application of stringent science to theories of causation may affect claims of disability, workers' compensation, and personal injury but should also help treating physicians' communications with their patients. "Physicians have the power to increase or decrease illness and disability with their words. In my opinion, we should provide patients with the most optimistic, positive, practical, and enabling illness concepts that are consistent with the best available scientific data." Although complaints of activity-related wrist pain are commonly associated with CTS, Ring said the true hallmark of the condition is numbness at night or when awakening in the morning. Pain without numbness is not characteristic of CTS.

Wrist Positions

In a prospective study of 37 patients,[180] researchers proposed the development of guidelines to help workers avoid wrist postures that may be associated with median nerve compression. Researchers with backgrounds in human factors and ergonomics found that as the wrist posture changes, pressure in the carpal canal can increase, which may be associated with the development of CTS. Based on this hypothesis, they considered 30 mm Hg the upper limit of normal pressure and elected to find the angle at which 75% of the individual's pressures remained below this maximum. (There is currently no science to support that the arbitrary limit of 30 mm Hg has a direct relationship to the onset of CTS.) The researchers found that sustained wrist positions should not exceed the following angles: extension, 32.7°; flexion, 48.6°; ulnar deviation, 14.5°; and radial deviation, 21.8°.

In a controlled trial study[181] of 36 people, researchers simultaneously measured changes in tactile threshold and discomfort ratings during prolonged wrist flexion in symptomatic patients from a rehabilitation clinic and from a control population. Prolonged (15 minutes) wrist flexion significantly increased tactile threshold and discomfort ratings above baseline levels in symptomatic and control populations. Of the symptomatic sample, 62% was found to have abnormal conduction latency. Tactile threshold in symptomatic subjects with normal conduction latency (n = 13) did not differ significantly from that in control subjects (n = 36) at baseline but showed significant elevation during wrist flexion. In contrast, subjects with abnormal conduction latency (n = 21) exhibited significant elevation relative to control subjects at baseline and throughout wrist flexion, as well as a slower recovery after flexion. Conduction latency correlated with baseline ($r = 0.52$; $P < .0001$) and 15-minute ($r = 0.67$; $P < .0001$) tactile threshold for the entire subject population, as well as 15-minute threshold ($r = 0.53$; $P = .013$) for the subpopulation with abnormal conduction latency. At 2.5 minutes after flexion, correlation was significant for whole ($r = 0.64$; $P < .0001$) and abnormal conduction latency ($r = 0.58$; $P = .0063$) samples. Regression slope of tactile threshold vs conduction latency was significantly greater than zero and did not differ significantly from linearity. The study demonstrates that increases in mechanosensory threshold and discomfort ratings during prolonged wrist flexion are more profound (and recovery less rapid) in patients with electrophysiologic evidence of injury.[181]

Interior Changes in CTS

Researchers at the Mayo Clinic, Rochester, Minn, studied light and scanning electron microscopic imaging of the subsynovial connective tissue from biopsy specimens of 11 patients (12 hands) with idiopathic CTS, 14 cadaver controls, and two cadavers with a history of CTS. The connective tissue is made up of three parts. The visceral synovial layer is an uninterrupted membrane that defines the bursa dorsally. The subsynovial connective tissue consists of fibrous bundles that run parallel to the tendon, interconnected by smaller fibrous fibers. It connects to the synovial membrane and the flexor tendons. The control tissue showed interconnections between all the parallel layers, whereas in patients with idiopathic CTS, these interconnections were absent, replaced with thicker parallel fibrous bundles. Similar changes were found in the cadaver CTS specimens. These pathologic changes in the patient and cadaver CTS specimens were most apparent close to the tendon and became progressively less severe in more superficial layers. It was postulated that during tendon motion, the loose fibers between adjacent layers are stretched, which results in these changes. The authors further concluded that because the most severe changes in the subsynovial connective tissue were found close to the tendon, these changes may be the result of a shearing injury.[181]

Carpal Tunnel Anatomy With Changing Wrist Positions

Researchers reported[182] on the use of magnetic resonance imaging to evaluate the shape of the carpal tunnel in the neutral position, 30° extension, and 30° flexion. Computerized reconstruction provided detailed anatomic visualization of the carpal tunnel and has created a framework to develop a biomechanical model thereof. Similar reconstruction of the tissue structures entering and passing through the carpal tunnel will enable evaluation and partitioning of median nerve injury mechanisms. Three-dimensional reconstruction of the carpal tunnels of 8 volunteers from the university community revealed the orientation of the carpal tunnel was not directly explained by external wrist angle. The average orientation of the carpal tunnel was extended in all postures, ranging from 25° ± 9° in extension, 13° ± 5° in neutral, and 4° ± 4° in flexion. Changing the orientation of the imaging plane to be perpendicular to the reconstructed carpal tunnel revealed that axial images overestimated the cross-sectional area by an average of nearly 10% in extension, 4% in neutral, and less than 1% in flexion. Further study will be required to relate this information into practical clinical practice.[182]

Biomarkers

A prospective study of 22 people with upper extremity musculoskeletal disorders due to overuse for no longer than 12 weeks were stratified according to the severity of symptoms and signs. Several biomarkers (interleukin-1β, tumor necrosis factor α, interleukin-6, and C-reactive protein) were studied with BMI and age as covariates. The authors concluded that early-onset, overuse-related musculoskeletal disorders may have an inflammatory component. Further research as to clinical application is appropriate.[183]

Ulnar Nerve Entrapment at Elbow (Cubital Tunnel Syndrome)

This syndrome is a complex of symptoms and signs resulting from compression of the ulnar nerve about the elbow that may result in numbness, paresthesias, and/or dysesthesias of the ring and little fingers plus weakness of grip. Because electrodiagnostic testing is considered the "gold standard" for diagnosis, the best risk factors studies include NCT/electromyography as the requirement for diagnosis.

Occupational Risk Factors for Ulnar Nerve Entrapment at the Elbow

The following are the proposed occupational risk factors:

- Combination of risk factors (e.g., force and repetition, force and posture)
- Vibration
- Highly repetitive work alone or in combination with other factors
- Forceful work
- Awkward postures
- Keyboard activities
- Cold environment
- Length of employment
- Dominant hand

There is *insufficient evidence* for all of the occupational risk factors.

Nonoccupational Risk Factors for Ulnar Nerve Entrapment at the Elbow

The following are the proposed nonoccupational risk factors:

- Age: some evidence; risk increases with increasing age
- BMI: some evidence; risk increases with higher BMI
- Gender: some evidence; risk increased for females
- Biopsychosocial factors: insufficient evidence
- Diabetes: insufficient evidence

Table 9-16 shows the results of the literature searches for ulnar nerve entrapment at the elbow, and Table 9-17 gives the representative references and comments.

TABLE 9-16	Results of Literature Search for Ulnar Nerve Entrapment at the Elbow
Step	**Results**
Step 1: Search all fields for the combination of	
Search 1: ulnar nerve entrapment elbow & causation	4 articles; in English but only 1 addressed workplace causation
Search 2: ulnar nerve elbow & causation	36 articles; 30 in English but only 2 addressed workplace causation
Search 3: ulnar nerve elbow & epidemiology	21 articles; 15 in English; 6 duplicate; only 2 addressed workplace causation*
Steps 2, 3 and 4	Completed; representative references provided

* Because of the limited number of articles, two English abstracts were added to the discussion sections but not used to calculate the strength of evidence.

TABLE 9-17	Representative References and Comments for Ulnar Nerve Entrapment at the Elbow
Risk Factor	**References and Comments**
Combination of risk factors (eg, force and repetition, force and posture)	Insufficient evidence. Residents of a health district where manual work is dominant had a higher male-specific incidence (57.1) than other areas [184]
Vibration	Insufficient evidence. Non-English article[185]
Highly repetitive work alone or in combination with other factors	None
Forceful work	Insufficient evidence
Awkward postures	3-year prospective survey: holding a tool in position the only predictive biomechanical factor (OR, 4.1; 95% CI, 1.4-12.0)[186]
Keyboard activities	Insufficient evidence

TABLE 9-17 Representative References and Comments for Ulnar Nerve Entrapment at the Elbow (continued)

Risk Factor	References and Comments
Cold environment	Insufficient evidence
Length of employment	Insufficient evidence
Dominant hand	Insufficient evidence
Age	Insufficient evidence. Increasing age for men ($P = .008$),[187]; increasing trend with each decade of age[184]
BMI	Insufficient evidence. Obesity[186]; increasing BMI for men,[187] decreasing BMI for women (OR, 2.3; 95% CI, 1.3-4.2 for BMI $\leq$22.0 vs >22.0)[187]
Gender	Insufficient evidence. Electrodiagnostic criteria for males (OR, 6.9; 95% CI, 2.4-20.4; $P < .001$)[187]
Biopsychosocial factors	Insufficient evidence. Data confirm the mutual influences of individual factors, physical and psychological factors, and workplace factors in occurrence of painful disorders related to occupational activity; therapeutic approach must involve physical, psychological, and social evaluation (non-English article)[188]
Smoking	Insufficient evidence. Electrodiagnostically confirmed ulnar mononeuropathy at the elbow, case-control study, cigarette smoking increases risk[189]
Diabetes	Insufficient evidence.

Confounders

In a 3-year prospective survey, the annual incidence was estimated at 0.8% per person-year,[186] and a 3-year prospective survey found that obesity increased the risk of ulnar nerve entrapment at the elbow (OR, 4.3; 95% CI, 1.2-16.2), as did the presence of medial epicondylitis, CTS, radial tunnel syndrome, and cervicobrachial neuralgia.[186] In a retrospective study to identify newly diagnosed cases on the basis of clinical symptoms or signs and slowing of motor conduction velocity of the ulnar nerve across the elbow or surgical evidence of nerve compression in the elbow region during 5-year period from 1995 to 1999, 311 cases

(112 females and 199 males; mean age, 56 years; range, 15-86 years) the mean annual crude incidence was 24.7 cases per 100 000 person-years, and the standardized incidence was 20.9. The sex-specific incidences were 32.7 for men and 17.2 for women[184]; there was no association between prevalence of compressive mononeuropathies and age of the patient or time since onset of injury following chronic paraplegia.[190]

Scrutiny of the aforementioned literature reviewed leads to the following conclusions: (1) A myth has been perpetuated from one review to another implicating repetivitive strain injury (RSI) as a cause for ulnar nerve entrapment in workers. (2) Reviews on RSI and ulnar nerve entrapment cite no credible medical literature to support this myth. (3) Case reports and cadaver studies provide tenuous support for ulnar nerve entrapment in high-force situations such as pitching and throwing in baseball. (4) The only prospective, high-quality study showed no causal relationship between RSI and ulnar nerve entrapment. In summary, no causal relationship between repetitive elbow motions and ulnar neuropathy at the elbow in industrial workers has been demonstrated in the medical literature.[191]

Shoulder Tendinitis, Impingement, and Rotator Cuff Tears

Impingement syndrome of the shoulder occurs when soft tissues, the subacromial bursa, rotator cuff (primarily supraspinatus), and, perhaps, the long head of the biceps tendons are pinched between structures above—the acromion, coracoacromial ligament, and/or distal clavicle—and the greater tuberosity below. This occurs during shoulder elevation (abduction and/or flexion) between 70° and 120°. This compression can cause subacromial bursitis and tendinitis of the supraspinatus or perhaps long head of biceps, plus abrasion and attenuation of the tendon, predisposing it to tears. Tendinitis may also be a precursor to or a cause and an effect of impingement because an inflamed, swollen, and, hence, enlarged tendon occupies more of the subacromial space. Impingement most often occurs in persons whose work or avocational pursuits involve repetitive abduction and/or flexion and is usually manifested by pain on and limitation of shoulder elevation.

The most common causes of impingement are downward projections of the acromion and/or distal clavicle. The former may consist of congenital or developmental variations in shape and slope, such as a curved or hooked acromion. An acromion and a distal clavicle may also become spurred with aging, generally due to degenerative arthritis of the acromioclavicular joint. If the osteophytes project inferiorly, they often impinge on and abrade the underlying bursa and tendon.

The prevalence and determinants of clinically diagnosed chronic rotator cuff tendinitis and self-reported nonspecific shoulder pain were studied in Finland during a 2000 health survey. A representative sample of 8028 persons aged 30 to 64 years who had held a job during the preceding 12 months demonstrated a 2.0% prevalence of chronic rotator cuff tendinitis (78/3909 subjects) vs 11.6% for nonspecific shoulder pain (410/3525 subjects).[192]

The lack of universally agreed-on inclusion criteria for study of the conditions labeled shoulder bursitis, tendinitis, and impingement has hampered population studies.[193] This is further confounded by the determination that pain was related to the tasks with the highest estimated daily loads, but a history of and current pain were associated with higher scores on the psychological scales, suggesting an interaction between physical and psychological factors. These findings support the hypotheses that excessive cumulative daily loads contribute to work-related shoulder conditions and that shoulder-arm pain seems related to psychological factors.[194]

Similar concerns about epidemiologic conclusions were acknowledged by Bernard et al because the majority of studies used observation or measurement of job characteristics to compare workers in jobs with higher levels of exposure with workers with lower levels of exposure for onset of symptoms.[109]

Occupational Risk Factors for Shoulder Tendinitis, Impingement, and Rotator Cuff Tears

The following are proposed occupational risk factors for shoulder tendinitis, impingement, and rotator cuff tears:

- Combination of risk factors (e.g., force and repetition, force and posture): some evidence
- Vibration: insufficient evidence
- Highly repetitive work alone or in combination with other factors: some evidence
- Forceful work: insufficient evidence
- Awkward postures: some evidence; sustained shoulder postures with more than 60° of flexion or abduction[109]
- Keyboard activities: insufficient evidence
- Cold environment: insufficient evidence
- Length of employment: insufficient evidence
- Dominant hand: insufficient evidence

Nonoccupational Risk Factors for Shoulder Tendinitis, Impingement, and Rotator Cuff Tears

The following are proposed nonoccupational risk factors for shoulder tendinitis, impingement, and rotator cuff tears:

- Age: strong evidence
- BMI: strong evidence; higher BMI increases risk
- Sex: insufficient evidence
- Biopsychosocial factors: strong evidence
- Diabetes: insufficient evidence

Table 9-18 shows the results of the literature searches for shoulder tendinitis, impingement, and rotator cuff tears, and Table 9-19 gives the representative references and comments.

TABLE 9-18	Results of Literature Search for Shoulder Tendinitis, Impingement, and Rotator Cuff Tears
Step	**Results**
Step 1: search all fields for the combination of	
Search 1: shoulder tendinitis & causation	19 articles, with 1 non-English and 12 after 1996.
Search 2: shoulder tendinitis & causation	26 articles, with 6 non-English and 20 after 1996; of these, 17 duplicates from first search.
Search 3: shoulder impingement & causation	30 articles, with 12 non-English and 15 after 1996; of these, 12 duplicates from first or second search; resulted in 18 articles for review with 2 prospective cohort, 3 cross-sectional, and 13 epidemiologic studies*
Steps 2, 3 and 4	were completed. Representative references are provided.

* Available studies were added to the 20 epidemiologic studies used in the July 1997 Musculoskeletal Disorders and Workplace Factors: A Critical Review of Epidemiologic Evidence for Work-related Musculoskeletal Disorders of the Neck, Upper Extremity, and Low Back.[109]

TABLE 9-19	Representative References for Shoulder Tendinitis, Impingement, and Rotator Cuff Tears

Risk Factor	Reference and Comments
Combination of risk factors (eg, force and repetition, force and posture)	Combination of factors when comparing workers in jobs with higher exposure to workers with lower exposure found increased risks for symptoms[109]; prospective cohort study, workplace factors (not well defined) increased risk[152]; cross-sectional study for shoulder loads and frequency of movement, shoulder tendinitis higher among exposed workers (adjusted OR, 3.1; 95% CI, 1.3-3)[195]; cross-sectional study to evaluate effect of individual characteristics and workplace factors (physical and psychosocial) on neck and shoulder pain with pressure tenderness in the muscles, association with high repetitiveness (prevalence ratio, 1.8; 95% CI, 1.1-2.9), high force (prevalence ratio, 2.0,; 95% CI, 1.2-3.3), and high repetitiveness and high force (prevalence ratio, 2.3; 95% CI, 1.4-4.0)[196]; 4-y prospective cohort study to quantify relative contribution of work-related physical, psychosocial workplace, and individual factors and aspects of somatization to the onset of neck or shoulder pain, 14.1% participants reported neck or shoulder pain of new onset; among these, 82 (1.7%) also had clinical signs of substantial muscle tenderness[197]
Vibration	Insufficient evidence for a positive association between vibration and shoulder tendinitis based on currently available epidemiologic studies[109]
Highly repetitive work alone or in combination with other factors	Cross-sectional study of historical cohort of 1591 workers, shoulder impingement syndrome ratio of 5.27 with a 95% CI among current workers; authors concluded "intensive work" is a contributor[198]; cross-sectional study to evaluate the effect of individual characteristics and workplace factors (physical and psychosocial) on neck or shoulder pain with pressure tenderness in the muscles, prevalence of neck or shoulder pain with pressure tenderness, 7.0% among participants performing repetitive work and 3.8% among referents[186]; 4-y prospective cohort study, high shoulder repetition related to being a future symptom case[197]

TABLE 9-19 Representative References for Shoulder Tendinitis, Impingement, and Rotator Cuff Tears (continued)

Risk Factor	Reference and Comments
Forceful work	Insufficient evidence[109]; epidemiologic study concluded physical work exposures, e.g., repetitive and forceful movements, important source of risk among manual workers[199]
Awkward postures	Sustained shoulder postures with >60° of flexion or abduction increased risks for symptoms[109]; case study of betel pepper cultivation (job activities that include prolonged static posture and repetitive motion), shoulder impingement significantly higher among cullers than among noncullers (0.45 vs 0.15,; $P = .011$)[117]
Keyboard activities	Epidemiologic study using questionnaires to study frequent computer users, self-reported pain with a prevalence of moderate-to-severe pain in the neck and right shoulder of 4.1% and 3.4%, respectively, and 1-y incidence rates for no or minor baseline symptoms of 1.5% and 1.9%, respectively; at baseline, prevalence rate ratio for neck pain, 1.7 (95% CI, 1.1-2.6) for mouse use >25 h/wk; for right shoulder pain, increased from 1.6 (95% CI, 1.1-2.4) for 15-19 h/wk to 2.5 (95% CI, 1.4-4.3) for >30 h/wk of mouse use; for tension neck syndrome, increased from 3.5 (95% CI, 1.0-12.0) for 25-29 h/wk to 4.7 (95% CI, 1.2-18.0) for >30 h/wk of mouse use; RR for new neck pain, 1.8 (95% CI, 0.8-3.9) for keyboard use ≥15 h/w and increased to 2.4 (95% CI, 0.8-6.8) for ≥30 h/w; new right shoulder pain associated with mouse use >20 h/wk (RR, 1.9; 95% CI, 1.0-3.5, and RR, 3.3; 95% CI, 1.2-8.9) and keyboard use >15 h/wk (RR, 2.2; 95% CI, 1.0-4.9)[200]
Cold environment	Insufficient evidence[109]
Length of employment	Insufficient evidence[109]
Dominant hand	Insufficient evidence[109]
Age	Prospective cohort study, age older than 40 y increased risk[152]

TABLE 9-19 Representative References for Shoulder Tendinitis, Impingement, and Rotator Cuff Tears (continued)

Risk Factor	Reference and Comments
BMI	Prospective cohort study, BMI >30 increased risk[152]; frequency-matched case-control study, 311 patients 53-77 years old underwent arthroscopy and rotator cuff and/or other repair of shoulder; showed association between increasing BMI and shoulder repair surgery; highest ORs for men (OR, 3.13; 95% CI, 1.29-7.61) and women (OR, 3.51; 95% CI, 1.80-6.85) were for people with BMI of ≥35.0 kg/m[201]
Sex	Cross-sectional study, increased risk for female sex (prevalence ratio, 1.8; CI, 1.2-2.8)[196]
Biopsychosocial factors	Strong evidence[109]; cross-sectional study, strongest work-related psychosocial risk was high job demands (prevalence ratio, 1.8; CI, 1.2-2.7)[196]; 4-y prospective cohort study, high job demands associated with future symptoms and high distress level predicted subsequent neck or shoulder pain[197]; consistent evidence that shoulder pain associated with biomechanical, physiologic, and psychosocial issues[109]; prospective cohort study, previous shoulder or neck discomfort increased risk[152]; specific examples of workplace psychosocial factors include monotonous work, time pressure, high workload, lack of peer support, and poor supervisor-employee relationship[202]; population study on shoulder tendinitis, symptoms related to burnout (adjusted OR, 1.7; 95% CI, 1.4-2.2); depression (among women, adjusted OR, 1.8 [95% CI, 1.1-2.9] for mild depression and 3.0 [95% CI, 1.6-5.6] for severe depression); and inability to express one's feelings (alexithymia), 0.0 (adjusted OR, 1.6; 95% CI, 1.1,-2.5)[192]
Diabetes	Population study on shoulder tendinitis, no relationship between rotator cuff tendinitis and work-related cumulative loading on the shoulder, age, and type 1 diabetes mellitus (adjusted OR, 8.8; 95% CI, 1.9-40.3)[192]

Confounders

A prospective cohort study found a history of CTS increased risk.[152] A cross-sectional study found previous neck or shoulder injury also increased risk (prevalence ratio, 2.6; CI, 1.6-4.1).[196] A cross-sectional study found increased risk for low-pressure pain threshold (prevalence ratio, 1.6; CI, 1.1-2.3).[196]

Reduced health-related quality of life is associated with subjective pain and clinical signs from the neck and shoulders.[196] An epidemiologic follow-up study showed that 50% of workers recovered within 10 months (95% CI, 6-14 months) of the onset of shoulder tendinitis in a cross-sectional sample of industrial and service workers. This estimate is most likely biased toward too high a value. Recovery was strongly reduced by older age.

Physical workplace exposures and perceived psychosocial job characteristics during the period preceding diagnosis seem to be unimportant prognostic factors.[203] A retrospective study analyzed 760 open rotator cuff repairs and related them to the profession and occupational load. Rotator cuff repairs were performed in 472 males who had no evidence of a traumatic origin. After statistical analysis ($P < .001$), significantly more patients were working in agriculture, forestry, and the building industry than in the general population. The authors concluded that the data suggest that working exposure increases the risk or leads to the clinical manifestation of rotator cuff tears. Although a detailed analysis of individual physical exposure is not available, the statistical results indicate that rotator cuff tears must be taken into consideration as a result of ergonomic exposure.[204]

A prospective cohort study followed up 501 active workers for an average of 5.4 years. Incident cases were defined as workers who were asymptomatic at baseline testing and had no history of shoulder tendinitis. The cumulative incidence in this cohort was 24.3%, or 4.5% annually. The factors with the highest predictive value for identifying a person likely to develop shoulder tendinitis in the near future included age older than 40 years, a BMI of more than 30, a complaint at baseline of shoulder or neck discomfort, a history of CTS, and a job with a higher shoulder posture rating. The risk profile identifies ergonomic and personal health factors as risks, and both categories of factors may be amenable to prevention strategies.[152]

A retrospective study found that power lifting showed twice the injury rate of bodybuilding for shoulder tendinitis.[205] A retrospective review of National Football League quarterbacks showed that the vast majority of shoulder injuries occurred as a result of direct trauma (82.3%) and fewer than 15% were overuse injuries resulting from the actual throwing motion.[206] The determinants of specific musculoskeletal disorders differ from those of subjective complaints without clinical findings. Such complaints may be indicators of adverse psychological and psychosocial factors rather than an underlying pathologic condition.[192]

References

1. Abe Y, Watson HK, Renaud S. Flexor tendon sheath ganglion: analysis of 128 cases. *Hand Surg.* 2004;9:1-4.

2. Jacobs LG, Govaers KJ. The volar wrist ganglion: just a simple cyst? *J Hand Surg [Br].* 1990;15:342-346.

3. Hindocha S, John S, Stanley JK, Watson SJ, Bayat A. The heritability of Dupuytren's disease: familial aggregation and its clinical significance. *J Hand Surg [Am].* 2006;31:204-210.

4. Logan AJ, Mason G, Dias J, Makwana N. Can rock climbing lead to Dupuytren's disease? *Br J Sports Med.* 2005;39:639-644.

5. Brenner P, Krause-Bergmann A, Van VH. Dupuytren contracture in North Germany; epidemiological study of 500 cases [in German]. *Unfallchirurg.* 2001;104:303-311.

6. Bennett B. Dupuytren's contracture in manual workers. *Br J Ind Med.* 1982;39: 98-100.

7. Liss GM, Stock SR. Can Dupuytren's contracture be work-related? review of the evidence. *Am J Ind Med.* 1996;29:521-532.

8. Thomas PR, Clarke D. Vibration white finger and Dupuytren's contracture: are they related? *Occup Med (Lond).* 1992;42:155-158.

9. Bovenzi M. Italian Study Group on Physical Hazards in the Stone Industry. Hand-arm vibration syndrome and dose-response relation for vibration induced white finger among quarry drillers and stonecarvers. *Occup Environ Med.* 1994; 51:603-611.

10. Cocco PL, Frau P, Rapallo M, Casula D. Occupational exposure to vibration and Dupuytren's disease: a case-controlled study [in Italian]. *Med Lav.* 1987;78:386-392.

11. Dasgupta AK, Harrison J. Effects of vibration on the hand-arm system of miners in India. *Occup Med (Lond).* 1996;46:71-78.

12. Stock SR. Workplace ergonomic factors and the development of musculoskeletal disorders of the neck and upper limbs: a meta-analysis. *Am J Ind Med.* 1991;19:87-107.

13. de la Caffinière JY, Wagner R, Etscheid J, Metzger F. Manual labor and Dupuytren disease: the results of a computerized survey in the field of iron metallurgy [in French]. *Ann Chir Main.* 1983;2:66-72.

14. Hindocha S, Stanley JK, Watson S, Bayat A. Dupuytren's diathesis revisited: evaluation of prognostic indicators for risk of disease recurrence. *J Hand Surg [Am].* 2006;31:1626-1634.

15. Arkkila PE, Kantola IM, Viikari JS, Ronnemaa T, Vahatalo MA. Dupuytren's disease in type 1 diabetic patients: a five-year prospective study. *Clin Exp Rheumatol.* 1996;14:59-65.

16. Carson J, Clarke C. Dupuytren's contracture in pensioners at the Royal Hospital Chelsea. *J R Coll Physicians Lond.* 1993;27:25-27.

17. Geoghegan JM, Forbes J, Clark DI, Smith C, Hubbard R. Dupuytren's disease risk factors. *J Hand Surg [Br].* 2004;29:423-426.

18. Saboeiro AP, Porkorny JJ, Shehadi SI, Virgo KS, Johnson FE. Racial distribution of Dupuytren's disease in Department of Veterans Affairs patients. *Plast Reconstr Surg.* 2000;106:71-75.

19. Zerajic D, Finsen V. Dupuytren's disease in Bosnia and Herzegovina: an epidemiological study. *BMC Musculoskelet Disord.* 2004;5:1-10. http://www.biomedcentral.com/1471-2474/5/10. Accessed July 15, 2007.

20. Lockshin MD. Endocrine origins of rheumatic disease: diagnostic clues to interrelated syndromes. *Postgrad Med.* 2002;111:87-88, 91-92.

21. Rayan GM, Moore J. Non–Dupuytren's disease of the palmar fascia. *J Hand Surg [Br].* 2005;30:551-556.

22. Elsner G, Nienhaus A, Beck W. Arthroses of the finger joints and thumb saddle joint and occupationally related factors [in German]. *Gesundheitswesen.* 1995;57:786-791.

23. Haara MM, Heliovaara M, Kroger H, et al. Osteoarthritis in the carpometacarpal joint of the thumb: prevalence and associations with disability and mortality. *J Bone Joint Surg Am* 2004; 86-A:1452-1457.

24. Valentino M, Rapisarda V. Rhizarthrosis of the thumb in ironing workers [in Italian]. *Med Lav.* 2002;93:80-86.

25. Wilder FV, Barrett JP, Farina EJ. Joint-specific prevalence of osteoarthritis of the hand. *Osteoarthritis Cartilage.* 2006;14:953-957.

26. Jonsson H, Manolescu I, Stefansson SE, et al. The inheritance of hand osteoarthritis in Iceland. *Arthritis Rheum.* 2003;48:391-395.

27. Yoshida S, Aoyagi K, Felson DT, et al. Comparison of the prevalence of radiographic osteoarthritis of the knee and hand between Japan and the United States. *J Rheumatol.* 2002;29:1454-1458.

28. Solovieva S, Vehmas T, Riihimaki H, Luoma K, Leino-Arjas P. Hand use and patterns of joint involvement in osteoarthritis; a comparison of female dentists and teachers. *Rheumatology (Oxford).* 2005;44:521-528.

29. Dahaghin S, Bierma-Zeinstra SM, Ginai AZ, et al. Prevalence and pattern of radiographic hand osteoarthritis and association with pain and disability (the Rotterdam study). *Ann Rheum Dis.* 2005;64:682-687.

30. Glass LS, ed. *Occupational Medicine Practice Guidelines.* 2nd ed. Beverly, MA: OEM Press; 2004:259.

31. Amano M, Umeda G, Nakajima H, Yatsuki K. Characteristics of work actions of shoe manufacturing assembly line workers and a cross-sectional factor-control study on occupational cervicobrachial disorders. *Sangyo Igaku.* 1988;30:3-12.

32. Tanaka S, Petersen M, Cameron L. Prevalence and risk factors of tendinitis and related disorders of the distal upper extremity among US workers: comparison to carpal tunnel syndrome. *Am J Ind Med.* 2001;39:328-335.

33. Armstrong TJ, Fine LJ, Goldstein SA, Lifshitz YR, Silverstein BA. Ergonomic considerations in hand and wrist tendinitis. *J Hand Surg [Am].* 1987;12A:830-837.

34. Gorsche R, Wiley JP, Renger R, et al. Prevalence and incidence of stenosing flexor tenosynovitis (trigger finger) in a meat-packing plant. *J Occup Environ Med.* 1998;40:556-560.

35. Luopajarvi T, Juorinka I, Virolainen M, Holmberg M. Prevalence of tenosynovitis and other injuries of the upper extremities in repetitive work. *Scand J Work Environ Health.* 1979;5:48-55.

36. Roto P, Kivi P. Prevalence of epicondylitis and tenosynovitis among meatcutters. *Scand J Work Environ Health.* 1984;10:203-205.

37. Saour S, Leong SC. Frozen-food-related hand injuries. *Ann Plast Surg.* 2006;57: 18-19.

38. Sungpet A, Suphachatwong C, Kawinwonggowit V. The association of age, sex and the number of sides of carpal tunnel syndrome. *J Med Assoc Thai.* 1999;82:220-223.

39. Neubauer E, Junge A, Pirron P, Seemann H, Schiltenwolf M. HKF-R 10: screening for predicting chronicity in acute low back pain (LBP): a prospective clinical trial. *Eur J Pain.* 2006;10:559-566.

40. Poirier JL, Hèrisson C, Guillot B, et al. Diabetic cheiroarthropathy [in French]. *Rev Rhum Mal Osteoartic.* 1989;56:511-517.

41. Benedetti A, Noacco C, Simonutti M, Taboga C. Diabetic trigger finger [letter]. *N Engl J Med.* 1982;306:1552.

42. Strom L. Trigger finger in diabetes. *J Med Soc N J.* 1977;74:951-954.

43. Kazuki K, Okada T, Naka Y. Case of trigger finger related to an intertendinous connection between the flexor tendons. *J Hand Surg [Br].* 2005;30:513-514.

44. Sherman PJ, Lane LB. The palmar aponeurosis pulley as a cause of trigger finger: a report of two cases. *J Bone Joint Surg Am.* 1996;78:1753-1754.

45. Matricali GA, Verstreken J. Anomalous origin of a lumbrical muscle as cause of a trigger finger. *Acta Orthop Belg.* 1993;59:315-316.

46. Bartell TH, Shehadi SI. Trigger finger secondary to anomalous lumbrical insertion: a case report and review of the literature. *Plast Reconstr Surg.* 1991;87:354-357.

47. Moon WN, Suh SW, Kim IC. Trigger digits in children. *J Hand Surg [Br].* 2001;26:11-12.

48. De Smet L, Steenwerckx A, Van Ransbeeck H. The so-called congenital trigger digit: further experience. *Acta Orthop Belg.* 1998;64:306-308.

49. Morales L, Pans S, Paridaens R, et al. Debilitating musculoskeletal pain and stiffness with letrozole and exemestane: associated tenosynovial changes on magnetic resonance imaging. *Breast Cancer Res Treat.* 2007;104:87-91.

50. Conner DE, Kolisek FR. Vibration-induced carpal tunnel syndrome. *Orthop Rev.* 1986;15:447-452.

51. Hayashi M, Uchiyama S, Toriumi H, et al. Carpal tunnel syndrome and development of trigger digit. *J Clin Neurosci.* 2005;12:39-41.

52. Harada K, Nakashima H, Teramoto K, et al. Trigger digits–associated carpal tunnel syndrome: relationship between carpal tunnel release and trigger digits. *Hand Surg.* 2005;10:205-208.

53. Fujiwara M. A case of trigger finger following partial laceration of flexor digitorum superficialis and review of the literature. *Arch Orthop Trauma Surg.* 2005;125:430-432.

54. Al Harthy A, Rayan GM. Phalangeal osteochondroma: a cause of childhood trigger finger. *Br J Plast Surg.* 2003;56:161-163.

55. Rankin EA, Reid B. An unusual etiology of trigger finger: a case report. *J Hand Surg [Am].* 1985;10:904-905.

56. Cakir M, Samanci N, Balci N, Balci MK. Musculoskeletal manifestations in patients with thyroid disease. *Clin Endocrinol (Oxf).* 2003;59:162-167.

57. Guyon MA, Honet JC. Carpal tunnel syndrome or trigger finger associated with neck injury in automobile accidents. *Arch Phys Med Rehabil.* 1977;58:325-327.

58. Ryzewicz M, Wolf JM. Trigger digits: principles, management, and complications. *J Hand Surg [Am].* 2006;31:135-146.

59. Rossi C, Cellocco P, Margaritondo E, Bizzarri F, Costanzo G. De Quervain disease in volleyball players. *Am J Sports Med.* 2005;33:424-427.

60. Reinstein L. de Quervain's stenosing tenosynovitis in a video games player. *Arch Phys Med Rehabil.* 1983;64:434-435.

61. Bystrom S, Hall C, Welander T, Kilbom A. Clinical disorders and pressure-pain threshold of the forearm and hand among automobile assembly line workers. *J Hand Surg [Br].* 1995;20B:782-790.

62. Kuorinka IA, Koskinen P. Occupational rheumatic diseases and upper limb strain in manual jobs in a light mechanical industry. *Scand J Work Environ Health.* 1979;5:39-47.

63. McCormack RR, Inman RD, Wells A, Berntsen C, Imbus HR. Prevalence of tendinitis and related disorders of the upper extremity in a manufacturing workforce. *J Rheumatol.* 1990;17:958-964.

64. Kurppa K, Viikari-Juntura E, Kuosma E, Huuskonen M, Kivi P. Incidence of tenosynovitis or peritendinitis and epicondylitis in a meat-processing factory. *Scand J Work Environ Health.* 1991;17:32-37.

65. Shiraishi N, Matsumura G. Anatomical variations of the extensor pollicis brevis tendon and abductor pollicis longus tendon: relation to tenosynovectomy. *Okajimas Folia Anat Jpn.* 2005;82:25-29.

66. Nishijo K, Kotani H, Miki T, Senzoku F, Ueo T. Unusual course of the extensor pollicis longus tendon associated with tenosynovitis, presenting as de Quervain disease: a case report. *Acta Orthop Scand.* 2000;71:426-428.

67. Jackson WT, Viegas SF, Coon TM, et al. Anatomical variations in the first extensor compartment of the wrist: a clinical and anatomical study. *J Bone Joint Surg Am.* 1986;68:923-926.

68. Leslie WD. The scintigraphic appearance of de Quervain tenosynovitis. *Clin Nucl Med.* 2006;31:602-604.

69. Chien AJ, Jacobson JA, Martel W, Kabeto MU, Marcantonio DR. Focal radial styloid abnormality as a manifestation of de Quervain tenosynovitis. *AJR Am J Roentgenol.* 2001;177:1383-1386.

70. Andersen JH, Gaardboe O. Prevalence of persistent neck and upper limb pain in a historical cohort of sewing machine operators. *Am J Ind Med.* 1993;24:677-687.

71. Baron S, Milliron M, Habes D, Fidler A. Hazard evaluation and technical assistance report: Shoprite Supermarkets, New Jersey-New York. Cincinnati, OH: US Dept of Health and Human Services, Public Health Services, Centers for Disease Control, National Institute for Occupational Safety and Health; 1991:1-16.

72. Burt S, Hornung R, Fine L. Hazard evaluation and technical assistance report: Newsday, Inc., Melville, NY. Cincinnati, OH: US Dept of Health and Human Services, Public Health Service, Centers for Disease Control, National Institute for Occupational Safety and Health; 1990:1-16.

73. Chiang HC, Chen S, Yu H, Ko Y. The occurrence of carpal tunnel syndrome in frozen food factory employees. *J Med Sci.* 1990;6:73-80.

74. Shiri R, Viikari-Juntura E, Varonen H, Heliovaara M. Prevalence and determinants of lateral and medial epicondylitis: a population study. *Am J Epidemiol.* 2006;164:1065-1074.

75. Haahr JP, Andersen JH. Prognostic factors in lateral epicondylitis: a randomized trial with one-year follow-up in 266 new cases treated with minimal occupational intervention or the usual approach in general practice. *Rheumatology (Oxford).* 2003;42:1216-1225.

76. Walker-Bone K, Cooper C. Hard work never hurt anyone: or did it? A review of occupational associations with soft tissue musculoskeletal disorders of the neck and upper limb. *Ann Rheum Dis.* 2005;64:1391-1396.

77. Gruchow HW, Pelletier D. An epidemiologic study of tennis elbow: incidence, recurrence, and effectiveness of prevention strategies. *Am J Sports Med.* 1979;7:234-238.

78. Engel J. Tennis: dynamics of racket-grip interaction. *J Hand Surg [Am].* 1995;20(3 pt 2):S77-S81.

79. Carroll R. Tennis elbow: incidence in local league players. *Br J Sports Med.* 1981;15:250-256.

80. Bovenzi M, Zadinin A, Franzinelli A, Borgogni F. Occupational musculoskeletal disorders in the neck and upper limbs of forestry workers exposed to hand-arm vibration. *Ergonomics.* 1991;34:547-562.

81. Chang MH, Wei SJ, Chiang HL, et al. The cause of slowed forearm median conduction velocity in carpal tunnel syndrome: a palmar stimulation study. *Clin Neurophysiol.* 2002;113:1072-1076.

82. Hennig EM, Rosenbaum D, Milani TL. Transfer of tennis racket vibrations onto the human forearm. *Med Sci Sports Exerc.* 1992;24:1134-1140.

83. Chiang HC, Ko Y, Chen S, et al. Prevalence of shoulder and upper-limb disorders among workers in the fish-processing industry. *Scand J Work Environ Health.* 1993;19:126-131.

84. Moore JS, Garg A. Upper extremity disorders in a pork processing plant: relationships between job risk factors and morbidity. *Am Ind Hyg Assoc J.* 1994;55:703-715.

85. O'Sullivan LW, Gallwey TJ. Upper-limb surface electro-myography at maximum supination and pronation torques: the effect of elbow and forearm angle. *J Electromyogr Kinesiol.* 2002;12:275-285.

86. Landis J, Keselman I, Murphy CN. Comparison of electromyographic (EMG) activity of selected forearm muscles during low grade resistance therapeutic exercises in individuals diagnosed with lateral epicondylitis. *Work.* 2005;24:85-91.

87. Hughes RE, Silverstein BA, Evanoff BA. Risk factors for work-related musculoskeletal disorders in an aluminum smelter. *Am J Ind Med.* 1997;32:66-75.

88. Waugh EJ, Jaglal SB, Davis AM, Tomlinson G, Verrier MC. Factors associated with prognosis of lateral epicondylitis after 8 weeks of physical therapy. *Arch Phys Med Rehabil.* 2004;85:308-318.

89. Ritz BR. Humeral epicondylitis among gas and waterworks employees. *Scand J Work Environ Health.* 1995;21:478-486.

90. Dimberg L. The prevalence and causation of tennis elbow (lateral humeral epicondylitis) in a population of workers in an engineering industry. *Ergonomics.* 1987;30:573-579.

91. Hakim AJ, Cherkas LF, Spector TD, MacGregor AJ. Genetic associations between frozen shoulder and tennis elbow: a female twin study. *Rheumatology (Oxford).* 2003;42:739-742.

92. Ruch DS, Papadonikolakis A, Campolattaro RM. The posterolateral plica: a cause of refractory lateral elbow pain. *J Shoulder Elbow Surg.* 2006;15:367-370.

93. Murray-Leslie C, Wright V. Carpal tunnel syndrome and tennis elbow [letter]. *Br Med J.* 1976;2:526.

94. Murray-Leslie CF, Wright V. Carpal tunnel syndrome, humeral epicondylitis, and the cervical spine: a study of clinical and dimensional relations. *Br Med J.* 1976;1:1439-1442.

95. Kristenson H, Johnell O. Minor orthopaedic disease: registration for alcoholism and serum gamma-glutamyltransferase in men. *Drug Alcohol Depend.* 1985;15:405-408.

96. Vicenzino B, Paungmali A, Buratowski S, Wright A. Specific manipulative therapy treatment for chronic lateral epicondylalgia produces uniquely characteristic hypoalgesia. *Man Ther.* 2001;6:205-212.

97. Zeisig E, Ohberg L, Alfredson H. Extensor origin vascularity related to pain in patients with Tennis elbow. *Knee Surg Sports Traumatol Arthrosc.* 2006;14: 659-663.

98. Kay NR. Litigants' epicondylitis. *J Hand Surg [Br].* 2003;28:460-464.

99. World Health Organization. Identification and control of work-related diseases. Geneva, Switzerland: World Health Organization; 1985:1-85. Technical report series No. 714.

100. Louis DS, Calkins ER, Harris PG. Carpal tunnel syndrome in the work place. *Hand Clin.* 1996;12:305-312.

101. Katz JN, Larson MG, Fossel AH, Liang MH. Validation of a surveillance case definition of carpal tunnel syndrome. *Am J Public Health.* 1991;81:189-193.

102. Szabo RM, Madison M. Carpal tunnel syndrome as a work-related disorder. In: American Academy of Orthopaedic Surgeons. *Repetitive Motion Disorders of the Upper Extremity.* Rosemont, IL: American Academy of Orthopaedic Surgeons; 1995:421-434.

103. Melhorn JM. Occupational orthopaedics: the future: a how to manual. In: Melhorn JM, Zeppieri JP, eds. *Workers' Compensation Case Management: A Multidisciplinary Perspective.* Rosemont, IL: American Academy of Orthopaedic Surgeons; 1999:407-448.

104. Melhorn JM, Talmage JB, Fries BE, Zeppieri JP. Impairment evaluations for the upper extremities using the AMA Guides. In: Melhorn JM, Strain RE Jr, eds. *Occupational Orthopaedics and Workers' Compensation: A Multidisciplinary Perspective.* Rosemont, IL: American Academy of Orthopaedic Surgeons; 2002:351-442.

105. Melhorn JM. Occupational orthopaedics: chronic musculoskeletal pain. In: Melhorn JM, DiPaola J, eds. *8th Annual Occupational Orthopaedics and Workers' Compensation: A Multidisciplinary Perspective.* Rosemont, IL: American Academy of Orthopaedic Surgeons; 2006. Ch. 1, 49-102.

106. Melhorn JM, Freeman GC. When the forms don't work. In: Melhorn JM, DiPaola J, eds. *8th Annual Occupational Orthopaedics and Workers' Compensation: A Multidisciplinary Perspective.* Rosemont, IL: American Academy of Orthopaedic Surgeons; 2006. Ch. 26: 701-711.

107. Aronoff GM, Rallagher RM, Feldman JB. Biopsychosocial evaluation and treatment of chronic pain. In: Raj PP, ed. *Practical Management of Pain.* St Louis, MO: Mosby; 2001:156-165.

108. Gatchel RJ. Psychosocial factors that can influence the self-assessment of function. In: *Workers' Compensation Symposium 2002.* San Francisco, CA: California Workers' Compensation Commission; 2002:51-55.
109. US Department of Health and Human Services. Musculoskeletal Disorders and Workplace Factors: A Critical Review of Epidemiologic Evidence for Work-Related Musculoskeletal Disorders of the Neck, Upper Extremity, and Low Back. Cincinnati, OH: National Institute for Occupational Safety and Health; 1997.
110. Jianmongkol S, Kosuwon W, Thumroj E, Sumanont S. Prevalence of carpal tunnel syndrome in workers from a fishnet factory in Thailand. *Hand Surg.* 2005;10:67-70.
111. Palmer KT, Calnan M, Wainwright D, et al. Upper limb pain in primary care: health beliefs, somatic distress, consulting and patient satisfaction. *Fam Pract.* 2006;23:609-617.
112. Bahou YG. Carpal tunnel syndrome: a series observed at Jordan University Hospital (JUH), June 1999-December 2000. *Clin Neurol Neurosurg.* 2002;104:49-53.
113. Osorio AM, Ames RG, Jones JA, et al. Carpal tunnel syndrome among grocery store workers. *Am J Ind Med.* 1994;25:229-245.
114. Silverstein B, Fine L, Stetson D. Hand-wrist disorders among investment casting plant workers. *J Hand Surg [Am].* 1987;12:838-844.
115. Barnhart S, Demers PA, Miller M. Carpal tunnel syndrome among ski manufacturing workers. *Scand J Work Environ Health.* 1991;17:46-52.
116. Silverstein B, Welp E, Nelson N, Kalat J. Claims incidence of work-related disorders of the upper extremities: Washington state, 1987 through 1995. *Am J Public Health.* 1998;88:1827-1833.
117. Wang LY, Pong YP, Wang HC, et al. Cumulative trauma disorders in betel pepper leaf-cullers visiting a rehabilitation clinic: experience in Taitung. *Chang Gung Med J.* 2005;28:237-246.
118. Frost P, Andersen JH, Nielsen VK. Occurrence of carpal tunnel syndrome among slaughterhouse workers. *Scand J Work Environ Health.* 1998;24:285-292.
119. Chiang HC, Chen SS, Yu HS, Ko YC. The occurrence of carpal tunnel syndrome in frozen food factory employees. *Gaoxiong Yi Xue Ke Xue Za Zhi.* 1990;6:73-80.
120. Loslever P, Ranaivosoa A. Biomechanical and epidemiological investigation of carpal tunnel syndrome at workplaces with high risk factors. *Ergonomics.* 1993;36:537-554.
121. Roquelaure Y, Mechali S, Dano C, et al. Occupational and personal risk factors for carpal tunnel syndrome in industrial workers. *Scand J Work Environ Health.* 1997;23:364-369.
122. Tanaka S, Wild DK, Cameron LL, Freund E. Association of occupational and non-occupational risk factors with the prevalence of self-reported carpal tunnel syndrome in a national survey of the working population. *Am J Ind Med.* 1997;32:550-556.
123. Nathan PA, Meadows KD, Istvan JA. Predictors of carpal tunnel syndrome: an 11-year study of industrial workers. *J Hand Surg [Am].* 2002;27A:644-651.
124. Chatterjee DS. Workplace upper limb disorders: a prospective study with intervention. *J Occup Environ Med.* 1992;42:129-136.
125. Chatterjee DS. Exploratory electromyography in the study of vibration-induced white finger in rock drillers. *Br J Ind Med.* 1982;39:89-97.

126. Nathan PA, Meadows KD, Doyle LS. Occupation as a risk factor for impaired sensory conductions of the median nerve at the carpal tunnel. *J Hand Surg [Br]*. 1988;13B:167-170.

127. Nathan PA, Keniston RC, Myers LD. Longitudinal study of median nerve sensory conduction in industry: relationship to age, gender, hand dominance, occupational hand use, and clinical diagnosis. *J Hand Surg [Am]*. 1992;17A:850-851.

128. Ferrero MG, Pescarmona G. The carpal tunnel syndrome: etiologic and prognostic role of biological and professional risk factors. *Minerva Ortop Traumatol*. 2001; 52:4-5. In: Diagnosis, Causation and Treatment of Carpal Tunnel Syndrome: An Evidence-Based Assessment. Fertl, E., C. Wober, et al. A Background Paper Prepared for Alberta's Workers' Compensation Board. May 2004: 43. www.wcb. ab.ca/pdfs/CTS_Bkg_Paper.pdf. Accessed July 15, 2007.

129. Babski-Reeves K, Crumpton-Young L. Comparisons of measures for quantifying repetition in predicting carpal tunnel syndrome. *Int J Ind Ergon*. 2002;30:1-6

130. DeKrom M, Kester ADM, Knipschild PG, Spaans F. Risk factors for carpal tunnel syndrome. *Am J Epidemiol*. 1990;132:1102-1110.

131. Cosgrove JL, Chase PM, Mast NJ, Reeves R. Carpal tunnel syndrome in railroad workers. *Am J Phys Med Rehabil*. 2002;81:101-107.

132. Nathan PA, Keniston RC, Myers LD, Meadows KD. Obesity as a risk factor for slowing of sensory conduction of the median nerve in industry; a cross-sectional and longitudinal study involving 429 workers. *J Occup Med*. 1992;34:379-383.

133. Rules and regulations. *Fed Regist*. 2006;65:68511-68560. Small Business Administration: Office of Advocacy—Ergonomics and Small Business: Rules and regulations.

134. Bleecker ML. Medical surveillance for carpal tunnel syndrome in workers. *J Hand Surg [Am]*. 1987;12A:845-848.

135. Winn FJ Jr, Habes DJ. Carpal tunnel area as a risk factor for carpal tunnel syndrome. *Muscle Nerve*. 1990;13:254-258.

136. Tan M, Tan U. Correlation of carpal tunnel size and conduction velocity of the sensory median and ulnar nerves of male and female controls and carpet weavers. *Percept Mot Skills*. 1998;87:1195-1201.

137. Boz C, Ozmenoglu M, Altunayoglu V, Velioglu S, Alioglu Z. Individual risk factors for carpal tunnel syndrome: an evaluation of body mass index, wrist index and hand anthropometric measurements. *Clin Neurol Neurosurg*. 2004;106:294-299.

138. Moghtaderi A, Izadi S, Sharafadinzadeh N. An evaluation of gender, body mass index, wrist circumference and wrist ratio as independent risk factors for carpal tunnel syndrome. *Acta Neurol Scand*. 2005;112:375-379.

139. Stallings SP, Kasdan ML, Soergel TM, Corwin HM. A case-control study of obesity as a risk factor for carpal tunnel syndrome in a population of 600 patients presenting for independent medical examination. *J Hand Surg [Am]*. 1997;22A:211-215.

140. Werner RA, Franzblau A, Gell N, et al. Incidence of carpal tunnel syndrome among automobile assembly workers and assessment of risk factors. *J Occup Environ Med*. 2005;47:1044-1050.

141. Delaney K. Two fellows violate expert witness SOPs. *AAOS Now*. 2007;1:1-3.

142. Liu CW, Chen TW, Wang MC, et al. Relationship between carpal tunnel syndrome and wrist angle in computer workers. *Kaohsiung J Med Sci*. 2003;19:617-623.

143. Andersen JH, Thomsen JF, Overgaard E, et al. Computer use and carpal tunnel syndrome: a 1-year follow-up study. *JAMA.* 2003;289:2963-2969.

144. Clarke Stevens J, Witt JC, Smith BE, Weaver AL. The frequency of carpal tunnel syndrome in computer users at a medical facility. *Neurology.* 2001;56:1568-1570.

145. Nordstrom DL, Vierkant RA, DeStefano F, Layde PM. Risk factors for carpal tunnel syndrome in a general population. *Occup Environ Med.* 1997;54:734-740.

146. Nathan PA, Keinston RC, Meadows KD. Keyboarding as a risk factor for carpal tunnel syndrome: comparing clerical workers to managers in eight industries. In: American Society for Surgery of the Hand Annual Meeting. Englewood, CO, American Society for Surgery of the Hand; 1993:78-79.

147. Hadler NM. A keyboard for "Daubert." *J Occup Environ Med.* 1996;38:469-476.

148. Garland FC, Garland CF, Doyle EJ, et al. Carpal tunnel syndrome and occupation in US Navy enlisted personnel. *Arch Environ Health.* 1996;51:395-407.

149. Rempel D, Tittiranonda P, Burastero S, Hudes M, So Y. Effect of keyboard keyswitch design on hand pain. *J Occup Environ Med.* 1999;41:111-119.

150. Falck B, Aarnio P. Left-sided carpal tunnel syndrome in butchers. *Scand J Work Environ Health.* 1983;9:291-297.

151. Nathan PA, Keniston RC, Myers LD, Meadows KD. Obesity as a risk factor for slowing of sensory conduction of the median nerve in industry: a cross-sectional and longitudinal study involving 429 workers. *J Occup Environ Med.* 1992;34:379-383.

152. Werner RA, Franzblau A, Gell N, Ulin SS, Armstrong TJ. A longitudinal study of industrial and clerical workers: predictors of upper extremity tendonitis. *J Occup Rehabil.* 2005;15:37-46.

153. Winn FJ Jr, Putz-Anderson V. Vibration thresholds as a function of age and diagnosis of carpal tunnel syndrome: a preliminary report. *Exp Aging Res.* 1990;16:221-224.

154. Bland JD. The relationship of obesity, age, and carpal tunnel syndrome: more complex than was thought? *Muscle Nerve.* 2005;32:527-532.

155. Becker J, Nora DB, Gomes I, et al. An evaluation of gender, obesity, age and diabetes mellitus as risk factors for carpal tunnel syndrome. *Clin Neurophysiol.* 2002;113:1429-1434.

156. Nathan PA, Meadows KD, Doyle LS. Relationship of age and sex to sensory conduction of the median nerve at the carpal tunnel and associations of slowed conduction with symptoms. *Muscle Nerve.* 1988;11:1149-1153.

157. Nathan PA, Keniston RC. Carpal tunnel syndrome and its relation to general physical condition. *Hand Clin.* 1993;9:253-261.

158. Radecki P. Carpal tunnel syndrome: effects of personal factors and associated medical conditions. *Phys Med Rehabil Clin N Am.* 1997;8:419-437.

159. Bland JD, Rudolfer SM. Clinical surveillance of carpal tunnel syndrome in two areas of the United Kingdom, 1991-2001. *J Neurol Neurosurg Psychiatry.* 2003;74:1674-1679.

160. Schottland JR, Kirschberg GJ, Fillingim R. Median nerve latencies in poultry processing workers: an approach to resolving the role of industrial "cumulative trauma" in the development of carpal tunnel syndrome. *J Occup Environ Med.* 1991;33:627-630.

161. Roquelaure Y, Mariel J, Dano C, Fanello S, Penneau-Fontbonne D. Prevalence, incidence and risk factors of carpal tunnel syndrome in a large footwear factory. *Int J Occup Med Environ Health.* 2001;14:357-367.

162. Bernard BP. Carpal tunnel syndrome: evidence for work-relatedness. In: Bernard BP, ed. *Musculoskeletal Disorders and Workplace Factors.* Cincinnati, OH: National Institute for Occupational Safety and Health; 1997:1-67.

163. Nathan PA, Istvan JA, Meadows KD. A longitudinal study of predictors of research-defined carpal tunnel syndrome in industrial workers: findings at 17 years. *J Hand Surg [Br].* 2005;30:593-598.

164. Werner RA, Albers JW, Franzblau A, Armstrong TJ. The relationship between body mass index and the diagnosis of carpal tunnel syndrome. *Muscle Nerve.* 1994;17:632-636.

165. Nathan PA, Takigawa K, Keniston RC, Meadows KD, Lockwood RS. Slowing of sensory conduction of the median nerve and carpal tunnel syndrome in Japanese and American industrial workers. *J Hand Surg [Br].* 1994;19B:30-34.

166. Kouyoumdjian JA, Morita MP, Rocha PR, Miranda RC, Gouveia GM. Wrist and palm indexes in carpal tunnel syndrome. *Arq Neuropsiquiatr.* 2000;58:625-629.

167. Ferry S, Hannaford P, Warskyj M, Lewis M, Croft P. Carpal tunnel syndrome: a nested case-control study of risk factors in women. *Am J Epidemiol.* 2000;151:566-574.

168. Gell N, Werner RA, Franzblau A, Ulin SS, Armstrong TJ. A longitudinal study of industrial and clerical workers: incidence of carpal tunnel syndrome and assessment of risk factors. *J Occup Rehabil.* 2005;15:47-55.

169. Leclerc A, Franchi P, Cristofari MF, et al. Carpal tunnel syndrome and work organisation in repetitive work: a cross sectional study in France. Study Group on Repetitive Work. *Occup Environ Med.* 1998;55:180-187.

170. Leclerc A, Landre MF, Chastang JF, Niedhammer I, Roquelaure Y. Upper-limb disorders in repetitive work. *Scand J Work Environ Health.* 2001;27:268-278.

171. Guyatt G, Rennie D. *User's Guides to the Medical Literature: A Manual for Evidence-Based Clinical Practice.* Chicago, IL: AMA Press; 2002:1-736.

172. Stevens JC, Beard CM, O'Fallon WM. Conditions associated with carpal tunnel syndrome. *Mayo Clin Proc.* 1992;67:541-543.

173. Singh R, Gamble G, Cundy T. Lifetime risk of symptomatic carpal tunnel syndrome in type 1 diabetes. *Diabet Med.* 2005;22:625-630.

174. Braddom RL. Familial carpal tunnel syndrome in three generations of a black family. *Am J Phys Med.* 1985;64:227-234.

175. Pascual E, Giner V, Arostegui A, et al. Higher incidence of carpal tunnel syndrome in oophorectomized women. *Br J Rheumatol.* 1991;30:60-62.

176. Kutluhan S, Akhan G, Demirci S, et al. Carpal tunnel syndrome in carpet workers. *Int Arch Occup Environ Health.* 2001;74:454-457.

177. Nathan PA, Keniston RC, Lockwood RS, Meadows KD. Tobacco, caffeine, alcohol, and carpal tunnel syndrome in American industry: a cross-sectional study of 1464 workers. *J Occup Environ Med.* 1996;38:290-298.

178. Yagev Y, Carel RS, Yagev R. Assessment of work-related risks factors for carpal tunnel syndrome. *Isr Med Assoc J.* 2001;3:569-571.

179. Ring D. Carpal tunnel syndrome causation. In: 74th Annual Meeting of the American Academy of Orthopaedic Surgeons at San Diego, CA; February 16, 2007. Rosemont, IL: American Academy of Orthopaedic Surgeons; 2007:1-2.

180. Keir PJ, Bach JM, Hudes M, Rempel DM. Guidelines for wrist posture based on carpal tunnel pressure thresholds. *Hum Factors.* 2007;49:88-99.

181. Sesek RF, Khalighi M, Bloswick DS, Anderson M, Tuckett RP. Effects of prolonged wrist flexion on transmission of sensory information in carpal tunnel syndrome. *J Pain.* 2007;8:137-151.

182. Mogk JP, Keir PJ. Evaluation of the carpal tunnel based on 3-D reconstruction from MRI. *J Biomech.* 2006. http://www.ncbi.nlm.nih.gov/sites/entrez?db= pubmed&list_uids=17166503&cmd=Retrieve&indexed=google. Accessed July 14, 2007.

183. Carp SJ, Barbe MF, Winter KA, Amin M, Barr AE. Inflammatory biomarkers increase with severity of upper-extremity overuse disorders. *Clin Sci (Lond).* 2007;112:305-314.

184. Mondelli M, Giannini F, Ballerini M, Ginanneschi F, Martorelli E. Incidence of ulnar neuropathy at the elbow in the province of Siena (Italy). *J Neurol Sci.* 2005;234:5-10.

185. Saito K, Kumashiro M, Niioka T, Fujimoto S, Shibano N. The recent status of vibration hazards among workers at the state forests in Hokkaido [in Japanese; authors' transl]. Abstract. *Sangyo Igaku.* 1980;22:348-354.

186. Descatha A, Leclerc A, Chastang JF, Roquelaure Y. Incidence of ulnar nerve entrapment at the elbow in repetitive work. *Scand J Work Environ Health.* 2004;30:234-240.

187. Richardson JK, Green DF, Jamieson SC, Valentin FC. Gender, body mass and age as risk factors for ulnar mononeuropathy at the elbow. *Muscle Nerve.* 2001;24:551-554.

188. Pellieux S, Fouquet B, Lasfargues G. Ulnar nerve tunnel syndrome of the elbow and an occupational disorder: analysis of socio-professional and physical parameters [in French]. *Ann Readapt Med Phys.* 2001;44:213-220.

189. Richardson JK, Jamieson SC. Cigarette smoking and ulnar mononeuropathy at the elbow. *Am J Phys Med Rehabil.* 2004;83:730-734.

190. Davidoff G, Werner R, Waring W. Compressive mononeuropathies of the upper extremity in chronic paraplegia. *Paraplegia.* 1991;29:17-24.

191. Katz RT. Ulnar neuropathy at the elbow due to repetition: myth or reality? *Guides Newsletter.* September October 2006:1-12.

192. Miranda H, Viikari-Juntura E, Heistaro S, Heliovaara M, Riihimaki H. A population study on differences in the determinants of a specific shoulder disorder versus nonspecific shoulder pain without clinical findings. *Am J Epidemiol.* 2005;161:847-855.

193. Helliwell PS, Bennett RM, Littlejohn G, Muirden KD, Wigley RD. Towards epidemiological criteria for soft-tissue disorders of the arm. *Occup Med (Lond).* 2003;53:313-319.

194. Helliwell PS, Mumford DB, Smeathers JE, Wright V. Work related upper limb disorder: the relationship between pain, cumulative load, disability, and psychological factors. *Ann Rheum Dis.* 1992;51:1325-1329.

195. Frost P, Bonde JP, Mikkelsen S, et al. Risk of shoulder tendinitis in relation to shoulder loads in monotonous repetitive work. *Am J Ind Med.* 2002;41:11-18.

196. Andersen JH, Kaergaard A, Frost P, et al. Physical, psychosocial, and individual risk factors for neck/shoulder pain with pressure tenderness in the muscles among workers performing monotonous, repetitive work. *Spine.* 2002;27:660-667.

197. Andersen JH, Kaergaard A, Mikkelsen S, et al. Risk factors in the onset of neck/shoulder pain in a prospective study of workers in industrial and service companies. *Occup Environ Med.* 2003;60:649-654.

198. Frost P, Andersen JH. Shoulder impingement syndrome in relation to shoulder intensive work. *Occup Environ Med.* 1999;56:494-498.

199. Melchior M, Roquelaure Y, Evanoff B, et al. Why are manual workers at high risk of upper limb disorders? The role of physical work factors in a random sample of workers in France (the Pays de la Loire study). *Occup Environ Med.* 2006;63:754-761.

200. Brandt LP, Andersen JH, Lassen CF, et al. Neck and shoulder symptoms and disorders among Danish computer workers. *Scand J Work Environ Health.* 2004;30:399-409.

201. Wendelboe AM, Hegmann KT, Gren LH, et al. Associations between body-mass index and surgery for rotator cuff tendinitis. *J Bone Joint Surg Am.* 2004;86-A:743-747.

202. Hales TR, Bernard BP. Epidemiology of work-related musculoskeletal disorders. *Orthop Clin North Am.* 1996;27:679-709.

203. Bonde JP, Mikkelsen S, Andersen JH, et al. Prognosis of shoulder tendonitis in repetitive work: a follow up study in a cohort of Danish industrial and service workers. *Occup Environ Med.* 2003;60:E8-E10.

204. Rolf O, Ochs K, Bohm TD, et al. Rotator cuff tear: an occupational disease? An epidemiological analysis [in German]. *Z Orthop Ihre Grenzgeb.* 2006;144:519-523.

205. Goertzen M, Schoppe K, Lange G, Schulitz KP. Injuries and damage caused by excess stress in body building and power lifting [in German]. *Sportverletz Sportschaden.* 1989;3:32-36.

206. Kelly BT, Barnes RP, Powell JW, Warren RF. Shoulder injuries to quarterbacks in the National Football League. *Am J Sports Med.* 2004;32:328-331.

CHAPTER 10

Lower Limb

Kenneth P. Subin, MD, MPH, and Christopher R. Brigham, MD

There are a variety of conditions affecting the lower limb that can become disabling in the workplace environment, such as osteoarthritis of the knee and hip, meniscal disorders, and plantar fasciitis. This chapter focuses on the risk factors of these disorders and evidence for industrial causation.

Osteoarthritis

Burden

The term *arthritis* refers to joint inflammation and is used to describe more than 100 rheumatic conditions such as osteoarthritis, rheumatoid arthritis, and gout.[1] The most commonly diagnosed form of arthritis is osteoarthritis, which is estimated to affect more than 20 million adults in the United States.[1] Worldwide, the knee is the joint most commonly affected by osteoarthritis.[2] Arthritis is the most prevalent chronic condition in the United States, the most commonly reported cause of disability, and the third leading cause of self-reported work limitation (8.2 million adults aged 18-64 years).[3] The total indirect costs, or lost earnings, attributable to arthritis and other rheumatic conditions were estimated in 2003 to be $47.0 billion.[1]

Definition

Osteoarthritis is defined by the Subcommittee on Osteoarthritis of the American College of Rheumatology Diagnostic and Therapeutic Criteria Committee as "A heterogeneous group of conditions that lead to joint symptoms and signs which are associated with defective integrity of articular cartilage, in addition to related changes in the underlying bone at the joint margins."[2] The condition is associated with joint pain, swelling, and motion loss and is characterized by "focal areas of loss of articular cartilage within synovial joints, associated with hypertrophy of bone (osteophytes and subchondral bone sclerosis) and thickening of the capsule."[2] There are many classification schemes of osteoarthritis, but the most commonly applied method is based on the radiographic appearance of the joint proposed by Kellgren and Lawrence.[2] This method grades the severity of arthritis of a joint on a 0 – 4 scale based on the presence of radiographic hallmarks of osteoarthritis including joint space narrowing, sclerosis, and cyst formation. The score is determined by comparing the subject to a standard atlas of radiographs where a score of 0 indicates the absence of arthritis, 1 is doubtful narrowing of joint space, 2 is minimal evidence of arthritis with possible joint space narrowing, 3 is moderate arthritis with definite joint space narrowing and some sclerosis, and 4 is severe arthritis. Other classifications require clinical criteria such as pain in the involved joint.[2]

Most studies of the causative relationship between arthritis of the knee and work-related activities have focused on arthritis affecting the tibiofemoral joint. Some studies defined the outcome variable as radiographic evidence of arthritis, whereas others assessed for symptomatic arthritis. Many studies have defined workplace exposure by job title, whereas others have attempted to define the specific activities involved in the job activities, such as frequency of knee bending, climbing, heavy lifting, and walking. The difficulty in identifying the activities associated with the development of arthritis of the knee is controlling for known confounders such as age, previous trauma, genetics, and job duration while also considering the "healthy worker effect" where there is a tendency towards reduced morbidity and mortality in occupational cohorts when compared to the general population. that can distort these associations.

Tibiofemoral Joint

Conclusions on Nonoccupational Risk Factors

The proposed nonoccupational risk factors are as follows:

- **Age:** Accepted risk factor, very strong evidence; risk increases with age[4,5]
- **Overweight or obese:** Accepted risk factor, very strong evidence[6-9]; odds ratio (OR), 1.10 (95% confidence interval [CI], 1.05-1.16) for body mass index (BMI) as continuous variable among men and women requiring total knee arthroplasty (TKA); evidence for dose-response relationship among women[4]; OR, 3.0 (95% CI, 1.9-4.5)[10]; evidence for dose-response relationship for both sexes[11-13]
- **Previous trauma:** Accepted risk factor, strong evidence[6,7]; OR, 3.44 (95% CI, 1.74-6.8) among men requiring TKA; OR, 1.51 (95% CI 1.05-2.17) among men and women requiring TKA[14]; for Japanese women, OR, 5.0 (95% CI, 2.44-10.23) with history of knee injury[9]; OR, 4.5 (95% CI, 3.0-6.8) for both sexes[11]; for Chinese men, OR, 12.1 (95% CI, 3.4-42.5) and women, OR, 7.6 (95% CI, 3.8-15.2)[15]; OR, 8.0 (95% CI, 2.0-32.0), P = .003[5,16]
- **Previous meniscectomy or meniscus injury:** Accepted risk factor, strong evidence[6,7]; OR, 9.7 (95% CI, 3.5-26.7)[10]; degenerative meniscal tears, OR, 1.9 (95% CI, 1.1-3.5)[12]; total meniscectomy, OR, 3.6 (95% CI, 1.4-9.4)[12]
- **Family history:** Accepted risk factor, further analysis required[7,17,18].
- **Female:** Accepted risk factor, further analysis required[4,7,19,20]; OR, 2.4 (95% CI, 1.2-4.6)[12]
- **Physical exercise:** Insufficient evidence for protective effect, further analysis required; OR, 0.59 (95% CI, 0.38-0.91) for low levels of exercise and OR, 0.41 (95% CI, 0.2-0.81) for higher levels of exercise[14,16]
- **Cigarette smoking:** Insufficient evidence for protective effect, further analysis required[4,15]

Conclusions on Occupational Risk Factors

The evidence for occupational risk factors is as follows:

- **Jumping:** Insufficient evidence[21]
- **Kneeling:** Some evidence[5,6,11,14,22]
- **Lifting:** Insufficient evidence[6,11,15,21,23]
- **Sitting:** Insufficient evidence as protective effect[6,9,11,21]
- **Squatting and knee bending:** Some evidence[4,6,11,14,21]
- **Standing and walking:** Insufficient evidence[6,11,21]
- **Combination risk factors:** Some evidence: Kneeling and squatting with heavy lifting[11]; squatting, kneeling, climbing[6]; knee bending and heavy physical demand[10,20]

Literature Searches and Representative References for Osteoarthritis of the Knee

Table 10-1 shows the results for the literature searches for osteoarthritis of the knee, and Table 10-2 shows representative references and comments.

TABLE 10-1 Literature Searches for Osteoarthritis of the Knee*

Search No. / Search Terms	Result
1/osteoarthritis & knee & occupational diseases	0 results
2/osteoarthritis & knee & accidents, occupational	0 results
3/osteoarthritis & knee & etiology	133 results; 0 applicable by abstract review
4/knee osteoarthritis & occupational	50 results; 15 chosen by abstract review
5/knee osteoarthritis & causation	234 results; 13 chosen by abstract review
6/knee osteoarthritis & Work	86 results; 9 chosen by abstract review

* Search limits were English language and human in all searches.

TABLE 10-2	Representative References and Comments for Osteoarthritis of the Knee

Risk Factor	References and Comments
Climbing	Among men, OR, 3.06 (95% CI, 1.25-7.46) for development of severe osteoarthritis (OA) requiring TKA when exposed to medium level of climbing but no dose-response relationship[14]; OR, 1.73 (95% CI, 1.13-2.66) for development of severe OA requiring TKA when exposed ≥2 h/d; among men, climbing more than 30 times per day for more than 1 y associated with OR of 2.3 (95% CI, 1.3-4.0) for development of knee OA[11]; Chinese women climbing ≥15 flights per day, OR, 5.1 (95% CI, 2.5-10.2)[15]
Jumping	Among men, after adjusting for confounders and other physical load activities, OR, 2.0 (95% CI, 1.2-3.3) for development of severe OA requiring TKA[21]
Kneeling, squatting, knee bending	Among men, after adjusting for confounders and other physical load activities, OR, 2.0 (95% CI, 1.1-3.6) for development of severe OA requiring TKA[21]; OR, 2.45 (95% CI, 1.21-4.97) for men exposed to much knee bending to some knee bending and OR, 3.49 (95% CI, 1.22-10.52) for women[4]; among both sexes, statistically significant association between kneeling and/or squatting for more than 1 h/d for more than 1 y; also, increased risk with kneeling or squatting for period of 1-9.9 y but no dose-response relationship[11]; systematic literature review: strong and consistent evidence to support that kneeling and/or squatting associated with increased risk of developing OA in the knees[22]; comparison study between carpet/floor layers and painters, statistically significant increase (P < .01) in degenerative changes of the knee by radiographic examination of carpet/floor layers compared with painters[5]

TABLE 10-2 Representative References and Comments for
Osteoarthritis of the Knee (continued)

Risk Factor	References and Comments
Lifting	Insufficient evidence; among men, although cumulative lifetime heavy lifting had statistically significant association with severe knee OA requiring TKA (OR, 2.5 for "medium exposure" [95% CI, 1.5 - 4.4]; OR, 3.0 for "heavy exposure" [95% CI, 1.6-5.5]), after adjusting for other physical load factors and confounders, no statistically significant association between lifting and knee OA; no association found in women[21]; increased risk among both sexes lifting ≥25 kg more than 10 times per week for more than 20 y[11]; for Chinese men lifting >10 kg more than 10 times per week, OR, 5.4 (95% CI, 2.4-12.4) and for women, OR, 2.0 (95% CI, 1.2-3.1)[15]
Sitting	Protective effect noted among Japanese women in occupations with sitting ≥2 h/d (OR, 0.43 [95% CI, 0.23-0.78])[9]; OR, 0.5 (95% CI, 0.3-0.7) for development of symptomatic OA of the knee compared with weight-bearing knee-bending work[10]
Standing	Insufficient evidence, mixed results; protective effect noted with medium to high levels of standing compared with low levels[14]
Walking	Among both sexes, walking more than 2 mi/d associated with risk of knee OA[11]
Combination of risk factors	
Knee bending and heavy physical demand	Strong evidence for radiographic evidence of OA in men; adjusted OR, 2.22 (95% CI, 1.38-3.58) for work involving knee bending and at least medium demand compared with no bending in combination with, at most, light-demand work; test for trend "suggested" dose-response relationship with increased exposure time to bending and at least medium-demand work resulted in increased rates of OA; mean ± SD attributable risk of OA to knee bending and physical demands, 14.7% ± 4.9% and 15.4% ± 7.2% for severe OA; no association found for work activity and symptomatic OA[20].

TABLE 10-2 Representative References and Comments for Osteoarthritis of the Knee (continued)

Risk Factor	References and Comments
Squatting, kneeling, climbing	When examined individually and adjusted for BMI and presence of Heberden nodes, each activity statistically significant (squatting >30 min/d, OR, 6.9 [95% CI, 1.8-26.4]; kneeling >30 min/d, OR, 3.4 [95% CI, 1.3-9.1]; climbing stairs >10 flights per day, OR, 2.7 [95% CI, 1.2-6.1); no statistically significant association found after adjusting for each activity; further analysis revealed interaction between heavy lifting (>25 kg) and kneeling, squatting, or climbing (OR, 5.4 [95% CI, 1.4-21.0])[6]
Kneeling/squatting with heavy lifting	Among both sexes, OR, 3.0 (95% CI, 1.7-5.4) for development of OA of the knee[11]

Hip Joint

Conclusions on Nonoccupational Risk Factors

The evidence for nonoccupational risk factors is as follows:
- **Age:** Accepted risk factor; risk increases with age[24]
- **Overweight or obese:** Accepted risk factor[25,26]; OR, 1.7 (95% CI, 1.3-2.4) for a BMI of 28.0 or more and trend $P < .001$[19,26-29]
- **Previous trauma:** Accepted risk factor[15,25]; OR, 4.3 (95% CI, 2.2-8.4) among people with OA of the hip who had history of hip injury[19,27,28,30,31]
- **Congenital and developmental disorders:** Accepted risk factor[26-28,30]
- **Genetic predisposition evidenced by Heberden nodes:** Strong evidence, further investigation required; OR, 3.4 (95% CI, 1.2-10)[24]; OR, 1.6 (95% CI, 1.2-2.2)[19,25-27,30]
- **Smoking:** Insufficient evidence to support protective effect; OR, 0.4 (95% CI, 0.2-0.9) among men with OA of the hip who are current smokers; no similar finding among women[26]

Conclusions on Occupational Risk Factors

The evidence for occupational risk factors is as follows:
- **Climbing:** Insufficient evidence[15,25,32]
- **Jumping:** Insufficient evidence[32,33]
- **Kneeling:** Insufficient evidence[25,27]
- **Lifting:** Some evidence[15,24,25,27,33]
- **Sitting:** Insufficient evidence as a protective factor[27]
- **Squatting:** Insufficient evidence[25,27]
- **Standing and walking:** Insufficient evidence[25,27]

Literature Searches and Representative References for Osteoarthritis of the Hip

Table 10-3 shows the results for the literature searches for osteoarthritis of the hip, and Table 10-4 shows representative references and comments.

TABLE 10-3 Literature Searches for Osteoarthritis of the Hip*

Search No./Search Terms	Results
1/osteoarthritis & hip & occupational	84 results; 14 chosen by abstract review
2/osteoarthritis & hip & work	101 results; none chosen by abstract review
3/osteoarthritis & hip & causation	299 results; none additional chosen by abstract review
4/osteoarthritis & hip & industrial	2 results; neither chosen by abstract review

* Search limits were English language and human in all searches.

TABLE 10-4	Representative References and Comments for Osteoarthritis of the Hip
Risk Factor	**References and Comments**
Climbing	For men awaiting total hip arthroplasty for severe OA of the hip, OR, 2.3 (95% CI, 1.1-4.9) exposed to climbing more than 30 flights of stairs for 10-19.9 y compared with men who had never done such climbing; no statistically significant trend with increasing duration of exposure to climbing[25]; for women awaiting THA for primary OA of the hip, OR, 2.1 (95% CI, 1.2-3.6) with high exposure to work activity before age 50 y that required stair climbing compared with women with low exposure[32]; study of Chinese subjects, OR, 12.5 (95% CI, 1.5-104.3) for men climbing at least 15 flights of stairs per day in main employment before onset of hip pain and diagnosed with OA of the hip; no association found in women[15]
Jumping	For women awaiting THA for primary OA of the hip, OR, 2.1 (95% CI, 1.1-4.2) high exposure to work activity before age 50 y that required jumps or movements between different levels compared with women who had low exposure[32]; for men who had received THA for idiopathic OA, OR, 1.83 (95% CI, 1.06-3.14) for medium vs low exposure to jumping activity before age 49 y; no statistically significant association found in men with high vs low exposure[33]
Kneeling	No statistically significant association[25,27]

CHAPTER 10

TABLE 10-4 Representative References and Comments for Osteoarthritis of the Hip (continued)

Risk Factor	References and Comments
Lifting	For men awaiting THA for severe OA of the hip, OR, 2.3 (95% CI, 1.2-4.2) exposed to regular heavy lifting of ≥10 kg for at least 10 y before age 30 y compared with men who had never done such lifting; for subjects exposed to lifting ≥25 kg for at least 10 y before age 30 y, OR, 2.7 (95% CI, 1.4-5.1), and OR, 2.3 (95% CI, 1.3-4.4) if lifting this weight for at least 20 y up to 10 y before study; although not presented as statistically significant, there was a trend toward increasing risk with prolonged duration of exposure and maximum weight exposure; for men awaiting THA for severe OA of the hip, OR, 3.0 (95% CI, 1.5-6.3) if exposed to lifting 25-49 kg and OR, 2.9 (95% CI, 1.3-6.4) if exposed to lifting at least 50 kg for at least 10 y before age 30 y, compared with men who lifted <10 kg; OR, 3.2 (95% CI, 1.6-6.5) for men who lifted at least 50 kg for at least 10 y up to 10 y before the study[25]; for Japanese men and women awaiting THA for severe OA of the hip, OR, 3.5 (95% CI, 1.3-9.7) if exposed to lifting >25 kg during first employment and OR, 4.1 (95% CI, 1.1-15.2) if exposed to lifting >50 kg during main employment compared with subjects who had no similar lifting jobs[27]; study of Chinese subjects, OR, 2.4 (95% CI, 1.1-5.3) for women lifting at least 10 kg more than 10 times per week in main employment before onset of hip pain and diagnosed with OA of the hip; no association found in men[15]; for men with radiographic evidence of OA of the hip or history of hip replacement, OR, 2.5 (95% CI, 1.1-5.7) that they were exposed to at least 20 y of lifting at least 25.4 kg in their occupations[24]; for men who had received THA for idiopathic OA, OR, 1.84 (95% CI, 1.12-3.03) for men with high vs low exposure to heavy lifting (tons) before age 49 y and OR, 2.4 (95% CI, 1.5-3.83) for men with high vs low exposure to lifting >40 kg[33]
Sitting	Study of Japanese men and women awaiting THA for severe hip OA, sitting offered protective effect from development of OA of the hip, OR, 0.5 (95% CI, 0.3-0.9)[27]
Squatting	No statistically significant association[25,27]
Standing and walking	No statistically significant association[25,27]

TABLE 10-4 Representative References and Comments for Osteoarthritis of the Hip (continued)

Risk Factor	References and Comments
Other	Occupational activities grouped into light, intermediate, and heavy work: heavy work, "heavy work standing," "work walking," or "work kneeling or crouching"; light work, sitting and "light work standing"; for men with radiographic evidence of OA of the hip, consistent increased probability of exposure to heavy work vs light work when controlling for confounding factors including certain sports activities; conclusions cannot be drawn for specific physical movements and risk for OA of the hip[34]

Meniscal Disorders

Burden

In addition to various arthritic disorders, a common cause of knee pain is injuries to the meniscus. It has been reported that between 11.1% and 31.5% of asymptomatic people have degenerative meniscal changes in the knee.[35] Studies have suggested that the highest incidence occurs in men between 20 and 49 years of age and 70% of hospital cases are the result of acute injuries, often sports-related injuries.[36] Although acute meniscal tears are common in athletic injuries and there is an estimated fourfold increase in the risk of subsequent development of osteoarthritis of the knee after injury and surgical treatment,[36] there is little published in the literature regarding the population burden of symptomatic degenerative meniscal disorders and economic impact of this potentially disabling condition.

Conclusions on Nonoccupational Risk Factors

The evidence for nonoccupational risk factors is as follows:
- **Overweight or obese:** Strong evidence, further analysis required; for men and women between the ages of 25 and 59 years diagnosed with meniscal tears during arthroscopy, OR, 2.3 (95% CI, 1.5-3.4) with a BMI of 24.1 to 27.0 and OR, 1.7 (95% CI, 1.2-2.6) with a BMI of 27.0 or more; the higher BMI category associated only with degenerative meniscal lesions and not acute tears (OR, 4.7 [95% CI, 1.9-11.2])[36]; dose-response relationship was statistically significant in men and women with history of meniscal surgery[35]

■ **Sporting activities:** Strong evidence, further analysis required; for men between the ages of 20 and 59 years who underwent meniscectomy, OR, 6.9 (95% CI, 3.5-13.3) that they were exposed to playing soccer at least 5 times per year when knee symptoms first developed; OR, 3.4 (95% CI, 1.5-7.8) for men playing rugby and OR, 2.1 (95% CI, 1.2-3.6) for men playing other sports[37]; for men and women between the ages of 25 and 59 years diagnosed with meniscal tears during arthroscopy, OR, 3.7 (95% CI, 2.1-6.6) that they played soccer during the 12 months before onset of knee symptoms

Conclusions on Occupational Risk Factors

The evidence for occupational risk factors is as follows:
- **Climbing:** Insufficient evidence[36]
- **Driving:** Insufficient evidence[36]
- **Kneeling:** Insufficient evidence[36,37]
- **Lifting:** Insufficient evidence[36]
- **Sitting:** Insufficient evidence[36]
- **Squatting:** Insufficient evidence[36,37]
- **Standing:** Insufficient evidence[36]
- **Walking:** Insufficient evidence[36]

Literature Searches and Representative References for Meniscal Disorders of the Knee

Table 10-5 shows the results for the literature searches for meniscal disorders of the knee, and Table 10-6 shows representative references and comments.

TABLE 10-5   Literature Searches for Meniscal Disorders of the Knee*

Search No. and Search Terms	Results
1/menisci, tibial & causation	53 results; 3 original articles chosen by abstract review
2/menisci, tibial & occupational	23 results; none chosen by abstract review
3/menisci, tibial & etiology	592 results; none chosen by abstract review
4/menisci, tibial & risk factors	50 results; none chosen by abstract review

* Search limits were English language and human in all searches.

TABLE 10-6	References and Comments for Meniscal Disorders of the Knee
Risk Factor	**References and Comments**
Climbing	OR, 2.7 (95% CI, 1.8-4.1) for men and women exposed to climbing more than 30 flights of stairs in an average workday who had arthroscopically diagnosed meniscal injuries[36]
Driving	OR, 2.3 (95% CI, 1.4-3.8) for men and women exposed to >4 h of driving in an average workday who had arthroscopically diagnosed meniscal injuries[36]
Kneeling	For men between the ages of 20 and 59 y who underwent meniscectomy, OR, 2.5 (95% CI, 1.3-4.8) that they were exposed to >1 h of kneeling in an average workday when before onset of knee symptoms[37]; OR, 2.6 (95% CI, 1.6-4.3) for men and women exposed to >1 h of kneeling in an average workday who had arthroscopically diagnosed meniscal injuries[36]
Lifting	Statistically significant association between having arthroscopically diagnosed meniscal injuries in men and women and history of lifting >10 kg, 25 kg, and 50 kg more than 10 times in an average workday; no dose-response relationship noted between the categories of weight lifting[36]
Sitting	No statistically significant association[36]
Squatting	For men between the ages of 20 and 59 y who underwent meniscectomy, OR, 2.5 (95% CI, 1.2-4.9) that they were exposed to >1 h of squatting in an average workday when before onset of knee symptoms[37]; OR, 2.2 (95% CI, 1.4-3.6) for men and women exposed to >1 h of squatting in an average workday who had arthroscopically diagnosed meniscal injuries[36]
Standing	No statistically significant association[36]
Walking	OR, 1.8 (95% CI, 1.2-2.7) for men and women exposed to walking >2 mi in an average workday who had arthroscopically diagnosed meniscal injuries[36]

Plantar Fasciitis and Heel Pain

Burden

Chronic plantar heel pain is one of the most common foot disorders and has been estimated to account for 15% of all adult foot complaints requiring medical care.[38] Approximately 2 million people are affected in the United States each year and approximately 10% of the population during a lifetime, usually adults older than 40 years.[38] Although many risk factors have been proposed in the literature, there is limited conclusive evidence to support most hypotheses.

Conclusions on Nonoccupational Risk Factors

The evidence for nonoccupational risk factors is as follows:

- **Overweight or obese:** Insufficient evidence, further analysis required; several case-control studies found statistically significant difference in BMI between cases of chronic plantar heel pain and controls without this condition in a nonathletic population; similar results not found in an athletic population[38]; OR, 2.0 (95% CI, 1.28-3.08) for people with BMI of 25.0 to 30 compared with a BMI of less than 25.0 and OR, 5.6 (95% CI, 1.9-16.6) for people with a BMI of more than 30 compared with a BMI of less than 25.0[39]
- **Age:** Insufficient evidence, further analysis required; in some studies, statistically significant increased age between cases with chronic plantar heel pain and controls in athletic and nonathletic populations[38]
- **Ankle motion:** Insufficient evidence, further analysis required; mixed results with respect to ankle dorsiflexion motion and association with chronic plantar heel pain[38]; decreased ankle dorsiflexion of uninvolved limb significantly associated with diagnosis of plantar fasciitis with possible dose-response relationship[39]
- **Static foot posture:** Insufficient evidence, further analysis required; mixed results with respect to static foot posture and association with chronic plantar heel pain[38]
- **Calcaneal spur:** Insufficient evidence, further analysis required[38]
- **Jogging:** Insufficient evidence, further analysis required[39]

Conclusions on Occupational Risk Factors

For standing and walking, there is *insufficient evidence.*[38,39]

Literature Search and Representative References for Plantar Fasciitis and Heel Pain

A search for the term fasciitis, plantar with the limits English and human, provided 179 results, of which 2 articles were chosen by abstract review.

For standing and walking, subjects diagnosed with plantar fasciitis were 3.6 times more likely to have self-reported working on their feet a majority of the workday compared with subjects who did not work on their feet (95% CI, 1.3-10.1).[39]

References

1. Arthritis – Overview, Arthritis Basics, http://www.cdc.gov/arthritis/arthritis/index. htm. Accessed March 18, 2007.
2. Arthritis – Data and Statistics – Arthritis Related Statistics, Data and Statistics, http://www.cdc.gov/arthritis/data_statistics/arthritis_related_statistics.htm. Accessed March 18, 2007.
3. Symmons, D., Mathers, C., Pfleger, B. (2006). *Global Burden of osteoarthritis in the year 2000*, http://www.who.int/healthinfo/statistics/bod_osteoarthritis.pdf. Accessed March 18, 2007.
4. MMWR, *Racial/Ethnic Differences in the Prevalence and Impact of Doctor-Diagnosed Arthritis --- United States, 2002*, February 11, 2005, 54(05); 119-123, http://www.cdc.gov/mmwr/preview/mmwrhtml/mm5405a3.htm, Accessed March 18, 2007.
5. MMWR, *National and State Medical Expenditures and Lost Earnings Attributable to Arthritis and Other Rheumatic Conditions --- United States, 2003,* January 12, 2007, 56(01); 4-7, http://www.cdc.gov/mmwr/preview/mmwrhtml/mm5601a2. htm?s_cid=mm5601a2_e. Accessed March 18, 2007.
6. Holmberg S, Thelin A, Thelin N. Is there an increased risk of knee osteoarthritis among farmers? A population-based case-control study. *International Archives of Occupational & Environmental Health.* 2004;77:345-350.
7. Cooper C, McAlindon T, Coggon D, Egger P, Dieppe P. Occupational activity and osteoarthritis of the knee. *Annals of Rheumatic Diseases.* 1994;53:90-93.
8. Neame RL, Muir K, Doherty S, Doherty M. Genetic risk of knee osteoarthritis: a sibling study. *Annals of Rheumatic Diseases.* 2004;63:1022-1027.
9. Felson DT, Hannan MT, Naimark A, Berkeley J, Gordon G, Wilson PWF, Anderson J. Occupational physical demands, knee bending, and knee osteoarthritis: Results from the Framingham Study. *The Journal of Rheumatology.* 1991;18:1587-92.
10. Sandmark H, Hogstedt, C Vingard, E. Primary osteoarthrosis of the knee in men and women as a result of lifelong physical load from work. *Scandinavian Journal of Work, Environment and Health.* 2000;26 (1):20-25.

11. Manninen P, Heliovaara M, Riihimaki H, Suomalainen O. Physical workload and the risk of severe knee osteoarthritis. *Scandinavian Journal of Work, Environment and Health.*2002;28(1):25-32.

12. Davis MA, Neuhaus JM Ettinger, WH Muller. Body fat distribution and osteoarthritis. *American Journal of Epidemiology.*1990;32:701-707.

13. Anderson JJ, Felson DT. Factors associated with osteoarthritis of the knee in the First National Health and Nutrition Examination Survey (Hanes I). *American Journal of Epidemiology.* 1988;128 (1):179-89.

14. Yoshimura N, Nishioka S, Kinoshita H, et al. Risk factors for knee osteoarthritis in Japanese women: Heavy weight, previous joint injuries, and occupational activities. *The Journal of Rheumatology.* 2004;31:157-62.

15. Sahlström A, Montgomery F. Risk analysis of occupational factors influencing the development of arthrosis of the knee. *European Journal of Epidemiology.* 1997;13:675-79.

16. McMillan G, Nichols L. Osteoarthritis and meniscus disorders of the knee as occupational diseases of miners. *Occupational and Environmental Medicine.* 2005;62:567-75.

17. Rossignol M, Leclerc A, Allaert FA, et al. Primary osteoarthritis of hip, knee, and hand in relation to occupational exposure. *Occupational and Environmental Medicine.* 2005;62:772-77.

18. Coggon D, Croft P, Kellingray S, Barrett D, McLaren M, Cooper C. Occupational physical activities and osteoarthritis of the knee. *Arthritis and Rheumatism.* 2000;43(7):1443-9.

19. Lau EC, Cooper C, Lam D, Chan VNH, Tsang KK, Sham A. Factors Associated with Osteoarthritis of the Hip and Knee in Hong Kong Chinese: Obesity, Joint Injury, and Occupational Activities. *American Journal of Epidemiology.* 2000;152:855-62.

20. Englund M, Lohmander LS. Risk Factors for Symptomatic Knee Osteoarthritis Fifteen to Twenty-Two Years after Meniscectomy. *Arthritis and Rheumatism.* 2004; 50(9):2811-19.

21. Sutton AJ, Muir KR, Mockett S, Fentem P. A case-control study to investigate the relation between low and moderate levels of physical activity and osteoarthritis of the knee using data collected as part of the Allied Dunbar National Fitness Survey. *Annals of the Rheumatic Diseases.* 2001;60:756-64.

22. Cimmino MA, Parodi M. *Risk Factors for Osteoarthritis. Seminars in Arthritis and Rheumatism.* 2005;34(6)(suppl 2):29-34.

23. Felson D. An update on the pathogenesis and epidemiology of osteoarthritis. *Radiologic Clinics of North America.* 2004;42:1-9.

24. Coggon D, Kellingray S, Inskip H, Croft P, Campbell L, Cooper C. Osteoarthritis of the Hip and Occupational Lifting. *American Journal of Epidemiology.* 1998;147(6):523-28.

25. Yoshimura N, Sasaki S, Iwasaki K, et al. Occupational Lifting is Associated with Hip Osteoarthritis: A Japanese Case-Control Study. *The Journal of Rheumatology.* 2000;27:434-40.

26. Vingård E, Alfredsson L, Malchau H. Osteoarthrosis of the hip in women and its relation to physical load at work and in the home. *Annals of the Rheumatic Diseases.* 1997;56:293-98.

27. Cooper C, Campbell L, Byng P, Croft P, Coggon D. Occupational activity and the risk of hip osteoarthritis. *Annals of the Rheumatic Diseases.* 1996;55(9):680-2.
28. Cooper C, Inskip H, Croft P, et al. Individual Risk Factors for Hip Osteoarthritis: Obesity, Hip Injury, and Physical Activity. *American Journal of Epidemiology.* 1998;147(6):516-22.
29. Ford G, Hegmann K, White G, Holmes E. Associations of Body Mass Index with Meniscal Tears. *American Journal of Preventive Medicine.* 2005;28(4):364-68.
30. Croft P, Coggon D, Cruddas M, Cooper C. Osteoarthritis of the hip: an occupational disease in farmers. *British Medical Journal.* 1992;304: 1269-71.
31. Mahomed N. Does Occupational Lifting Cause Hip Osteoarthritis? *The Journal of Rheumatology.* 2000;27(2):292-93.
32. Vignon E, Valat J, Rossignol M, et al. Osteoarthritis of the knee and hip and activity: a systematic international review and synthesis (OASIS). *Joint Bone Spine.* 2006;73:442-55.
33. Croft P, Cooper C, Wickman C, Coggon D. Osteoarthritis of the hip and occupational activity. *Scandinavian Journal of Work, Environment and Health.*1992;18 (1):59-63.
34. Vingård E, Hogstedt C, Alfredsson L, Fellenius E, Goldie I, Koster M. Coxarthrosis and physical work load. *Scandinavian Journal of Work, Environment and Health.* 1991;17(2):104-9.
35. Wearing SC, Henning EM, Byrne NM, Steele JR, Hills AP. Musculoskeletal disorders associated with obesity: a biomechanical perspective. *Obesity Reviews.* 2006;7:239-50.
36. Baker P, Reading I, Cooper C, Coggon D. Knee disorders in the general population and their relation to occupation. *Occupational and Environmental Medicine.* 2003;60:794-97.
37. Baker P, Coggon D, Reading I, Barrett D, McLaren M, Cooper C. Sports Injury, Occupational Physical Activity, Joint laxity, and Meniscal Damage. *The Journal of Rheumatology.* 2002; 29(3):557-63.
38. Kivimäki J, Riihimäki H, Hänninen K. Knee disorders in carpet and floor layers and painters. *Scandinavian Journal of Work, Environment and Health.* (1992); 18 (5):310-6.
39. Roach K, Persky V, Miles T, Budiman-Mak E. Biomechanical Aspects of Occupation and Osteoarthritis of the Hip: A Case-Control Study. *The Journal of Rheumatology.* 1994;21(12):2334-40.
40. Irving DB, Cook JL, Menz HB. Factors associated with chronic plantar heel pain: a systematic review. *Journal of Science and Medicine in Sport.* 2006;9(1-2):11-22.
41. Riddle D, Pulisic M, Pidcoe P, Johnson R. Risk Factors for Plantar Fasciitis: A Matched Case-Control Study. *The Journal of Bone and Joint Surgery.* 2003; 85-A (5): 872-77.
42. Li C, Sung F. A review of the healthy worker effect in occupational epidemiology. *Occupational Medicine.* 1999;49(4):225-229.

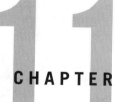

CHAPTER

Musculoskeletal Disorders

William Edward Ackerman, III, MD, and J. Mark Melhorn, MD

Criteria necessary to assess evidence for the work-relatedness of musculoskel-etal disorders have been discussed in previous chapters. This chapter reviews causation of work-related musculoskeletal pain, which is labeled as non-trau-matic soft tissue musculoskeletal disorders, cumulative trauma disorders, mus-culoskeletal disorders, and/or repetitive strain injury.[1] *Musculoskeletal pain* is defined as any pain that may involve the muscles, nerves, tendons, ligaments, bones, or joints.[2] The application of the aforementioned labels to musculoskel-etal pain that occurs in the workplace has led to speculation that there is direct causation between the workplace and the onset of musculoskeletal pain, despite studies demonstrating evidence to the contrary.[3] Efforts have been made by physicians to convert these labels for musculoskeletal pain into specific medical diagnoses. Examples of the attempted conversions are functional somatic syn-drome, myofascial pain syndrome (MPS), fibromyalgia, dystonia, and chronic fatigue syndrome (CFS). Even these diagnoses tend to be more of a label than a specific medical condition and these syndromes or labels are rarely determined as occupational-related conditions.

It must be remembered that occupational and environmental diseases frequently masquerade as routine medical disorders.[4] Symptoms of environmental diseases can be non-specific. A clinician may want to consider environmental issues as well. With non-specific disorders, a careful history should include a list of job titles and exposures to fumes, dusts, chemicals, loud noises, and radiation. Considerations of sources of exposure should also include the home surround-ings and exposure to hazardous agents.

Functional Somatic Syndromes

The term *functional somatic syndrome* has been applied to several related syn-dromes characterized more by symptoms, suffering, and disability than by con-sistently demonstrable tissue abnormalities. These syndromes include multiple chemical sensitivity syndrome, sick building syndrome, repetitive stress injury, side effects of silicone breast implants, Gulf War syndrome, chronic whiplash, CFS, irritable bowel syndrome, and fibromyalgia.[5] Patients with a functional somatic syndrome frequently have explicit, elaborated self-diagnoses, and their symptoms are often refractory to standard treatment. These syndromes have similar epidemiologic characteristics and are associated with a higher prevalence of psychiatric comorbid conditions.[5] Psychosocial factors can magnify a belief that one has a serious disease and that one's condition is disabling. Psychological factors may furthermore influence the somatic distress of patients with a func-tional somatic syndrome. The association of psychological trauma, posttrau-matic symptoms, psychological dissociation, and somatoform disorders is well documented.[6] When examining a patient with chronic pain, it is important to consider a possible psychological dimension and to investigate a history of previous psychological trauma. This approach can help identify possible contributions to and continued expression of some painful syndromes and aid in the recognition and treatment of psychiatric comorbid conditions. A literature search using the criteria outlined in Chapter 4 that included the key words "work-related" and "functional syndromes" yielded inconclusive consistent scientific evidence that functional somatic disorders are caused by occupational exposure.

Chronic nonspecific muscle pain, often labeled a musculoskeletal disorder, is commonly associated with the workplace. It can be difficult for clinicians interested in determining the work-relatedness of musculoskeletal pain to determine causation in many situations. Musculoskeletal disorders were evaluated in detail in 1997[7] by the National Institute for Occupational Safety and Health and described in the book, *Musculoskeletal Disorders and Workplace Factors: A Critical Review of Epidemiologic Evidence for Work-Related Musculoskeletal Disorders of the Neck, Upper Extremity, and Low Back.* The authors concluded that there was epidemiologic evidence to support an association but insufficient evidence to determine causation, and the association was significantly confounded by psychosocial issues.

In addition to musculoskeletal disorders, two common labels for nonspecific muscle pain (myalgia) that have a better medical definition for diagnosis include MPS and fibromyalgia pain syndrome. A *syndrome* is defined by *Mosby's Medical Dictionary,* sixth edition, as "a complex of signs and symptoms resulting from a common cause or appearing, in combination, to present a common picture of a disease or inherited abnormality." The MPS is described as overuse or muscle fatigues characterized by the presence of trigger points. *Fibromyalgia,* on the other hand, is a chronic, widespread muscle tenderness syndrome associated with central sensitization. Chronic sleep disturbances, fatigue, visceral pain, and interstitial cystitis are often described as accompanying fibromyalgia. Unfortunately, the labels myofascial pain and fibromyalgia are often used interchangeably; the syndromes should be considered distinct entities.[8] This interchangeability is but another confounder when studies are reviewed to determine the contribution of occupational exposures. Both syndromes are characterized by chronic muscle pain that may not improve until the underlying precipitating factors are diagnosed and treated.[9]

A literature review generated 680 articles for non-traumatic musculoskeletal pain risk factors, with 551 articles published after 1996. Of these, 256 articles discussed occupational risk factors, but only 85 discussed work-relatedness, of which 60 attributed symptoms to muscle overload or fatigue and the other 25 related symptoms to ergonomics or posture; none established direct causation. Individual risk factors for functional somatic syndromes include psychosocial issues, medicalization, female sex-specific syndromes, somatoform disorders, anxiety, and chronic depression.[10-12] No work-related factors for functional somatic syndromes were identified from a current literature search. As a result, there seems to be insufficient evidence to establish work-related causation for functional somatic syndromes.

Myofascial Pain Syndrome

The MPS is a common, localized painful musculoskeletal condition associated with trigger points. However, diagnostic criteria established in well-designed studies are lacking.[13] The *trigger point* is described as a focus of hyperirritability in the muscle that when compressed is painful and can cause referred pain and tenderness. The false assumption that many cases of nonspecific complaints affecting the musculoskeletal system may be ascribed to MPS makes clear the need for accurate diagnostic criteria.[13] The definitive pathogenesis of MPS is unknown, and no single diagnostic method with high sensitivity and specificity has consistently positive results in the presence of disease. Patients frequently complain of regional chronic pain, which varies in intensity and is most frequently found in the head, neck, shoulders, extremities, and low back. The MPS can be active or chronic. Active trigger points cause muscular pain and refer pain and tenderness to another area of the body when pressure is applied. Active trigger points are most frequently associated with a recent muscle strain, whereas latent trigger points are associated with chronic MPS. Latent trigger points cause pain when compressed, but they usually do not refer pain to other areas of the body.[14] Because of the lack of consistent, valid diagnostic tests, an accurate diagnosis of MPS must be based on clinical medical signs. For a medical sign to be diagnostically useful, independent examiners must be able to agree on its presence.[15]

Individual Risk Factors for MPS

Individual risk factors for MPS include the iliotibial band syndrome found in runners; structural or mechanical causes such as scoliosis; localized joint hypomobility; chest wall pain when athletes' bodies are subjected to sudden, large, indirect forces or overuse; stress fractures of the ribs caused by sporting activities associated with golf, rowing, and baseball pitching, in particular; and cycling and its association with the gluteus medius syndrome.[16-19]

Work-related risk factors for MPS include neck sprain, mechanical or muscular neck pain, and postural neck pain related to improper ergonomics at an employee's work station.[20] The MPS can be caused by recurrent overuse, resulting in microtrauma to muscle tissue. Local pain and tenderness, weakness, inflammation, and limited function are common findings in an overuse syndrome.[21] Performing artists often sustain a variety of neuromusculoskeletal problems that interfere with the ability to play or perform. Many of these conditions occur as a result of overuse.[22]

The diagnosis of MPS is complex, and there is a lack of a consistent valid diagnostic test for accurate diagnosis. A review of the medical literature using MPS and risk factors as search terms returned 39 articles. Analysis of these articles implicated posture and muscle trauma as general risk factors, whereas only eight articles discussed occupational risk factors. Muscle trauma was usually associated with recent cervical sprain or strain injuries.[23,24] The majority of articles acknowledge that the incidence of work-related MPS has rapidly increased during the last 20 years; there seems to be a strong contribution from psychosocial factors and non–work-related medical conditions.[25] The single most common diagnostic factor for workers'compensation-eligible MPS of the upper limb was a triggering event for nonspecific musculoskeletal pain. This finding is consistent with physical examination findings that often show no measurable tissue damage or inflammatory response. Further support for non-occupational causation can be seen in the seasonal variability of MPS, which is diagnosed more commonly during the winter months. The incidence of depression is also higher during winter months.[26] Abnormal posture is considered a risk factor for the perpetuation of myofascial pain.[76] Therefore, people who adopt poor postural habits for sitting, standing, or sleeping add to their risk outside the occupational environment. Furthermore, these postural habits are frequently independent of any preexisting structural physical abnormalities. Failure to correct postural habits may lead to chronic MPS.[27]

One clinical study of repetitive motion in sewing machine operators compared with nurses aides and home-helpers reported a statistically significant relationship between myofascial pain and years as a sewing machine operator. The authors also reported the finding that muscle palpation to be a reproducible examination consistent with trigger points with kappa values that approximated 0.70.[28] This conclusion for reproducible examination results would be inconsistent with findings of the majority of other studies. Furthermore, this study did not address preemployment, individual, or psychosocial risk factors.

Fibromyalgia

The American College of Rheumatology established the diagnostic criteria for fibromyalgia in 1990.[29] The diagnosis is established for an individual patient when the American College of Rheumatology criteria are met. These criteria include a chronic, widespread muscular pain of at least three months' duration above and below the diaphragm on both sides of the body and painful tender points in at least 11 of 18 locations.[29] Fibromyalgia is a chronic syndrome characterized by diffuse or specific muscle, joint, or bone pain; fatigue; and depression. Fibromyalgia can be a debilitating disorder also characterized by sleep disturbances and skin sensitivity. There are no genetic or biochemical markers and patients often have other comorbid diseases, such as migraines, interstitial cystitis, and irritable bowel syndrome.

Fibromyalgia is seen in 3% to 6% of the general population and is most commonly diagnosed in people between the ages of 20 and 50 years. Fibromyalgia is a common, chronic, widespread pain syndrome mainly affecting women.[30] Although the pathogenesis of fibromyalgia is not completely understood, varieties of neuroendocrine disturbances, and abnormalities of autonomic function have been implicated.[31]

Individual Risk Factors for Fibromyalgia

Exposure of a genetically predisposed person to a host of environmental stressors is presumed to lead to the development of fibromyalgia.[32] Fibromyalgia overlaps with several related syndromes, collectively comprising the spectrum of the functional somatic disorder. Fibromyalgia is characterized by a strong familial aggregation. Recent evidence suggests a role for polymorphisms of genes in the serotoninergic, dopaminergic, and catecholaminergic systems.[33] Although the diagnosis of fibromyalgia includes the presence of 11 of 18 trigger points, many patients with early symptoms might not fit this definition.[34] There is evidence of increased corticotropin-releasing hormone and substance P in the spinal fluid and serum of patients with fibromyalgia, and increased levels of interleukins 6 and 8 in the serum.[35]

Histologic muscle abnormalities of membranes, mitochondria, and fiber type have been well described at the light microscopic and ultrastructural levels in tissue samples from isolated tender areas associated with fibromyalgia.[36] The observed abnormalities in muscles affected by fibromyalgia are consistent with neurologic findings and disturbances in the hypothalamic-pituitary-adrenal axis.[36]

For work-related risk factors for fibromyalgia using the search criteria of fibromyalgia and occupational risk factors, no adequate epidemiologic studies were found for review. Most articles pertaining to fibromyalgia are anecdotal reports or small case series. There is insufficient evidence to indicate a causal relationship among workplace exposure, trauma in general, and the development of fibromyalgia. Isolated cases in which a reported association exists between work and fibromyalgia are occasionally published. For example, fibromyalgia was described in a population of assembly-line workers in Brazil.[37] Fibromyalgia was largely associated with symptoms of patients with repetitive strain injuries as opposed to coworkers with non-repetitive strain injuries. This study, however, did not identify whether any of the subjects had a history of fibromyalgia, the criteria used to determine fibromyalgia, or the impact of psychosocial issues.

A prospective study reviewed the association between occupational stress and the incidence of newly diagnosed fibromyalgia.[38] Stress, as indicated by high workload, low decision latitude, and being a victim of workplace bullying, was assessed. The authors concluded that stress is a contributing factor in the development of fibromyalgia in the workplace but that workplace stress does not cause fibromyalgia.[38] This information is further confused by reports that trauma to the soft tissue of the neck can result in an increased incidence of fibromyalgia compared with other injuries[39] and other study reports indicating aggravation of the symptoms of fibromyalgia by computer keyboard typing (37%), prolonged sitting (37%), prolonged standing and walking (27%), stress (21%), heavy lifting and bending (19%), and repeated moving and lifting (18%) but not with walking (19%), variable light sedentary work (15%), teaching (8%), light desk work (6%), or phone work (6%).[40]

Dystonia

Dystonia is defined as a postural disorder and may be associated with spasms in the musculature of the face, shoulders, neck, trunk, and limbs.[41] Little is known about the cause of idiopathic adult-onset dystonia. Possible individual risk factors include a genetic component,[42] an associated disease of the basal ganglia,[43] and psychosocial issues.[44] A search of the current medical literature for dystonia and risk factors returned 12 articles, of which 6 discussed activities or injury associations and 1 an occupational risk factor but was not relevant (with respect to strong evidence that supports occupational causation). Of the six, five discussed musicians and one an electrical injury.[45-50]

Individual Risk Factors for Dystonia

Literature search results support the idea that environmental and genetic factors may be important in the cause of adult-onset dystonia.[51,52] In musicians, unintended muscle synergies, postures, and movement patterns can develop as attempts are made to increase the speed and fluency of movements. These findings may seem to represent an aberrant outcome of normal motor learning with physiologic correlates that mimic neuropathologically based dystonia. However, stage fright and psychological tension frequently generate somatoform disorders and may contribute to the chronicity of physical disabilities in musicians.[48] Head or facial trauma with loss of consciousness, a family history of dystonia, and a family history of postural tremor independently increased the risk of developing adult-onset dystonia.[53] For work-related risk factors for dystonia, there is insufficient information available; a medical literature search returned one match. This article was not relevant.

Chronic Fatigue Syndrome

Chronic fatigue syndrome is characterized by severe fatigue and other nonspecific symptoms. Chronic fatigue syndrome was defined as an entity in 1988 by the US Centers for Disease Control and Prevention as quoted in a systematic review article by Maquet et al. [54] The prevalence of CFS ranges from 0.2% to 0.7% in the general population.[54] Fatigue is a common, nonspecific, subjective symptom associated with several medical and psychiatric illnesses. Chronic fatigue syndrome causes disturbances of normal activities of daily living. There is uncertainty about the cause of CFS, but there is a high prevalence of psychiatric comorbidity.[55] An accurate diagnosis of CFS (as a specific medical entity) is difficult to make even in the presence of the reported disabling complaint of fatigue. The different etiologic factors showing some degree of involvement in CFS might suggest that this syndrome is a multifactorial condition. An epidemiologic study of CFS has been published.[56] The study found that somatization was the strongest predictor of both new and chronic fatigue with an unknown cause.

Individual risk factors for CFS include elevations in cerebrospinal fluid protein levels and cerebral spinal fluid cytokine levels compared with a control group, which may suggest a viral cause.[57] For occupational factors, six journal articles were identified.[58-63] There is insufficient epidemiologic information to establish causation between work-related risk factors for CFS.

A review of the literature with reference to CFS risk factors and epidemiology returned 533 articles, of which 38 addressed the epidemiology of the syndrome and 11 specifically addressed psychosocial causes of CFS. Most studies indicated that the number of somatization symptoms and a history of dysphoric episodes were the two strongest predictors of new-onset fatigue and recurrent chronic fatigue.[64,65] In addition, people who reported a history of unexplained fatigue at baseline and during the follow-up were at increased risk for a new onset of major depression compared with people who never reported such fatigue.[64,65] It was concluded from this study that somatization was the strongest predictor of new and chronic fatigue. Adverse experiences during childhood and maternal overprotection may increase the risk for CFS in adulthood.[64,65] People with CFS reported significantly higher levels of childhood trauma and psychopathology.[66]

Acute and Chronic Pain

Acute and chronic pain have been the topic of many articles and books. The purpose of this section is not to review or debate the cause of acute or chronic pain but to analyze the possible occupational association or work-relatedness of acute and chronic pain. The International Association for the Study of Pain has defined *pain* as "an unpleasant sensory and emotional experience associated with actual or potential tissue damage, or described in terms of such damage." Pain results in learning, which makes repetition of a painful situation less likely. The differences between acute and chronic pain are many and varied.[67] Acute pain is a symptom of injury or illness that can be modulated by treating its cause.[68] Work-related acute pain usually has a specific traumatic cause or injury. Acute pain can be beneficial because it warns and protects a person after an injury.

It remains unclear why chronic pain develops in some people. Chronic pain in arthritic diseases is related to ongoing joint destruction. However, progress in the understanding of chronic pain with neuropathic features has been hindered by a lack of epidemiologic research.

The causes of the transition from acute to chronic pain and the development of disability need to be identified.[69] Psychological distress, however, has been found to influence the risk of such a transition.[70] Psychophysiologic mechanisms may affect whether acute pain becomes chronic and can furthermore be associated with the long-term consequences of chronic pain. The influence of occupational factors such as job satisfaction, low workplace support, and physical workload may be related to the transition from acute to chronic pain.[70] For chronic pain and work-relatedness, a significant negative relationship was reported between people receiving workers' compensation benefits and outcome that was mediated by a worker's pessimistic belief in the ability to return to his or her former occupation.[71] The outcome study concluded that the origin of the pessimistic belief may be the result of the occurrence of the initial severe pain with inadequate pain management following a work-related injury that caused the injured worker to stay away from his or her occupation for fear of re-injury and the recurrence of severe pain. Pain sensations that are normally appraised to signal a threat of injury or disability may be maintained and amplified in some people, resulting in the development of chronic pain.[72] Psychological factors that may be associated with the workplace may interfere with the person's ability to cope and, therefore, decrease his or her tolerance to other occupational risk factors.[72]

Individual Risk Factors for Acute and Chronic Pain

Each person is unique, and how he or she experiences pain is unique.[73] A person's pain threshold and a person's sensitivity to a painful stimulus varies among individuals. In general, when a traumatic event occurs in the workplace (occupational exposure) and subsequent musculoskeletal injury occurs, tissue damage or change is seen on physical examination or traditional medical imaging studies and the pain will respond to the appropriate medical intervention, which may require individual variations in dose and duration of treatment. Learned behaviors and social influence modify the expression of pain by each person who may experience a similar injury.[74] People with chronic neuropathic pain are more likely to be female, divorced, living in rental units, unable to work, and smokers and have minimal education. Neuropathic pain can occur as a result of injury or disease to the nerve tissue itself.

Work-Related Risk Factors for Acute and Chronic Pain

There is insufficient evidence to demonstrate a relationship between occupational exposures related to physical demands and chronic pain. The influence of occupational factors such as job satisfaction and low workplace support may be related to the transition from acute to chronic pain.[70][71] It was previously mentioned that workers' compensation recipients with high initial work-injury pain followed by a history of surgery and severe postoperative pain fared worse than a similar group of workers' compensation recipients without severe pain with severe post surgical pain. This study also compared non-worker's compensation findings for patients who had high initial pain and a history of painful surgery and these results were similar to those for workers' compensation recipients without pain or surgery.[71] Psychological factors in the workplace may interfere with behavioral buffer mechanisms that can decrease a person's pain tolerance.[72]

Summary

Determination of work-relatedness for causation of musculoskeletal disorders should be based on sound science. Currently, there is little evidence that occupational exposure is the primary contribution to the development of musculoskeletal pain as described in this chapter. This lack of evidence is confounded by the difficulty assigning a specific medical diagnosis to a condition that is primarily determined by subjective symptoms and has led to conflicting conclusions by many authors. On occasion, a disease label is assigned to a person by exclusion after other disease entities have been ruled out by objective tests. Environmental factors must enter into a clinician's differential diagnosis.

Table 11-1 summarizes the evidence for work-relatedness for this chapter.

TABLE 11-1	Musculoskeletal Disorders and Work-Relatedness
Disorder	**Evidence for Work-Relatedness***
Functional somatic syndromes, musculoskeletal disorders, cumulative trauma disorders, and repetitive strain injury	Insufficient
Myofascial pain syndrome	Some in specific cases
Fibromyalgia	Insufficient
Chronic fatigue syndrome	Insufficient
Dystonia	Insufficient
Acute pain	Evidence in some cases
Chronic pain	Insufficient evidence

* See Chapter 4 for the methods used for literature review and determining the strength evidence of work-relatedness.

References

1. Melhorn JM. Workers' compensation: top ten most controversial treatments. In: *IAIABC 32nd International Workers Compensation College.* Madison, WI: International Association of Industrial Accident Boards and Commissions; 2005. Ch. 6: 1-26.

2. Melhorn JM. Upper extremity: RTW by consensus documents. In: *8th Annual Occupational Orthopaedics and Workers' Compensation: A Multidisciplinary Perspective.* Rosemont, IL: American Academy of Orthopaedic Surgeons; 2006. Ch. 7: 187–218.

3. Vender MI, Kasdan ML, Truppa KL. Upper extremity disorders: a literature review to determine work-relatedness. *J Hand Surg [Am].* 1995;20A:534-541.

4. Goldman RH, Peters JM. The occupational and environmental health history. *JAMA.* 1981;246:2831-2836. Fukuda K, Straus SE, Hickie I, et al; Fukuda K, Straus SE, Hickie I, et al: The chronic fatigue syndrome: a comprehensive approach to its definition and study. International Chronic Fatigue Syndrome Study Group. Ann Intern Med 121:953-959, 1994. International Chronic Fatigue Syndrome Study Group. The chronic fatigue syndrome: a comprehensive approach to its definition and study. 1994;121:953-959.

5. Barsky AJ, Borus JF. Functional somatic syndromes. *Ann Intern Med.* 1999;130:910-921.

6. El-Hage W, Lamy C, Goupille P, et al. Fibromyalgia: a disease of psychic trauma. *Presse Med.* 2006; 35:1683-1689.

7. National Institute for Occupational Safety and Health. *Musculoskeletal Disorders and Workplace Factors: A Critical Review of Epidemiologic Evidence for Work-Related Musculoskeletal Disorders of the Neck, Upper Extremity, and Low Back.* Washington, DC: The National Academies Press.

8. Pearce JM. Myofascial pain, fibromyalgia or fibrositis? *Eur Neurol.* 2004;52:67-72.

9. Gerwin RD. A review of myofascial pain and fibromyalgia: factors that promote their persistence. *Acupunct Med.* 2005;23:121-134.

10. Kroenke K. Patients presenting with somatic complaints: epidemiology, psychiatric comorbidity and management. *Int J Methods Psychiatr Res.* 2003;12:34-43.

11. Staudenmayer H. Psychological treatment of psychogenic idiopathic environmental intolerance. *Occup Med.* 2000;15:627-646.

12. Velasco S, Ruiz MT, Alvarez-Dardet C. Attention models to somatic symptoms without organic cause: from physiopathologic disorders to malaise of women [in Spanish]. *Rev Esp Salud Publica.* 2006;80:317-333.

13. Pongratz DE, Spath M. Myofascial pain syndrome: frequent occurrence and often misdiagnosed [in German]. *Fortschr Med.* 1998;116:24-29.

14. Diakow PR. Differentiation of active and latent trigger points by thermography. *J Manipulative Physiol Ther.* 1992;15:439-441.

15. Gerwin RD, Shannon S, Hong CZ, et al. Interrater reliability in myofascial trigger point examination. *Pain.* 1997;69:65-73.

16. Fredericson M, Wolf C. Iliotibial band syndrome in runners: innovations in treatment. *Sports Med.* 2005;35:451-459.

17. Green BN, Johnson CD, Maloney A. Effects of altering cycling technique on gluteus medius syndrome. *J Manipulative Physiol Ther.* 1999;22:108-113.

18. Gregory PL, Biswas AC, Batt ME. Musculoskeletal problems of the chest wall in athletes. *Sports Med.* 2002;32:235-250.
19. Yap EC. Myofascial pain: an overview. *Ann Acad Med Singapore.* 2007;36:43-46.
20. Kirchhoff G, Kirchhoff C, Buhmann S, et al. A rare differential diagnosis to occupational neck pain: bilateral stylohyoid syndrome. *J Occup Med Toxicol.* 2006;1:14.
21. Sheon RP. Repetitive strain injury. 2: diagnostic and treatment tips on six common problems. The Goff Group. *Postgrad Med.* 1997;102:72-78, 81, 85 passim.
22. Rosen NB. Myofascial pain: the great mimicker and potentiator of other diseases in the performing artist. *Md Med J.* 1993;42:261-266.
23. Oliveira A, Gevirtz R, Hubbard D. A psycho-educational video used in the emergency department provides effective treatment for whiplash injuries. *Spine.* 2006;31:1652-1657.
24. Dommerholt J. Persistent myalgia following whiplash. *Curr Pain Headache Rep.* 2005;9:326-330.
25. Downs DG. Nonspecific work-related upper extremity disorders. *Am Fam Physician.* 1997;55:1296-1302.
26. Gallagher RM, Marbach JJ, Raphael KG, et al. Myofascial face pain: seasonal variability in pain intensity and demoralization. *Pain.* 1995;61:113-120.
27. Edwards J. The importance of postural habits in perpetuating myofascial trigger point pain. *Acupunct Med.* 2005;23:77-82.
28. Andersen JH, Gaardboe O. Musculoskeletal disorders of the neck and upper limb among sewing machine operators: a clinical investigation. *Am J Ind Med.* 1993;24:689-700.
29. Wolfe F, Smythe HA, Yunus MB, et al. The American College of Rheumatology 1990 Criteria for the Classification of Fibromyalgia: report of the Multicenter Criteria Committee. *Arthritis Rheum.* 1990;33:160-172.
30. Weir PT, Harlan GA, Nkoy FL, et al. The incidence of fibromyalgia and its associated comorbidities: a population-based retrospective cohort study based on International Classification of Diseases, 9th Revision codes. *J Clin Rheumatol.* 2006;12:124-128.
31. Staud R. Fibromyalgia pain: do we know the source? *Curr Opin Rheumatol.* 2004;16:157-163.
32. Neeck G, Crofford LJ. Neuroendocrine perturbations in fibromyalgia and chronic fatigue syndrome. *Rheum Dis Clin North Am.* 2000;26:989-1002.
33. Buskila D, Sarzi-Puttini P, Ablin JN. The genetics of fibromyalgia syndrome. *Pharmacogenomics.* 2007;8:67-74.
34. Lucas HJ, Brauch CM, Settas L, Theoharides TC. Fibromyalgia: new concepts of pathogenesis and treatment. *Int J Immunopathol Pharmacol.* 2006;19:5-10.
35. Anisman H, Baines MG, Berczi I, et al. Neuroimmune mechanisms in health and disease, 2: disease. *CMAJ.* 1996;155:1075-1082.
36. Park JH, Niermann KJ, Olsen N. Evidence for metabolic abnormalities in the muscles of patients with fibromyalgia. *Curr Rheumatol Rep.* 2000;2:131-140.
37. Gallinaro AL, Feldman D, Natour J. An evaluation of the association between fibromyalgia and repetitive strain injuries in metalworkers of an industry in Guarulhos, Brazil. *Joint Bone Spine.* 2001;68:59-64.

CHAPTER 11

38. Kivimaki M, Leino-Arjas P, Virtanen M, et al. Work stress and incidence of newly diagnosed fibromyalgia: prospective cohort study. *J Psychosom Res.* 2004;57:417-422.

39. Buskila D, Neumann L. Musculoskeletal injury as a trigger for fibromyalgia/ posttraumatic fibromyalgia. *Curr Rheumatol Rep.* 2000;2:104-108.

40. Waylonis GW, Ronan PG, Gordon C. A profile of fibromyalgia in occupational environments. *Am J Phys Med Rehabil.* 1994;73:112-115.

41. Fahn S, Eldridge R. Definition of dystonia and classification of the dystonic states. *Adv Neurol.* 1976;14:1-5.

42. Bressman S. Genetics of dystonia. *J Neural Transm Suppl.* 2006;70;489-495.

43. Jinnah HA, Hess EJ. A new twist on the anatomy of dystonia: the basal ganglia and the cerebellum? *Neurology.* 2006;67:1740-1741.

44. Lim VK, Altenmuller E, Bradshaw JL. Focal dystonia: current theories. *Hum Mov Sci.* 2001;20:875-914.

45. Hoppmann RA. Instrumental musicians' hazards. *Occup Med.* 2001;16:619-631.

46. Moreano B. Pianist's cramp and other musicians' diseases: suddenly the body does not play its part [in German]. *MMW Fortschr Med.* 2005;147:4-5.

47. Frucht SJ. Focal task-specific dystonia in musicians. *Adv Neurol.* 2004;94:225-230.

48. Schuppert M, Altenmuller E. Occupation-specific illnesses in musicians [in German]. *Versicherungsmedizin.* 1999;51:173-179.

49. Boonkongchuen P, Lees A. Case of torticollis occurring following electrical injury. *Mov Disord.* 1996;11:109-110.

50. Wilson FR, Wagner C, Homberg V. Biomechanical abnormalities in musicians with occupational cramp/focal dystonia. *J Hand Ther.* 1993;6:298-307.

51. Kaji R, Goto S, Tamiya G, et al. Molecular dissection and anatomical basis of dystonia: X-linked recessive dystonia-parkinsonism (DYT3). *J Med Invest.* 2005;52(suppl):280-283.

52. Crabb L. What is dystonia? *Prof Nurse.* 1994; 9:812-5.

53. Defazio G, Berardelli A, Abbruzzese G, et al. Possible risk factors for primary adult onset dystonia: a case-control investigation by the Italian Movement Disorders Study Group. *J Neurol Neurosurg Psychiatry.* 1998;64:25-32.

54. Maquet D, Demoulin C, Crielaard JM. Chronic fatigue syndrome: a systematic review. *Ann Readapt Med Phys.* 2006;49:337-347, 418-427.

55. Maoz D, Shoenfeld Y. Chronic fatigue syndrome [in Hebrew]. *Harefuah.* 2006;145:272-275.

56. Addington AM, Gallo JJ, Ford DE, Eaton WW. Epidemiology of unexplained fatigue and major depression in the community: the Baltimore ECA follow-up, 1981-1994. *Psychol Med.* 2001;31:1037-1044.

57. Natelson BH, Weaver SA, Tseng CL, Ottenweller JE. Spinal fluid abnormalities in patients with chronic fatigue syndrome. *Clin Diagn Lab Immunol.* 2005;12:52-55.

58. Huibers MJ, Kant IJ, Knottnerus JA, Bleijenberg G, Swaen GM, Kasl SV. Development of the chronic fatigue syndrome in severely fatigued employees: predictors of outcome in the Maastricht cohort study. *J Epidemiol Community Health.* 2004;58:877-882.

59. Huibers MJ, Kant IJ, Swaen GM, Kasl SV. Prevalence of chronic fatigue syndrome–like caseness in the working population: results from the Maastricht cohort study. *Occup Environ Med.* 2004;61:464-466.

60. Jason LA, Taylor SL, Johnson S, et al. Prevalence of chronic fatigue syndrome-related symptoms among nurses. *Eval Health Prof.* 1993;16:385-399.
61. Mounstephen A, Sharpe M. Chronic fatigue syndrome and occupational health. *Occup Med (Lond).* 1997;47:217-227.
62. Poulsen OM, Breum NO, Ebbehoj N, et al. Collection of domestic waste: review of occupational health problems and their possible causes. *Sci Total Environ.* 1995;170:1-19.
63. Tattam A. CFS: an occupational hazard for nurses? *Aust Nurs J.* 1994;2:21-22.
64. Romans S, Belaise C, Martin J, et al. Childhood abuse and later medical disorders in women: an epidemiological study. *Psychother Psychosom.* 2002;71:141-150.
65. Fisher L, Chalder T. Childhood experiences of illness and parenting in adults with chronic fatigue syndrome. *J Psychosom Res.* 2003;54:439-443.
66. Heim C, Wagner D, Maloney E, et al. Early adverse experience and risk for chronic fatigue syndrome: results from a population-based study. *Arch Gen Psychiatry.* 2006;63:1258-1266.
67. Auvenshine RC. Acute vs chronic pain. *Tex Dent J.* 2000;117:14-20.
68. Melhorn JM. Occupational orthopaedics: chronic musculoskeletal pain. In: Melhorn JM, DiPaola J, eds. *8th Annual Occupational Orthopaedics and Workers' Compensation: A Multidisciplinary Perspective.* Rosemont, IL: American Academy of Orthopaedic Surgeons; 2006.Ch. 2: 49-102.
69. Smith BH, Macfarlane GJ, Torrance N. Epidemiology of chronic pain, from the laboratory to the bus stop: time to add understanding of biological mechanisms to the study of risk factors in population-based research? *Pain.* 2007;127:5-10.
70. Cedraschi C, Allaz AF. How to identify patients with a poor prognosis in daily clinical practice. *Best Pract Res Clin Rheumatol.* 2005;19:577-591.
71. Burns JW, Sherman ML, Devine J, et al. Association between workers' compensation and outcome following multidisciplinary treatment for chronic pain: roles of mediators and moderators. *Clin J Pain.* 1995;11:94-102.
72. Knardahl S. Psychological and social factors at work: contribution to musculoskeletal disorders and disabilities. *G Ital Med Lav Ergon.* 2005;27:65-73.
73. Melhorn JM. Understanding and managing chronic non-malignant pain for the occupational orthopaedists. In: Melhorn JM, Strain RE Jr, eds. *Occupational Orthopaedics and Workers' Compensation: A Multidisciplinary Perspective.* Rosemont, IL: American Academy of Orthopaedics Surgeons; 2002;3-66.
74. Melhorn JM. The art of return to work (negotiating strategies). Presented at: 7th Annual WorkSafeBC Physicians' Education Conference; 2006; Victoria, BC, Canada: WorkSafeBC; 2006:1-65.
75. Eriksen J, Sjogren P. Epidemiological factors relating to long-term/chronic non-cancer pain in Denmark [in Danish]. *Ugeskr Laeger.* 2006;168:1947-1950.
76. Pope MH, Goh KL, Magnusson ML. Spine ergonomics, 2002;36(2)512-522.

CHAPTER 11

Suggested Reading

Han SC, Harrison P. Myofascial pain syndrome and trigger-point management. *Reg Anesth*. 1997;22:89-101.

Hubbard DR, Berkoff GM. Myofascial trigger points show spontaneous needle EMG activity. *Spine*. 1993;18:1803-1807.

Kruse RA Jr, Christiansen JA. Thermographic imaging of myofascial trigger points: a follow-up study. *Arch Phys Med Rehabil*. 1992;73:819-823.

Zautra AJ, Marbach JJ, Raphael KG, et al. The examination of myofascial face pain and its relationship to psychological distress among women. *Health Psychol*. 1995;14:223-231.

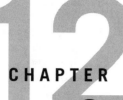

CHAPTER

Causation in Common Cardiovascular Problems

Elizabeth Genovese, MD and Mark H. Hyman, MD

This chapter reviews cardiovascular syndromes that have been commonly associated with occupational exposures. These include coronary artery disease (CAD), hypertension, cardiomyopathy, arrhythmias, and peripheral vascular disease, including venous thrombotic disease. A working knowledge of the evaluative testing for these conditions is found in many general internal medicine texts and has also been explored in Chapter 15 of *A Physician's Guide to Return to Work,* which readers are encouraged to review.[1]

Although there is a large body of literature regarding causation as it pertains to cardiovascular disease (CVD), most cardiovascular problems are not reflective of specific worksite factors. Indeed, even when there is a solid rationale for imputing the existence of a causal relationship between CVD and occupation, the workplace factor is rarely the sole cause of the disorder. Because one can not assess the contribution of occupational exposure to a given cardiovascular problem without knowing what other potentially etiologic factors were present, this chapter reviews commonly accepted causes of CVD and discusses the potential role of workplace factors in causing or contributing to injury. Special attention is given to relatively recent research into the effects of psychosocial factors, including stress, on cardiovascular risk. Infective endocarditis is not discussed; newly released guidelines are available for review.[2]

Cardiovascular Risk Factors

Common to the cardiovascular conditions are algorithms for assessing the impact of "conventional risk factors" and emerging literature on recently identified markers.[3] Caution must be exercised in identifying conditions or test abnormalities as representing true independent risk factors for CVD.[4,5]

Conventional Cardiovascular Risk Factors

Most evaluators identify advancing age, hypertension, diabetes mellitus, dyslipidemia, and cigarette smoking as traditional risk factors.[6,7] Closely articulated with these conditions are genetic risk, obesity, microalbuminuria, and lack of exercise.[1,8-10] Obesity is an important risk factor for CVD that also predicts general disability.[11,12] Obstructive sleep apnea, often caused by obesity, contributes to hypertension.[13] Black populations do not have increased genetic risk compared with white populations,[14] and genetics also do not predict whether an acute coronary syndrome will occur.[15] The metabolic syndrome has emerged as a diagnostic assimilation of the conventional risk factors and predicts development of CAD or diabetes (if not included in the definition), although not all agree on a precise definition.[16-18] Control of this constellation of metabolic risk factors seems to be uniquely controlled by the endocannabinoid system.[19] The metabolic syndrome has been noted occupationally in football lineman[20] and is associated with increased frailty.[21]

Poor diabetic control clearly raises the risk of CVD,[22] with a future heart attack as likely in a patient with diabetes as in one with a prior myocardial infarction.[23] Remediating the conventional or metabolic risk factors for CVD mandates dietary modification, exercise, weight loss, and, often, pharmacologic interventions. Most studies show a decrease in cardiovascular risk in conjunction with lifestyle modifications such as weight loss, dietary changes, and exercise, although this reduced risk is not found in all populations.[24-32] Once the diagnosis of coronary heart disease is made, secondary prevention of recurrence continues to require these same lifestyle interventions.[33,34] Although many of the conventional risk factors for heart disease can be reduced significantly by the effects of diet and exercise, the impact of lifestyle modification on hypertension is not as clear. Indeed, studies of the pathogenesis of hypertension continue to identify that the vast majority of cases do not have a clear cause.[35] The diabetic state seems to be primarily a genetically determined beta-cell impairment with an acquired environmental insulin resistance.[36-38] Various scoring systems based on these conventional risk factors have been developed to predict CVD[39,40]; these risk factors clearly account for most cases of cardiovascular disease[41,42] independent of any work-related factors.

Unconventional Cardiovascular Risk Factors

There is a growing body of medical literature identifying many novel risk factors for CVD, some of which are gaining greater acceptance in routine screening measures[1,4,43] (See Table 12-1 on p. 247). High levels of C-reactive protein, a nonspecific indicator for the known underlying inflammatory processes operating in CVD, have been associated with CAD; its value as a screening test is being scrutinized.[44-47] The concept of using a marker for systemic inflammation as a cardiovascular screening tool is consistent with reports in the literature demonstrating the risk of myocardial infarction (and stroke) to be highest during the first 3 days of systemic infection (after which it gradually decreases), presumably owing to concurrent inflammation or a prothrombotic effect of the infection.[48,49]

Alcohol consumption in moderate amounts (usually defined as fewer than two drinks per day for men, and one drink per day for women) seems to be protective against CVD; excess amounts contribute to it.[50-52] The relationship between coffee consumption and cardiac disease is complex because it has been shown to increase the risk of myocardial infarction and heart disease in a subgroup of patients who are slow caffeine metabolizers.[53,54] Other large prospective cohort

CHAPTER 12

studies have failed to demonstrate increased risk and have even demonstrated benefit, possibly owing to antioxidants found in coffee.[55-57] Antioxidant content is also the most likely explanation for the inverse relationship between cocoa,[58,59] black[60] or green[61] tea, and CVD. Combination therapy[62] or, possibly, only protease inhibitor antiretroviral therapy for human immunodeficiency virus infection,[63] cocaine,[64] environmental tobacco smoke,[65,66] psoriasis,[67] loss of height,[68] hormone replacement therapy using continuous conjugated equine estrogens and medroxyprogesterone,[69] selective estrogen receptor modulators,[70] testosterone deficiency,[71,72] migraine headaches,[73] and poor medical compliance [74] are associated with increased risk of cardiovascular, cerebrovascular, and/or vascular disease. Short-term hormone replacement therapy would seem to not increase CVD risk.[75] Nevertheless, guidelines for women now clearly emphasize the traditional approach of lifestyle modification.[76] Although the use of cyclooxygenase-2 inhibitors has been associated with CVD,[77] a recent meta-analysis indicated that nonselective nonsteroidal anti-inflammatory drugs, especially naproxen, have no significant adverse effect.[78] A siesta may lower the risk of CVD.[79] Air pollution has received significant growing attention as being etiologic not only in respiratory illness, but also as increasing the risk for CVD, with the particle size $PM_{2.5}$ being implicated in the pathogenesis.[80-86]

Occupational Risk Factors

Many occupational risk factors for ischemic CVD are present environmentally or reflect leisure activities. Separating occupational from nonoccupational risk factors can be difficult.

The relationship between exposure to carbon monoxide (CO) and CVD as a result of atmospheric pollution or passive inhalation of cigarette smoke has been described in the literature.[87-90] An association between the two due to work-related exposure is routinely described in standard occupational medicine textbooks.[91] For example, in a cohort of foundry workers followed up for 20 years, regular CO exposure was identified as one of the significant predictors of mortality from ischemic heart disease.[92] Levels of CO of 6% or higher were required to precipitate ischemia in people with known CAD.[93] Tunnel workers with higher CO exposure have shown increased risk of heart disease as opposed to bridge workers.[94] Myocardial infarction and decreased left ventricular ejection fraction have been described in people with normal coronary arteries and CO exposure.[95,96] Methylene chloride is a solvent that is converted metabolically to CO, and exposure to high levels is also associated with myocardial infarction. Alternatively, the maintenance of at least low endogenous levels of CO has a critical role in maintaining normal cardiovascular homeostasis.[97] Thus, although it is reasonable to describe high CO levels as a cause of acute cardiac dysfunction, the effect of long-term exposure on CVD has not been adequately studied.

The role of cadmium in atherosclerosis is attributed to cadmium-related prolif-eration of vascular smooth muscle.[98-100] Recent studies of carbon disulfide expo-sure have been consistent with findings described in earlier literature linking exposure to CVD,[101,102] although the size of this effect has been questioned.[103]

There is a large body of literature linking lead exposure to hypertension owing to its renal effects via alteration of the renin-angiotensin system and a direct effect on vascular smooth muscle.[104] Arsenic exposure due to contamination of drinking water or occupational sources has been linked to CAD and arrhythmias.[105-111]

Other occupational (and environmental) risk factors for CAD have been noted to include beryllium, organic solvents, organophosphates, and polycyclic aromatic compounds; however, research reports in the literature have not established a causal relationship with any of these substances.[112] Firefighters, who are often exposed to chemicals, as a cohort, have lower risk of heart disease but are at increased risk of death due to heart disease while performing duties of fire sup-pression or emergency response.[113] An association between noise exposure and hypertension has been noted[114,115]; however, the findings reported literature link-ing noise exposure to CAD have been mixed.[113, 116-118]

Stress, Psychosocial Factors, and Cardiovascular Risk

Uniform agreement would be expected regarding the relationship between expo-sure to acute stress through activation of the normal flight-or-fight mechanism and the development of a hypertensive response or myocardial ischemia.[119] An early onset of depression in myocardial infarction worsens outcomes,[120] whereas treatment or attention to stress and psychological factors, in particular depres-sion, generally has the opposite effect.[121-125] Psychosocial factors reflecting a poor childhood environment have been described as adversely affecting cardio-vascular risk, whereas pervasive positive personality factors can overcome poor environments or social support needs.[126-128]

Parallel research has explored the effects of chronic stress on cardiovascular risk. Our understanding of the mechanisms through which stress affects the previ-ously described biomarkers continues to evolve.[129] When examining the effects of chronic stress, Karasek,[130] Karasek et al,[131] and Theorell and Karasek[132] identi-fied job strain and stress as the combination of high psychological demands and low decision latitude, described as the "demand control" model. Psychological demands were determined by the quantity of work, mental requirements with time constraints, i.e., working fast and hard; and decision latitude was the ability to use personal creativity and skills to make decisions about one's work. Thus, higher psychological demands and lower decision latitude translated into the highest risk group. Siegrist[133] and Peter and Siegrist[134,135] offered an alternative model with characteristics similar to that of the model developed by Karasek and colleagues, called the "effort reward" model. In this model, job strain and stress were products of high job effort with low social reward. Belkic et al[136,137] expanded this area with research confirming the deleterious effects of certain types of stress within the work environment. However, the effects vary from person to person and are difficult to distinguish from nonoccupational stressors. For example, although job strain has been described as having its strongest impact on people from lower socioeconomic groups who display hostility, anger, time urgency or impatience, depression, and/or anxiety,[138,139] there is also a significant body of literature linking nonoccupational stressors to CVD.[140-144] The work of Landsbergis et al[145] indicates that the potential effects of stress, regardless of cause, on cardiovascular risk were equal to those of cholesterol and cigarettes. Part of the effect of stress was mediated by the effect on hypertension, with job strain, age, and body mass index the only reliable predictors. The average effect of job strain seemed to be an increase in the systolic blood pressure of **7** mm Hg but may be as high as 12 mm Hg (P.L. Schnall, personal verbal communication, ACOEM Meeting, Los Angeles, May 8, 2006). Baroreceptor reflex sensitivity may be the mechanism through which psychosocial factors affect CVD.[146-148] Shift work has also been associated with worsened cardiovascular risk,[149] although it is unclear whether shift work is a proxy for job stress.

Of equal note are the recent data on the effect of the same stress and psychosocial factors on diabetes. As was the case for CVD, the normal mechanisms of an acute stress response are well characterized and affect the blood glucose level through the pituitary-adrenal axis.[150] Data are showing an association among job stress, psychosocial factors, and worsened diabetic control.[151-153] Parallel to the hypertension and CVD discussion, treatment of depression seems to improve management of diabetes.[154] Similarly, shift work has been shown to be associated with risk of diabetes.[155] The bulk of the literature on these topics consists of observational studies that do not fully control for the impact of confounding factors on assessed outcomes. In particular, the degree of stress or other psychosocial factors that affect compliance with recommended lifestyle modifications and disease-management strategies is often unclear. Psychosocial and behavioral factors have also been invoked to explain the neuroendocrine adaptations that accompany the metabolic syndrome. Although the conclusion was that chronic stress may contribute to the metabolic syndrome, the need for confirmatory prospective studies is described.[156,157]

Observational and case-control studies suggest a possible relationship between chronic stress and hypertension, diabetes, or CVD in certain subpopulations.[158-162] Nevertheless, the impact of job stress as opposed to that of other risk factors is difficult to quantify. As noted previously, it would be reasonable to state that people who have more difficulty tolerating stress will experience problems in both their personal and occupational situations.

The degree to which stress develops as a result of work most likely represents a complex interaction between the work and nonwork environments superimposed on personality attributes and patterns of neurochemical response that reflect genetics, early childhood environment, socioeconomic strata, and the degree to which exposed people experience health care inequalities and inadequate social support.[113,163,164] Regardless, the weight of the evidence from all lines of research suggests that chronic stress contributes to cardiovascular risk in certain subgroups of people through hypertension or alterations in the adrenal cortical and medullary systems.

Cardiomyopathy and Heart Failure (HF)

There are many excellent reviews of the pathophysiology and the impact of cardiomyopathy and congestive heart failure (HF).[165] The current terminology favors using the term *heart failure* to reflect that many cases are not classic HF; a classification scheme has been advanced.[166] The risk of developing HF is substantial[167,168] and typically reflects the same risk factors that result in CAD.[169] Molecular[170] and familial genetic risks[171] are important considerations in this population. The ischemic process is usually followed by loss of functioning myocytes, fibrosis, and remodeling, with mitral valve involvement a greater risk.[172] The most common cause of nonischemic cardiomyopathy, up to 45% of cases, is alcohol use.[33] Methamphetamines are also etiologic in the development of HF.[173] Additional causes are hypertension, infection, and collagen vascular disease. Higher dosages of thiazolidinediones (antihyperglycemic agents) have also been shown to cause HF.[174] Probably the best-described occupational exposure would be cobalt.[175,176] An important diagnostic tool to differentiate cardiomyopathy from other causes of dyspnea, aid in monitoring treatment, and apply toward future clinical outcomes prediction is the NT-proB-type natriuretic peptide.[177-182] When determining the level of impairment and causes of cardiac limitations in HF, there is no relationship between the impairment and limitations and ejection fraction, cardiac index, pulmonary capillary wedge pressure, and peak metabolic performance (maximum oxygen consumption).[183] The actual cause of decreased exercise tolerance is skeletal muscle myopathy[184] due to an oxidative shift and altered mitochondrial content.[185] Optimal treatment will moderate risk and complications.[186-188] Recent literature has been focused on *heart failure with preserved ejection fraction,* formerly called *diastolic heart failure* or *diastolic dysfunction.*[192] The patients tend to have, at best, only marginally better survival than the systolic heart failure group [HF group][189-191] and require differential identification and treatment.[192]

Arrhythmia, Syncope, and Heart Rate Variability

The correlation of symptoms with rhythm disturbances is not straightforward,[193] with the risk for developing a specific rhythm disturbance influenced by the presence of underlying heart disease.[194] Thus, people at greatest risk of developing an arrhythmia generally have known ischemia or structural or congenital conduction system abnormalities. Other causes of arrhythmia include conventional and unconventional risk factors such as cigarette smoking, obesity, physical inactivity, alcohol consumption,[33] caffeine, stress, illicit drug use, cold preparations, weight loss products, and herbal products.[195] Air pollution can also trigger arrhythmias.[196]

A specific example of a disorder resulting in an arrhythmia is sick sinus syndrome, which is commonly idiopathic but has also been associated with many intrinsic structural diseases of the heart.[197] Although patients with left atrial enlargement, increased left ventricular wall thickness, HF, diabetes, thyroid disease, advancing age, excessive alcohol consumption,[198] obesity,[199,200] corticosteroid use,[201] bisphosphonate use,[202] and hypertension or elevated pulse pressure are at risk for atrial fibrillation,[203-205] there is a growing recognition of genetic and familial risk factors.[206-208] Most first-detected episodes resolve spontaneously.[209] Atrial fibrillation seems to be associated with an increased future risk of CAD in women.[210]

Ventricular arrhythmias are associated with risk profiles similar to those seen in patients with cardiomyopathy. Left ventricular dysfunction and long-term alcohol use also confer risk for persistent ventricular arrhythmias.[33,211] Syncope can be caused by the previously noted conventional risk factors[212]; however, the most common cause is unknown, followed by vasovagal causes.[213]

Heart rate variability (HRV) is the variation and fluctuation of the heartbeat in relation to the mean heart rate. The heart rate is controlled by the autonomic nervous system, and it can be a useful measure to identify patients at risk for arrhythmias.[214] Some risk factors affect the cardiovascular system through the HRV pathway. Heart rate variability is influenced by age, body temperature, posture, and respiratory rate.[215] Normally, HRV decreases during the day and increases at night. However, decreased daytime variability has been demonstrated in myocardial infarction,[216] HF,[217] diabetes,[218] renal failure,[219] stroke,[220] obesity,[221] alcoholism,[222] and air pollution.[223] Exposure to CO has also been shown to alter cardiac autonomic regulation.[224] Given the relationship between depression and outcome in patients after myocardial infarction and the potential use of depression as a possible useful indicator for functional somatic syndromes, the findings of decreased HRV in depression[225,226] are even more provocative.

Although acute intoxication due to occupational exposure to high ambient levels of CO or other exposures might reasonably result in arrhythmia, cigarette smoking, inadequate diet, excessive alcohol intake, and inactivity are modifiable behavioral risk factors implicated as the true, underlying, most common reasons for death in the United States, with sudden cardiac death due to arrhythmia the final common pathway.[227,228] Of patients who die of sudden cardiac death, 75% have CAD and more than 50% have acute thrombosis but never had previous symptoms. In people older than 35 years, the left ventricular ejection fraction remains the most important predictor of sudden cardiac death, whereas in patients younger than 35 years, hypertrophic cardiomyopathy accounts for the most common cause of sudden cardiac death.[229]

Peripheral Arterial Disease and Venous Thromboembolism

Peripheral arterial disease (PAD) is generally caused by the same CVD risk factors described earlier in the chapter.[230] The frequency of detection of PAD is increasing, especially in elderly people.[235] The occurrence of PAD has significant overlap with other CVD risk factors and conditions.[232] The natural history of the disease shows significant adverse events.[233,234] Peripheral arterial disease has been associated with urinary levels of cadmium, lead, barium, cobalt, cesium, molybdenum, antimony, thallium, and tungsten.[235]

The Virchow triad of stasis, trauma, and hypercoagulable states forms the classic risk factors for deep venous thrombosis (DVT). The first two criteria are often easily identified by history. Relevant coagulation disturbances include protein C deficiency, protein S deficiency, antithrombin lll deficiency, the presence of factor V Leiden, a prothrombin gene mutation, an elevated homocysteine level, the presence of antiphospholipid antibodies, or elevated levels of factors VIII, IX, and XI. These coagulation disturbances all must be identified via laboratory testing and cannot be accurately measured in patients who have already started warfarin therapy following an episode of venous thrombosis. The development of venous thrombosis generally reflects the interplay between genetic and environmental factors.[236] Nevertheless, when DVT develops following work-related trauma, after a work-related operative procedure, or owing to enforced inactivity in conjunction with a work injury, it is reasonable to indicate the thrombosis is work-related. Guidelines to assist in DVT diagnosis have been published.[237]

Assessing the Contribution
of Occupational Risk Factors to CVD

Genetics, hyperlipidemia, obesity, diabetes, hypertension, and inactivity are the classic, and primary, risk factors for CVD; genetics, obesity, lack of exercise, and in certain people, dietary factors are risk factors for hypertension. Although other "unconventional" risk factors may also be contributory, their relative impact is smaller. Many studies now explore risk factors for cardiovascular morbidity and mortality[238,239] in worker populations, confirming that these unique exposures are risk factors.[240,241] The role of chemical and toxic exposures has been decreasing (as a consequence of workplace precautions), whereas the precise impact of novel workplace cardiovascular risks such as job stress, and, to a lesser extent noise, remains under investigation. The degree to which they contribute to disease in a given person will vary and will be based on the number and severity of other risk factors superimposed on the degree to which the person is uniquely sensitive to these stressors. Special attention is required for evaluating public safety personnel, owing to not only jurisdictional laws that establish presumed risk, but also the acute, rare, high-demand nature of the work duties.[242-245]

In a person with an acute cardiovascular event, it is generally possible to ascertain whether workplace factors contributed to its occurrence at a specific time. The impact of these factors on later cardiovascular disease requires one to ascertain to what degree later disease reflects residual deficits from the "injury" or the effect of the underlying risk factors without which the acute stressor would not have had an impact. It would seem unreasonable to attribute CVD or hypertension to only workplace stress or noise in workers who clearly have other, more significant risk factors for disease. It would also seem unreasonable to attribute CVD to workplace stress in workers who do not have jobs characterized by high demand and low decision latitude. Although there seems to be a subgroup of workers for whom stress-related factors are sufficiently relevant as to invoke them as at least, in part, causal, optimal means of identifying these workers and separating the effects of these factors from those of other risk factors have not been fully identified.

TABLE 12-1	Examples of Risk Factors That Have Achieved "Independence" in Statistical Models for Various Cardiovascular Outcomes After Controlling for Other Cardiovascular Risk Factors*⁴

Risk Factors

Demographic factors
  Age
  Sex
  Race
Family history
  Myocardial infarction or premature
    atherosclerosis
  Sudden death
Anthropometric measures
  Body mass index
  Waist-to-hip ratio
Anatomic cardiovascular factors
  Carotid intima media thickness
  Left ventricular dysfunction
  Known coronary artery atherosclerosis
  Cerebrovascular disease
  Peripheral vascular disease
Markers of fluid/electrolyte homeostasis
  Angiotensin II
  B-type natriuretic peptide
  Genetic polymorphisms affecting the
    renin-angiotensin-aldosterone system
Electrocardiographic (ECG) findings
  Atrial fibrillation
  Left ventricular hypertrophy
  Bundle branch blocks
  Frequent premature ventricular
    contractions
  Nonsustained ventricular tachycardia
  QT-interval dispersion
  Other ECG abnormalities
Hemostatic variables
  Fibrinogen
  Tissue-type plasminogen activator
  Thrombomodulin
  Von Willebrand factor
  Plasminogen activator inhibitor-1
    (PAI-1)
  Factor VII
  Factor VIII
  D-dimer
  Plasmin-antiplasmin complex
  Platelet volume
  Platelet aggregation
  Genetic polymorphisms affecting
    thrombomodulin, platelet membrane
    glycoproteins, and PAI-1 activity

  Aspirin resistance
  CD40 ligand
Autonomic nervous system variables
  Heart rate variability
  Levels of catecholamines at rest or with
    exercise
  Heart rate recovery after exercise
  Chronotropic response to exercise
Markers of myocardial strain or damage
  Cardiac enzymes
Renal parameters
  Serum creatinine
  Dialysis-dependent renal failure
  Urinary albumin excretion or proteinuria
Pharmacotherapy
  Treatment with digoxin
  Treatment with antiarrhythmic drugs
Markers of oxidative stress
  Genetic polymorphisms in glutathione
    metabolism
  Low activity of glutathione peroxidase 1
  Advanced oxidation products
  Nitrotyrosine
Psychological factors
  Depression
  Inadequate relaxation
  Lack of social support
  Lack of a sense of personal control
  Impaired sleep
Lifestyle factors
  Tobacco abuse
  Dietary factors
  Physical exercise habits
  Alcohol consumption
Inflammatory factors
  Macrophage colony stimulating factor
  C-reactive protein
  Interleukin 6
  Lipoprotein-associated phospholipase A_2
  Tumor necrosis factor α
  Presence of connective tissue disease
  Pregnancy-associated plasma protein
  Genetic polymorphisms of matrix
    metaloproteinase
  Myeloperoxidase
  Placental growth factor

CHAPTER 12

TABLE 12-1 Examples of Risk Factors That Have Achieved "Independence" in Statistical Models for Various Cardiovascular Outcomes After Controlling for Other Cardiovascular Risk Factors[*4] (continued)

Physiologic parameters
  Systolic blood pressure
  Diastollic blood pressure
  Arterial pulse pressure
  Diurnal blood pressure variability
  Aortic pulse-wave velocity
  Peak workload with exercise
  Ventilatory response to exercise
  Arterial elasticity
Metabolic conditions and markers
  Plasma glucose
  Insulin resistance and hyperinsulinemia
  Diabetes mellitus
  Triglycerides
  Nonesterified (free) fatty acid
    concentrations
  High-density lipoprotein cholesterol
  Low-density lipoprotein (LDL) and LDL
    particle size
  Fasting cholesterol
  Lipoprotein(a)
  Leptin
  Adiponectin
  Genetic polymorphisms affecting lipid
    metabolism

Vascular endothelium-related factors
  Endothelin
  Endothelium-mediated vasodilatation
  Genetic polymorphisms in nitric oxide
    metabolism
Miscellaneous
  Lewis blood group phenotype
  γ-Glutamyltransferase
  serum calcium
  Serum potassium
  Albumin
  Soluble adhesion molecules
  Homocysteine and genetic
    polymorphisms of homocysteine
    metabolism
  Uric acid
  Serum ferritin
  Choline
  Headaches
  Enterolactone
  Sleep-disordered breathing
  Infection with *Mycoplasma pneumoniae*

ARCH INTERN MED. JAN. 24, 2005; 165; p: 141.

References

1. Hyman MH. Working with common cardiopulmonary problems. In: Talmage JB, Melhorn JM, eds. *A Physician's Guide to Return to Work.* Chicago, IL: AMA Press; 2005:233-266.
2. Wilson W, Taubert KA, Gewitz M, et al. Prevention of infective endocarditis: guidelines from the American Heart Association. *Circulation.* 2007. www. circahajournals.org. Accessed April 23, 2007.
3. Ridker PM, Buring JE, Rifai N, et al. Development and validation of improved algorithms for the assessment of global cardiovascular risk in women. *JAMA.* 2007;297:611-619.
4. Brotman DJ, Walker E, Lauer MS, et al. In search of fewer independent risk factors. *Arch Intern Med.* 2005;165:138-145.
5. Ware JH. The limitations of risk factors as prognostic tools. *N Engl J Med.* 2006;355:2615-2617.
6. Greenland P, Knoll MD, Stamler J, et al. Major risk factors as antecedents of fatal and nonfatal coronary heart disease events. *JAMA.* 2003;290:891-897.
7. Khot UN, Khot MB, Bajzer CT, et al. Prevalence of conventional risk factors in patients with coronary heart disease. *JAMA.* 2003;290:898-904.
8. Murabito JM, Pencina MJ, Nam RH, et al. Sibling cardiovascular disease as a risk factor for cardiovascular disease in middle-aged adults. *JAMA.* 2005;294:3117-3123.
9. Visscher TLS, Rissanen A, Seidell JC, et al. Obesity and unhealthy life-years in adult Finns. *Arch Intern Med.* 2004;164:1413-1420.
10. Moore LL, Visioni AJ, Qureshi MM, et al. Weight loss in overweight adults and the long-term risk of hypertension. *Arch Intern Med.* 2005;165:1298-1303.
11. Ostbye T, Dement JM, Krause KM. Obesity and workers' compensation. *Arch Intern Med.* 2007;167:766-773.
12. Al Snih S, Ottenbacher KJ, Markides KS, et al. The effect of obesity on disability vs. mortality in older Americans. *Arch Intern Med.* 2007;167:774-780.
13. Haentjens P, Van Meerhaeghe A, Moscariello A, et al. The impact of continuous positive airway pressure on blood pressure in patients with obstructive sleep apnea syndrome. *Arch Intern Med.* 2007;167:757-765.
14. Hozawa A, Folsom AR, Sharrett R, et al. Absolute and attributable risks of cardiovascular disease incidence in relation to optimal and borderline risk factors. *Arch Intern Med.* 2007;167:573-579.
15. Morgan TM, Krumholz HM, Lifton RP, et al. Nonvalidation of reported genetic risk factors for acute coronary syndrome in a large-scale replication study. *JAMA.* 2007;297:1551-1561.
16. Ferreira I, Twisk JWR, van Mechlen W. et al. Development of fatness, fitness, and lifestyle from adolescence to the age of 36 years. *Arch Intern Med.* 2005;165:42-48.
17. Galassi A, Reynolds K, He J. Metabolic syndrome and risk of cardiovascular disease: a meta-analysis. *Am J Med.* 2006;119:812-819.
18. Wannamethee SG, Shaper AJ, Lennon L, Morris RW. Metabolic syndrome vs Framingham Risk Score for prediction of coronary heart disease, stroke, and type 2 diabetes mellitus. *Arch Intern Med.* 2005;165:2644-2650.

CHAPTER 12

19. Smith SC. Modifying cardiovascular and metabolic risk factors: the role of the endocannabinoid system and cannabinoid receptors. *Am J Med.* 2007; 120(3A): S1-S34.

20. Damlo S. Retired lineman at high risk of cardiovascular problems. *Am Fam Physician.* 2007;75:969.

21. Barzilay JI, Blaum C, Moore T, et al. Insulin resistance and inflammation as precursors of frailty. *Arch Intern Med.* 2007;167:635-641.

22. Skyler JS. Diabetic complications: the importance of glucose control. *Endocrinol Metab Clin North Am.* 1996;25:243-254.

23. Haffner SM, Lehto S, Ronnemaa T, et al. Mortality from coronary heart disease in subjects with type 2 diabetes and in nondiabetic subjects with and without prior myocardial infarction. *N Engl J Med.* 1998;339:229-234.

24. Gulati M, Paddey DK, Armsdorf MF, et al. Exercise capacity and the risk of sudden death in women: the St. James Women Take Heart Project. *Circulation.* 2003;108:1554-1559.

25. Batty GD, Lee IM. Physical activity and coronary heart disease. *BMJ.* 2004;328:1089-1090.

26. Rauramaa R, Halonen P, Vaisanen SB, et al. Effects of aerobic physical exercise on inflammation and atherosclerosis in men: the DNASCO Study: a six-year randomized, controlled trial. *Ann Intern Med.* 2004;140:1007-1014.

27. Chobanian AV, Bakris GL, Black HR, et al. The seventh report of the Joint National Committee on Prevention, Detection, Evaluation, and Treatment of High Blood Pressure. *JAMA.* 2003;289:2560-2572.

28. Hill JO. What to do about the metabolic syndrome. *Arch Intern Med.* 2003;163:395-397.

29. Katzmarzyk PT, Church TS, Blair SN. Cardiorespiratory fitness attenuates the effects of the metabolic syndrome on all-cause and cardiovascular disease mortality in men. *Arch Intern Med.* 2004;164:1092-1097.

30. Turner RC, Cull CA, Frighi V, et al. Glycemic control with diet, sulfonylurea, metformin, or insulin in patients with type 2 diabetes mellitus. *JAMA.* 1999;281:2005-2012.

31. Diabetes Prevention Program Research Group. Reduction in the incidence of type 2 diabetes with lifestyle intervention or metformin. *N Engl J Med.* 2002;346:393-403.

32. Hu G, Lindstrom J, Valle TT, et al. Physical activity, body mass index, and risk of type 2 diabetes in patients with normal or impaired glucose regulation. *Arch Intern Med.* 2005;164:892-896.

33. Gatti JC. Exercise-based rehabilitation for coronary heart disease. *Am Fam Physician.* 2004;70:485-486.

34. Franco OH, de Laet C, Peeters A, et al. Effects of physical activity on life expectancy with cardiovascular disease. *Arch Intern Med.* 2005;165:2355-2360.

35. Oparil S, Zaman MA, Calhoun DA. Pathogenesis of hypertension. *Ann Intern Med.* 2003;139:761-776.

36. Polonsky KS, Sturis J, Bell GI. Non–insulin dependent diabetes mellitus: a genetically programmed failure of the beta cell to compensate for insulin resistance. *N Engl J Med.* 2005;334:777-783.

37. Gerich JE. Contributions of insulin-resistance and insulin-secretory defects to the pathogenesis of type 2 diabetes mellitus. *Mayo Clin Proc.* 2003;78:447-456.

38. Rother KI. Diabetes treatment: bridging the divide. *N Engl J Med.* 2007;356: 1499-1501.

39. Gidding SS, McMahan A, McGIll HC, et al. Prediction of coronary artery calcium in young adults using the pathobiological determinants of atherosclerosis in youth (PDAY) risk score. *Arch Intern Med.* 2006;166:2341-2347.

40. Woloshin S, Schwartz LM, Welch HG, et al. Risk charts: putting cancer in context. *J Natl Cancer Inst.* 2002;94:800-803.

41. Gundy SM, D'Agostino RB, Mosca L, et al. Cardiovascular risk assessment based on US cohort studies: findings from a National Heart, Lung, Blood Institute workshop. *Circulation.* 2001;104:491-496.

42. Stamler J. Low risk and the "no more than 50%" myth/dogma. *Arch Intern Med.* 2007;167:537-539.

43. Wang TJ, Gona P, Larson MG, et al. Multiple biomarkers for the prediction of first major cardiovascular events and death. *N Engl J Med.* 2006;355:2631-2639.

44. Smith GD, Timpson N, Lawlor DA. C-reactive protein and cardiovascular disease risk: still an unknown quantity? *Ann Intern Med.* 2006;145:70-72.

45. Lloyd-Jones DM, Liu K, Greenland P. Assessment of C-reactive protein in risk prediction for cardiovascular disease. *Ann Intern Med.* 2006;145:35-42.

46. Cook NR, Buring JE, Ridker PM. The effect of including C-reactive protein in cardiovascular risk prediction models in women. *Ann Intern Med.* 2006; 145:21-29.

47. Sesso HD, Buring JE, Rifai N. C-reactive protein and the risk of developing hypertension. *JAMA.* 2003;290:2945-2951.

48. Ridker PM, Hennekens CH, Buring JE, Kundsin R, Shih J. Baseline IgG antibody titers to *Chlamydia pneumoniae, Helicobacter pylori,* herpes simplex virus, and cytomegalovirus and the risk for cardiovascular disease in women. *Ann Intern Med.* 1999;131:573-577.

49. Smeeth L, Thomas SL, Hall AJ, Hubbard R, Farrington P, Vallance P. Risk of myocardial infarction and stroke after acute infection or vaccination. *N Engl J Med.* 2004; 351:2611-2618.

50. National institute on Alcohol Abuse and Alcoholism, US Department of Health and Human Services. *Tenth Special Report to the US Congress on Alcohol and Health.* Washington, DC: US Government. June 2000.

51. Beulens JWJ, Rimm EB, Ascherio A, et al. Alcohol consumption and risk for coronary heart disease among men with hypertension. *Ann Intern Med.* 2007146:10-19.

52. Castelnuovo AD, Costanzo S, Bagnardi V, et al. Alcohol dosing and total mortality in men and women. *Arch Intern Med.* 2006;166:2437-2445.

53. Cornelis MC, El-Sohemy A, Kabagambe EK, et al. Coffee, cyp1a2 genotype, and risk of myocardial infarction. *JAMA.* 2006;295:1135-1141.

54. Baylin A, Hernandez-Diaz S, Kabagambe EK, Siles X, Campos H. Transient exposure to coffee as a trigger of a first nonfatal myocardial infarction. *Epidemiology.* 2006;17:506-511.

55. Lopez-Garcia E, van Dam RRM, Willett WC, et al. Coffee consumption and coronary heart disease in men and women: a prospective cohort study. *Circulation.* 2006; 113:2045-2053.

56. Greenberg JA, Dunbar CC, Schnoll R, Kokolis R, Kokolis S, Kossotis J. Caffeinated beverage intake and the risk of heart disease mortality in the elderly: a prospective analysis. *Am J Clin Nutr.* 2007;85:392-398.

CHAPTER 12

57. Cornelis MC, El-Sohemy A. Coffee, caffeine, and coronary heart disease. *Curr Opin Lipidol.* 2007;18:13-19.

58. Buijesse B, Feskens EJM, Kok FL, et al. Cocoa intake, blood pressure, and cardiovascular mortality. *Arch Intern Med.* 2006;166:411-417.

59. Taubert D, Roesen R, Schomig E. Effect of cocoa and tea intake on blood pressure. *Arch Intern Med.* 2007;167:626-634.

60. Gardner EJ, Ruxton CH, Leeds AR. Black tea: helpful or harmful? A review of the evidence. *Eur J Clin Nutr.* 2007;61:3-18.

61. Kuriyama S, Shimazu T, Ohmori K, et al. Green tea consumption and mortality due to cardiovascular disease, cancer, and all causes in Japan: the Ohsaki study. *JAMA.* 2006;296:1255-1265.

62. Friis-Møller N, Sabin C, Weber R, et al; and the Data Collection on Adverse Events of Anti-HIV Drugs (DA) Study Group. Combination antiretroviral therapy and the risk of myocardial infarction. *N Engl J Med.* 2003;349:1993-2003.

63. The DAD Study Group. Class of antiretroviral drugs and the risk of myocardial infarction. *N Engl J Med.* 2007; 356:1723-1735.

64. Lai S, Lima JAC, Lai H, et al. Human immunodeficiency virus 1 infection, cocaine, and coronary calcification. *Arch Intern Med.* 2005;165:690-695.

65. Otsuka R, Watanabe H, Hirata K, et al. Acute effects of passive smoking on the coronary circulation in healthy young adults. *JAMA.* 2001; 286:436-441.

66. Stranges S, Bonner MR, Fucci F, et al. Lifetime cumulative exposure to secondhand smoke and risk of myocardial infarction in never smokers. *Arch Intern Med.* 2006;166:1961-1967.

67. Gelfand JM, Neimann Al, Shin DB, et al. Risk of myocardial infarction in patients with psoriasis. *JAMA.* 2006; 296:1735-1741.

68. Wannamethee SG, Shaper AG, Lennon L, Whincup PH. Height loss in older men; associations with total mortality and incidence of cardiovascular disease. *Arch Intern Med.* 2006; 166:2546-2552.

69. Manson JE, Hsia J, Johnson KC, et al. Estrogen plus progestin and the risk of coronary heart disease. *N Engl J Med.* 2003; 349:523-534.

70. Barrett-Connor E, Mosca L, Collins P, et al. Effects of raloxifene on cardiovascular events and breast cancer in postmenopausal women. *N Engl J Med.* 2006;355:125-137.

71. Jones RD, Nettleship JE, Kapoor D, Jones HT, Channer KS. Testosterone and atherosclerosis in aging men: purported association and clinical implications. *Am J Cardiovasc Drugs.* 2005;5:141-154.

72. Rosano GM, Cornoldi A, Fini M. Effects of androgens on the cardiovascular system. *J Endocrinol Invest.* 2005;28(3 suppl):32-38.

73. Kurth T, Gaziano JM, Cook NR, et al. Migraine and risk of cardiovascular disease in men. *Arch Intern Med.* 2007;167:795-801.

74. Simpson SH, Eurich DT, Majumdar SR, et al. A meta-analysis of the association between the adherence to drug therapy and mortality. *BMJ.* 2006;333:15-21.

75. Rossouw JE, Prentice RL, Manson JE, et al. Postmenopausal hormone therapy and risk of cardiovascular disease by age and years since menopause. *JAMA.* 2007;297:1465-1477.

76. Mosca L, Banka CL, Benjamin EJ, et al. 2007 guidelines preventing cardiovascular disease in women. American Heart Association. www.circ.ahajournal.org. Accessed April 23, 2007.

77. Kearney PM, Baigent C, Godwin J, et al. Do selective cyclo-oxygenase-2 inhibitors and traditional non-steroidal anti-inflammatory drugs increase the risk of atherosclerosis? *BMJ.* 2006;332:1302-1308.

78. Salpeter SR, Gregor P, Ormiston TM, et al. Meta-analysis: cardiovascular events associated with nonsteroidal anti-inflammatory drugs. *Am J Med.* 2006;119:552-559.

79. Naska A, Oikonomou E, Trichopoulou A, et al. Siesta in healthy adults and coronary mortality in the general population. *Arch Intern Med.* 2007;167:296-301.

80. Dominici F, Peng RD, Bell Ml, et al. Fine particulate air pollution and hospital admission for cardiovascular and respiratory diseases. *JAMA.* 2006;295:1127-1134.

81. Nel A. Air pollution–related illness: effects of particles. *Science.* 2005;308:804-807.

82. Sun Q, Wang A, Jin X, et al. Long-term air pollution exposure and acceleration of atherosclerosis and vascular inflammation in an animal model. *JAMA.* 2005;294:3003-3010.

83. Peters A. When myocardial infarction comes out of the not-so-blue air. *Circulation.* 2006;114:2430-2431.

84. Brook RD, Franklin B, Cascio W, et al. Air pollution and cardiovascular disease. *Circulation.* 2004;109:2655-2671.

85. Chuang KJ, Chan CC, Shiao GM, et al. Associations between submicrometer particles exposures and blood pressure and heart rate in patients with lung function impairments. *J Occup Environ Med.* 2005;47:1093-1098.

86. Miller KA, Siscovick DS, Sheppard L, et al. Long-term exposure to air pollution and incidence of cardiovascular events in women. *N Engl J Med.* 2007;356:447-458.

87. Maitre A, Bonneterre V, Huillard L, Sabatier P, de Gaudemaris R. Impact of urban atmospheric pollution on coronary disease. *Eur Heart J.* 2006;27:2275-2284.

88. Hedley AJ, McGhee SM, Repace JL, et al. Risks for heart disease and lung cancer from passive smoking by workers in the catering industry. *Toxicol Sci.* 2006;90:539-548.

89. McGrath JJ. Biological plausibility for carbon monoxide as a copollutant in PM epidemiologic studies. *Inhal Toxicol.* 2000;12(suppl 4):91-107.

90. Burnett RT, Cakmak S, Raizenne ME, et al. The association between ambient carbon monoxide levels and daily mortality in Toronto, Canada. *J Air Waste Manag Assoc.* 1998;48:689-700.

91. Zenz C, Dickerson OB, Horvath EP, eds. *Occupational Medicine.,* 3rd ed. St Louis, MO: Mosby; 1994.

92. Koskela RS, Mutanen P, Sorsa JA, Klockars M. Factors predictive of ischemic heart disease mortality in foundry workers exposed to carbon monoxide. *Am J Epidemiol.* 2000;152:628-632.

93. Adams KF, Koch G, Chatterjee B, et al. Acute elevation of blood carboxyhemoglobin to 6% impairs exercise performance and aggravates symptoms in patients with ischemic heart disease. *J Am Coll Cardiol.* 1988;12:900-909.

94. Stern FB, Halperin WE, Homung RW, et al. Heart disease mortality among bridge and tunnel officers exposed to carbon monoxide. *Am J Epidemiol.* 1988;128:1276-1288.

95. Marius-Nunez AL. Myocardial infarction with normal coronary arteries after acute exposure to carbon monoxide. *Chest.* 1990;97:491-494.

96. Kalay N, Ozdogru I, Cetinkaya Y, et al. Cardiovascular effects of carbon monoxide poisoning. *Am J Cardiol.* 2007;99:322-324.

CHAPTER 12

97. Durante W, Johnson FK, Johnson RA. Role of carbon monoxide in cardiovascular function. *J Cell Mol Med.* 2006;10:672-686.
98. Fujiwara Y, Watanabe S, Kaji T. Promotion of cultured vascular smooth muscle cell proliferation by low levels of cadmium. *Toxicol Lett.* 1998; 94:175-180.
99. Kishimoto T, Oguri T, Yamabe S, Tada M. Effect of cadmium injury on growth and migration of cultured human vascular endothelial cells. *Hum Cell.* 1996;9:43-48.
100. Kaji T, Ohkawara S, Inada M, Yamamoto C, Sakamoto M, Kozuka H. Alteration of glycosaminoglycans induced by cadmium in cultured vascular smooth muscle cells. *Arch Toxicol.* 1994;68:560-565.
101. Kotseva K, Braeckman L, De Bacquer D, Bulat P, Vanhoorne M. Cardiovascular effects in viscose rayon workers exposed to carbon disulfide. *Int J Occup Environ Health.* 2001;7:7-13.
102. Takebayashi T, Nishiwaki Y, Uemura T, et al. A six year follow up study of the subclinical effects of carbon disulphide exposure on the cardiovascular system. *Occup Environ Med.* 2004;61:127-134.
103. Sulsky SI, Hooven FH, Burch MT, Mundt KA. Critical review of the epidemiological literature on the potential cardiovascular effects of occupational carbon disulfide exposure. *Int Arch Occup Environ Health.* 2002;75:365-380.
104. Greenberg M, ed *Occupational, Industrial and Environmental Toxicology.* St. Louis. MO: Mosby; 1997.
105. Engel RR Smith AH. Arsenic in drinking water and mortality from vascular disease: an ecologic analysis in 30 counties in the United States. *Arch Environ Health.* 1994;49:418-427.
106. Chiou HY, Huang WI, Su CL, Chang SF, Hsu YH, Chen CJ. Dose-response relationship between prevalence of cerebrovascular disease and ingested inorganic arsenic. *Stroke.* 1997;28:1717-1723.
107. Lewis DR, Southwick JW, Ouellet-Hellstrom R, Rench J, Calderon RL. Drinking water arsenic in Utah: a cohort mortality study. *Environ Health Perspect.* 1999;107:359-365.
108. Tsai SM, Wang TN, Ko YC. Mortality for certain diseases in areas with high levels of arsenic in drinking water. *Arch Environ Health.* 1999;54:186-193.
109. Tseng CH, Chong CK, Tseng CP, et al. Long-term arsenic exposure and ischemic heart disease in arseniasis-hyperendemic villages in Taiwan. *Toxicol Lett.* 2003;137:15-21.
110. Mastin JP. Environmental cardiovascular disease. *Cardiovasc Toxicol.* 2005; 5:91-94.
111. Ferreccio C, Sancha AM. Arsenic exposure and its impact on health in Chile. *J Health Popul Nutr.* 2006;24:164-175.
112. European Heart Network. Social factors, work, stress and cardiovascular disease prevention in the European Union.. Brussels, Belgium: European Heart Network. July 1998.
113. Kales SN, Soteriades ES, Christophi CA, et al. Emergency duties and deaths from heart disease among firefighters in the United States. *N Engl J Med.* 2007;356:1207-1215.
114. Penney PJ, Earl CE. Occupational noise and effects on blood pressure: exploring the relationship of hypertension and noise exposure in workers. *AAOHN J.* 2004;52:476-480.

CHAPTER 12

115. Chang TY, Jain RM, Wang CS, et al. Effects of occupational noise exposure on blood pressure. *J Occup Environ Med.* 2003;45:1289-1296.
116. Virkkunen H, Harma M, Kauppinen T, Tenkanen L. The triad of shift work, occupational noise, and physical workload and risk of coronary heart disease. *Occup Environ Med.* 2006;63:378-386.
117. Virkkunen H, Kauppinen T, Tenkanen L. Long-term effect of occupational noise on the risk of coronary heart disease. *Scand J Work Environ Health.* 2005;31:291-299.
118. Melamed S, Kristal-Boneh E, Froom P. industrial noise exposure and risk factors for cardiovascular disease: findings from the CORDIS Study. *Noise Health.* 1999;1:49-56.
119. Habib KE, Gold PW, Chrousos GP. Neuroendocrinology of stress. *Endocrinol Metab Clin North Am.* 2001;30:695-728.
120. Parashar S, Rumsfeld JS, Spertus JA, et al. Time course of depression and outcome of myocardial infarction. *Arch Intern Med.* 2006;166:2035-2043.
121. Kivimaki M, Ferrie JE, Brunner E, et al. Justice at work and reduced risk of coronary heart disease among employees. *Arch Intern Med.* 2005;165:2245-2251.
122. Blumenthal JA, Sherwood A, Babyak MA, et al. Effects of exercise and stress management training on markers of cardiovascular risk in patients with ischemic heart disease. *JAMA.* 2005;293:1626-1634.
123. Writing Committee for the ENRICHD Investigators. Effects of treating depression and low perceived social support on clinical events after myocardial infarction: the Enhancing Recovery in Coronary Heart Disease Patients (ENRICHD) Randomized Trial. *JAMA.* 2003;289:3106-3116.
124. Whooley MA. Depression and cardiovascular disease. *JAMA.* 2006;295:2874-2881.
125. Lesperance F, Frasure-Smith N, Koszycki D, et al. Effects of citalopram and interpersonal psychotherapy on depression in patients with coronary artery disease. (CREATE). *JAMA.* 2007;297:367-379.
126. Kittleson MM, Meoni LA, Wang NY, et al. Association of childhood socioeconomic status with subsequent coronary heart disease in physicians. *Arch Intern Med.* 2006; 166:2356-2361.
127. Giltay EJ, Kamphuis NH, Kalmijn S, et al. Dispositional optimism and the risk of cardiovascular death. *Arch Intern Med.* 2006;166:431-436.
128. Mookadam F, Arthur H. Social support and its relationship to morbidity and mortality after acute myocardial infarction. *Arch Intern Med.* 2004;164:1514-1518.
129. Clays E, DeBacquer D, Delanghe J, et al. Associations between dimensions of job stress and biomarkers of inflammation and infection. *J Occup Environ Med.* 2005;47:878-883.
130. Karasek RA. Job demands, job decision latitude, and mental strain: implications for job redesign. *Admin Sci Quart.* 1979;24:285-308.
131. Karasek RA, Theorell T, Schwartz J, et al. Job, psychological factors and coronary heart disease. *Adv Cardiol.* 1982;29:62-67.
132. Theorell T, Karasek RA. Current issues relating to psychosocial job strain and cardiovascular disease research. *J Occup Health Psychol.* 1996;1:9-26.
133. Siegrist J. Adverse health effects of high-effort/low-reward conditions. *J Occup Health Psychol.* 1996;1:27-41.

CHAPTER 12

134. Peter R, Siegrist J. Threat to occupational status control and cardiovascular risk. *Isr J Med Sci.* 1996;32:179-184.

135. Peter R, Siegrist J. Chronic work stress, sickness absence, and hypertension in middle-managers: general or specific sociological explanations? *Soc Sci Med.* 1997;45:1111-1120.

136. Belkic KL, Schnall PL, Landsbergis PA, et al. Hypertension at the workplace: an occult disease? The need for worksite surveillance. In: Theorell T, ed. *Everyday biological stress mechanisms. (Adv Psychosom Med).* New York, NY: S Karger AG, 2001; 22:116-138.

137. Belkic KL, Landsbergis PA, Schnall PL, et al. Is job strain a major source of cardiovascular disease risk? *Scand J Work Environ Health.* 2004; 30:85-128.

138. Knox SS, Weidner G, Adelman A, et al. Hostility and physiological risk in the National Heart, Lung, and Blood Institute Family Heart Study. *Arch Intern Med.* 2004;164:2442-2448.

139. Bunker SJ, Colquhoun DM, Esler MD, et al. Stress and coronary heart disease: psychosocial risk factors. *Med J Aust.* 2003;178:272-276.

140. Pickering TG. Mental stress as a causal factor in the development of hypertension and cardiovascular disease. *Curr Hypertens Rep.* 2001;3:249-254.

141. Tennant C. Life stress and hypertension. *J Cardiovasc Risk.* 2001;8:51-56.

142. Garcia-Vera MP, Sanz J, Labrador FJ. Blood pressure variability and stress management training for essential hypertension. *Behav Med.* 2004;30:53-62.

143. Armario P, del Rey RH, Martin-Baranera M, Almendros MC, Ceresuela LM, Pardell H. Blood pressure reactivity to mental stress task as a determinant of sustained hypertension after 5 years of follow-up. *J Hum Hypertens.* 2003;17:181-186.

144. Williams RB, Barefoot JC, Schneiderman N. Psychosocial risk factors for cardiovascular disease: more than one culprit at work. *JAMA.* 2003;290:2190-2192.

145. Landsbergis PA, Schnall PL, Pickering TG, et al. Lower socioeconomic status among men in relation to the association between job strain and blood pressure. *Scand J Work Environ Health.* 2003;29:206-215.

146. Ducher M, Cerutti C, Chatellier G, Fauvel JP. Is high job strain associated with hypertension genesis? *Am J Hypertens.* 2006;19:694-700.

147. Ducher M, Fauvel JP, Cerutti C. Risk profile in hypertension genesis: a five-year follow-up study. *Am J Hypertens* 2006;19:775-781.

148. Lucini D, Mela GS, Malliani A, Pagnani M. Impairment in cardiac autonomic regulation preceding arterial hypertension in humans: insights from spectral analysis of beat-by-beat cardiovascular variability. *Circulation.* 2002;106: 2673-2679.

149. Van Amelsvoort LGPM, Schouten EG, Kok FJ. Impact of one year of shift work on cardiovascular disease risk factors. *J Occup Environ Med.* 2004;46:699-706.

150. Mizock BA. Alterations in carbohydrate metabolism during stress: a review of the literature. *Am J Med.* 1995;96:75-84.

151. Lynen F, Moreau M, Pelfrene E, et al. Job stress and prevalence of diabetes: results from the belstressstudy. *Arch Public Health.* 2003; 61:75-90.

152. Kumari M, Head J, Marmot M. Prospective study of social and other risk factors in the incidence of type 2 diabetes in the Whitehall ll study. *Arch Intern Med.* 2004;164:1873-1880.

CHAPTER 12

153. Carnethon MR, Biggs ML, Barzilay JI, et al. Longitudinal association between depressive symptoms and incident type 2 diabetes mellitus in older adults. *Arch Intern Med.* 2007;167:802-807.
154. Jackson JL, DeZee K, Berbano E. Can treating depression improve disease outcomes? *Ann Intern Med.* 2004;140:1054-1056.
155. Suwazono Y, Sakata K, Okubo Y, et al. Long-term longitudinal study on the relationship between alternating shift work and the onset of diabetes mellitus in male Japanese workers. *J Occup Environ Med.* 2006; 48:455-461.
156. Brunner EJ, Hemingway H, Walker BR, et al. Adrenocortical, autonomic, and inflammatory causes of the metabolic syndrome: nested case-control study. *Circulation.* 2002;106:2659-2665.
157. Hjemdahl P. Stress and the metabolic syndrome: an interesting but enigmatic association. *Circulation.* 2002;106:2634-2636.
158. Ranjit N, Diez-Roux AV, Shea S, et al. Psychosocial factors and inflammation in the multi-ethnic study of atherosclerosis. *Arch Intern Med.* 2007;167:174-181.
159. al'Absi M, Wittmers LE Jr. Enhanced adrenocortical responses to stress in hypertension-prone men and women. *Ann Behav Med.* 2003;25:25-33.
160. Harshfield GA, Grim CE. Stress hypertension: the "wrong" genes in the "wrong" environment. *Acta Physiol Scand Suppl.* 1997;640:129-132.
161. Sherwood A, Hinderliter AL, Light KC. Physiological determinants of hyperreactivity to stress in borderline hypertension. *Hypertension.* 1995;25:384-390.
162. Clays E, Leynen F, De Bacquer D, et al. High job strain and ambulatory blood pressure in middle-aged men and women from the Belgian job stress study. *J Occup Environ Med.* 2007;49:360-367.
163. Rozanski A, Blumenthal JA, Kaplan J. Impact of psychosocial factors on the pathogenesis of cardiovascular disease and implications for therapy. *Circulation.* 1999;99:2192-2217.
164. Kanjilal S, Gregg EW, Cheng YJ, et al. Socioeconomic status and trends in disparities in 4 major risk factors for cardiovascular disease among US adults, 1971-2002. *Arch Intern Med.* 2006;166:2348-2355.
165. Jessup M, Brozena S. Heart failure. *N Engl J Med.* 2003;348:2007-1018.
166. Hunt SA, Abraham WT, Chin MH, et al. ACC/AHA 2005 Guideline Update for the Diagnosis and Management of Chronic Heart Failure in the Adult: a report of the American College of Cardiology/American Heart Association Task Force on Practice Guidelines. *Circulation.* 2005;112:e154-e235. http://www.acc.org/clinical/guidelines/failure/index.pdf. Accessed December 17, 2006.
167. Lloyd-Jones DM, Larson MG, Leip EP, et al. Lifetime risk for developing congestive heart failure: the Framingham heart study. *Circulation.* 2002;106:3068-3072.
168. Levy D, Kenchaiah S, Larson MG, et al. Long-term trends in the incidence of and survival with heart failure. *N Engl J Med.* 2002;347:1397-1402.
169. Devereux RB, Roman MJ, Paranicas M, et al. A population-based assessment of left ventricular systolic dysfunction in middle-aged and older adults: the strong heart study. *Am Heart J.* 2001;141:439-446.
170. Small KM, Wagoner LE, Levin AM, Kardia SL, Liggett SB. Synergistic polymorphisms of beta1- and alpha2C-adrenergic receptors and the risk of congestive heart failure. *N Engl J Med.* 2002;347:1135-1142.

CHAPTER 12

171. Lee DS, Pencina MJ, Benjamin EJ, et al. Association of parental heart failure with risk of heart failure in offspring. *N Engl J Med.* 2006;355:138-147.

172. Aronson D, Goldsher N, Zukermann R, et al. Ischemic mitral regurgitation and risk of heart failure after myocardial infarction. *Arch Intern Med.* 2006;166: 2362-2368.

173. Yeo KK, Wijetunga M, Ito H, et al. The association of methamphetamine use and cardiomyopathy in young patients. *Am J Med.* 2007;120:165-171.

174. DREAM Investigators. Diabetes reduction assessment with ramipril and rosiglitazone. *Lancet.* 2006;368:1096-1105.

175. Barceloux DG. Cobalt. *J Toxicol Clin Toxicol.* 1999;37:201-206.

176. Seghizzi P, D'Adda F, Borleri D, Barbic F, Mosconi G. Cobalt myocardiopathy: a critical review of literature. *Sci Total Environ.* 1994;150:105-109.

177. Morrow DA, de Lemos JA, Blazing MA, et al. Prognostic value of serial B-type natriuretic peptide testing during follow-up of patients with unstable coronary artery disease. *JAMA.* 2005;294:2866-2871.

178. Battaglia M, Pewsner D, Juni P, et al. Accuracy of B-type natriuretic peptide tests to exclude congestive heart failure. *Arch Intern Med.* 2006;166:1073-1080.

179. Doust J, Lehman R, Glasziou P. The role of BNP testing in heart failure. *Am Fam Physician.* 2006;74:1893-1898.

180. Rothenbacher D, Koenig W, Brenner H. Comparison of N-terminal pro-B-natriuretic peptide, C-reactive protein, and creatinine clearance for prognosis in patients with known coronary heart disease. *Arch Intern Med.* 2006;166: 2455-2460.

181. De Lemos JA. The latest and greatest new biomarkers. *Arch Intern Med.* 2006;166:2428-2430.

182. Bibbins-Domingo K, Gupta R, Na B, et al. N-terminal fragment of the prohormone brain-type natriuretic peptide (NT-proBNP), cardiovascular events, and mortality in patients with stable coronary heart disease. *JAMA.* 2007;297: 169-176.

183. Wilson JR, Rayos G, Yeoh TK, et al. Dissociation between exertional symptoms and circulatory function in patients with heart failure. *Circulation.* 1995;92:47-53.

184. Mancini DM, Wilson JR, Bolinger L, et al. In vivo magnetic resonance spectroscopy measurement of deoxymyoglobin during exercise in patients with heart failure: demonstration of abnormal muscle metabolism despite adequate oxygenation. *Circulation.* 1994;90:500-508.

185. Drexler H, Riede U, Munzel T, et al. Alterations of skeletal muscle in chronic heart failure. *Circulation.*1992;85:1751-1759.

186. Desai AS, Fang JC, Maisel WH, Baughman KL. Implantable defibrillators for the prevention of mortality in patients with nonischemic cardiomyopathy. *JAMA.* 2004;292:2874-2879.

187. Amabile CM, Spencer AP. Keeping your patients with heart failure safe. *Arch Intern Med.* 2004;164:709-720.

188. Tandon P, McAlister FA, Tsuyuki RT, et al. The use of beta-blockers in a tertiary heart failure clinic. *Arch Intern Med.* 2004;164:769-774.

189. Owan TE, Hodge DO, Herges RM, et al. Trends in prevalence and outcome of heart failure with preserved ejection fraction. *N Engl J Med.* 2006;355:251-259.

190. Bhatia RS, Tu JV, Lee DS, et al. Outcome of heart failure with preserved ejection fraction in a population-based study. *N Engl J Med.* 2006;355:260-269.

CHAPTER 12

191. Aurigemma GP. Diastolic heart failure: a common and lethal condition by any name [editorial]. *N Engl J Med.* 2006;355:308-310.
192. Satpathy C, Mishra TK, Satpathy R, Satpathy HK, Barone E. Diagnosis and management of diastolic dysfunction and heart failure. *Am Fam Physician.* 2006;73:841-846.
193. Barsky AJ. Palpitations, arrhythmias and awareness of cardiac activity. *Ann Intern Med.* 2001;134:832-837.
194. Rubart M, Zipes DP. Genesis of cardiac arrhythmias: electrophysiologic considerations. In: Braunwald E., ed: *Heart Disease: A Textbook of Cardiovascular Medicine.* 6th ed. Philadelphia, PA: WB Saunders; 2001.
195. Abbott AV. Diagnostic approach to palpitations. *Am Fam Physician.* 2005;71: 743-750.
196. Berger A, Zareba W, Schneider A, et al. Runs of ventricular and supraventricular tachycardia triggered by air pollution in patients with coronary heart disease. *J Occup Environ Med.* 2006;48:1149-1158.
197. Adan V, Crown LA. Diagnosis and treatment of sick sinus syndrome. *Am Fam Physician.* 2003;67:1725-1732.
198. Frost L, Vetergaard P. Alcohol and risk of atrial fibrillation or flutter. *Arch Intern Med.* 2004;164:1993-1998.
199. Frost L, Hune LJ, Vestergaard P. Overweight and obesity as risk factors for atrial fibrillation or flutter: the Danish Diet, Cancer, and Health Study. *Am J Med.* 2005;118:489-495.
200. Dublin S, French B, Glazer NL, et al. Risk of new-onset atrial fibrillation in relation to body mass index. *Arch Intern Med.* 2006;166:2322-2328.
201. Van der Hooft CS, Heeringa J, Brusselle GG, et al. Corticosteroids and the risk of atrial fibrillation. *Arch Intern Med.* 2006;165:1016-1020.
202. Rosen CJ. Postmenopausal osteoporosis. *N Engl J Med.* 2005;353:595-603.
203. Benjamin EJ, Levy D, Vaziri SM, et al. Independent risk factors for atrial fibrillation in a population-based cohort: the Framingham Heart Study. *JAMA.* 1994;271:840-844.
204. Vaziri SM, Larson MG, Benjamin EJ, et al. Echocardiographic predictors of nonrheumatic atrial fibrillation; the Framingham Heart Study. *Circulation.* 1994;89:724-730.
205. Mitchell GF, Vasan RS, Keyes MJ, et al. Pulse pressure and the risk of new-onset atrial fibrillation. *JAMA.* 2007;297:709-715.
206. Fox CS, Parise H, D'Agostino RB, et al. Parental atrial fibrillation as a risk factor for atrial fibrillation in offspring. *JAMA.* 2004;291:2851-2855.
207. Olson TM, Michels VV, Ballew JD, et al. Sodium channel mutations and susceptibility to heart failure and atrial fibrillation. JAMA.2005;293:447-454.
208. Gollob MH, Jones DL, Krahn AD, et al. Somatic mutations in the connexin 40 gene (GJA5) in atrial fibrillation. *N Engl J Med.* 2006;354:2677-2688.
209. Dixon BJ, Bracha Y, Loecke SW, et al. Principal atrial fibrillation discharges by the new ACC/AHA/ESC classification. *Arch Intern Med.* 2005;165:1877-1881.
210. Miyasaka Y, Barnes ME, Gersh BJ, et al. Coronary ischemic events after first atrial fibrillation: risk and survival. *Am J Med.* 2007;120:357-363.
211. Miller JM, Zipes DP. Management of the patient with cardiac arrhythmias. In: Braunwald E., ed: *Heart Disease: A Textbook of Cardiovascular Medicine.* 6th ed. Philadelphia, PA: WB Saunders; 2001.

212. Ebell MH. Syncope: initial evaluation and prognosis. *Am Fam Physician.* 2006;74:1367-1370.

213. Soteriades ES, Evans JC, Larson MG, et al. Incidence and prognosis of syncope. *N Engl J Med.* 2002;347:878-885.

214. Dreifus LS, Agarwal JB, Botvinick EH, et al. Heart rate variability for risk stratification of life-threatening arrhythmias. J Am Coll Cardiol.1993; 22:948-50. Cardiovascular Technology Assessment Committee, American College of Cardiology. 1993.

215. Task Force of the European Society of Cardiology and the North American Society of Pacing and Electrophysiology. Heart rate variability: standards of measurement, physiological interpretation, and clinical use. *Circulation.* 1996;93:1043-1065.

216. Tsuji H, Larson MG, Venditti FJ, et al. Impact of reduced heart rate variability on risk for cardiac events: the Framingham Heart Study. *Circulation.* 1996;94:2850-2855.

217. Sopher SM, Smith ML, Eckberg DL, Fritsch JM, Dibner-Dunlap ME. Autonomic pathophysiology in heart failure: carotid baroreceptor-cardiac reflexes. *Am J Physiol.* 1990;259(3 pt 2):H689-H696.

218. Burger AJ, Aronson D. Effect of diabetes mellitus on heart rate variability in patients with congestive heart failure. *Pacing Clin Electrophysiol.* 2001;24:53-59.

219. Axelrod S, Lishner M, Oz O, et al. Spectral analysis of fluctuations in heart rate: an objective evaluation of autonomic nervous control in chronic renal failure. *Nephron.*1987;45:202-206.

220. Korpelianen JT, Sotaniemi KA, Huikuri HV, et al. Circadian rhythm of heart rate variability is reversibly abolished in ischemic stroke. *Stroke.* 1997;28:2150-2154.

221. Sajadieh A, Nielsen OW, Rasmussen V, et al. Increased heart rate and reduced heart-rate variability are associated with subclinical inflammation in middle-aged and elderly subjects with no apparent heart disease. *Eur Heart J.* 2004;25:363-370.

222. Malpas SC, Whiteside EA, Maling TJ. Heart rate variability and cardiac autonomic function in men with chronic alcohol dependence. *Br Heart J.* 1991;65:84-88.

223. Chen JC, Stone PH, Verrier RL, González-Hermosillo JA, et al. Personal coronary risk profiles modify autonomic nervous system responses to air pollution. *J Occup Environ Med.* 2006;48:1133-1142.

224. Riojas-Rodriguez H, Escamilla-Cejudo JA, et al. Personal PM2.5 and CO exposures and heart rate variability in subjects with known ischemic heart disease in Mexico City. *J Expo Sci Environ Epidemiol.* 2006;16:131-137.

225. Carney RM, Blumenthal JA, Freedland KE, et al. Low heart rate variability and the effect of depression on post–myocardial infarction mortality. *Arch Intern Med.* 2005;165:1486-1491.

226. Martinez-Lavin M, Hermosillo AG, Rosas M, et al. Circadian studies of autonomic nervous balance in patients with fibromyalgia: a heart rate variability analysis. *Arthritis Rheum.* 1998;41:1966-1971.

227. Goldenberg I, Jonas M, Tenenbaum A. et al. Current smoking, smoking cessation, and the risk of sudden cardiac death in patients with coronary artery disease. *Arch Intern Med.* 2003;163:2301-2305.

228. Mokdad AH, Marks JS, Stroup DF, et al. Actual causes of death in the United States, 2000. *JAMA.* 2004;291:10:1238-1245.

229. Myerburg RJ, Castellanos A. Cardiac arrest and sudden cardiac death. In: Zipes D, ed. *Braunwald's Heart Disease: A Textbook of Cardiovascular Medicine.* 7th ed. New York, NY: Saunders; 2005.
230. Wilson JF, Laine C, Goldmann D. In the clinic: peripheral arterial disease. *Ann Intern Med.* 2007;146:ITC3-1-ITC3-16.
231. Hiatt WR, Hoag S, Hamman RF. Effect of diagnostic criteria on the prevalence of peripheral arterial disease: the San Luis Valley diabetes study. *Circulation.* 1995;91:1472-1479.
232. Bhatt DL, Steg PG, Ohman EM, et al. International prevalence, recognition, and treatment of cardiovascular risk factors in outpatients with atherothrombosis. *JAMA.* 2006;295:180-189.
233. Weitz JI, Byrne J, Clagett GP, et al. Diagnosis and treatment of chronic arterial insufficiency of the lower extremities: a critical review. *Circulation.* 1996;102:3026-3049.
234. Steg PG, Bhatt DL, Wilson PW, et al. One year cardiovascular event rates in outpatients with atherothrombosis. *JAMA.* 2007;297:1197-1206.
235. Navas-Acien A, Selvin E, Sharrett AR, Calderon-Aranda E, Silbergeld E, Guallar E. Lead, cadmium, smoking, and increased risk of peripheral arterial disease. *Circulation.* 2004;109:3196-3201.
236. Brouwer JLP, Veeger NJGM, Kluin-Nelemans HC, et al. The pathogenesis of venous thromboembolism: evidence for multiple interrelated causes. *Ann Intern Med.* 2006;145:807-815.
237. Qaseem A, Snow V, Barry P, et al. Current diagnosis of venous thromboembolism in primary care: a clinical practice guideline from the American Academy of Family Physicians and the American College of Physicians. *Ann Intern Med.* 2007;146:454-458.
238. Lee DJ, Fleming LE, Gomez-Marin O, et al. Morbidity ranking of US workers employed in 206 occupations: the National Health Interview Survey (NHIS) 1986-1994. *J Occup Environ Med.* 2006;48:117-134.
239. Brechon F, Czernichow P, Leroy M, et al. Chronic diseases in self-employed French workers. *J Occup Environ Med.* 2005;47:909-915.
240. Ahola K, Honkonen T, Kivimaki M, et al. Contribution of burnout to the association between job strain and depression: the Health 2000 study. *J Occup Environ Med.* 2006;48:1023-1030.
241. Arena VC, Padiyar KR, Burton WN, et al. The impact of body mass index on short-term disability in the workplace. *J Occup Environ Med.* 2006;48:1118-1124.
242. Goldberg RL, Spilberg SW, Weyers SG, et al. *Medical Screening Manual for California Law Enforcement.* California Commission on Peace Officer Standards and Training (POST); Sacramento, CA:2004.
243. Holder JD, Stallings LA, Peeples L, et al. Firefighter heart presumption retirements in Massachusetts 1997-2004. *J Occup Environ Med.* 2006;48:1047-1053.
244. Hessl SM, Miller RJ, eds. Law enforcement worker health. *Clin Occup Environ Med.* 2003;3.
245. NFPA 1582 Standard on Medical Requirements for Fire Fighters and Information for Fire Department Physicians 2000 Edition. Quincy, MA: National Fire Protection Assn; 2000.

CHAPTER 12

CHAPTER 13

Causation in Common Pulmonary Problems

Elizabeth Genovese, MD, and Mark H. Hyman, MD

This chapter reviews the more common clinical syndromes encountered in work-related pulmonary evaluations and how to best evaluate whether they have been caused by specific occupational exposures. There are hundreds of substances potentially capable of leading to pulmonary symptoms or disease. It is not possible to provide an in-depth discussion of the evidence basis supporting the classification of each of these as possible pulmonary toxins or irritants. Instead, this chapter aims to familiarize clinicians with exposures and toxins that have been associated with respiratory disease and provide a general framework for assessing causal relationships between actual or putative exposures and respiratory disease. Detailed information about various toxins can be found at the Hazardous Substance Data Bank section of the Web site for Toxnet (http://toxnet.nlm.nih.gov/cgi-bin/sis/htmlgen?HSDB), the National Institute for Occupational Safety and Health (NIOSH) Web site(http://www.cdc.gov/niosh//topics/), Agency for Toxic Substances and Disease Registry Web site (http://www.atsdr.cdc.gov/), and the Haz-Map Web site (http://hazmap.nlm.nih.gov).

Evaluative testing for pulmonary conditions can include X-rays, spiral computed tomographic scanning, magnetic resonance imaging, and serologic or immunologic testing. However, pulmonary function tests (PFTs) are mandatory in the evaluation of most types of pulmonary disease because they allow quantification of lung function. Particularly for asthma, the forced vital capacity (FVC), forced expiratory volume in the first second of expiration (FEV_1), FEV_1/FVC, or forced expiratory flow $(FEF)_{25\%-75\%}$ (midexpiratory phase) can be used to assess the extent and reversibility (response to bronchodilators) of obstructive disease, whereas the FVC and the diffusing capacity of the lung for carbon monoxide (DLCO) can be used to evaluate the severity of restrictive disease. Bronchoprovocation testing with the potentially causative factor (especially in cases of reactive airways dysfunction syndrome [RADS]; see "Occupational Asthma") or nonspecific agents such as methacholine or histamine can be used to make a diagnosis of occupational asthma when symptoms are intermittent and in response to specific inhalations and when PFT results are unclear. Further information about the appropriate use of tests in the evaluation of occupational pulmonary disorders is available in most occupational medicine textbooks and also in Chapter 15 of *A Physician's Guide to Return to Work*, which readers are encouraged to review.[1]

Pulmonary Risk Factors

Cough, wheezing, and the clinical impression of pulmonary disease may reflect conditions such as congestive heart failure or pulmonary emboli or extrathoracic causes such as rhinitis with postnasal drip or gastroesophageal reflux disease.[2] Although infections are the most common cause of pulmonary symptoms,[3] work-related pulmonary disease is predominantly the result of inhalational exposures. It is often difficult to assess whether a given pulmonary condition is work-related because the degree to which a given inhalational exposure results in disease not only reflects the intensity, duration, and type of exposure, but also varies based on host factors such as genetic susceptibility, comorbid conditions, and lifestyle factors and habits (e.g., cigarette smoking). The concentration, durability, and chemical properties (reactivity) of the substance involved are also relevant; in cases of exposure to asbestos and manufactured vitreous fibers, information about fiber length and width relates to their penetrance and persistence.

The vast majority of work-related pulmonary conditions consequently require measurable environmental determinations, sometimes in conjunction with sequential testing of pulmonary function, to ascertain whether there has been sufficient exposure to affect the lungs.[4] This area of investigation overlaps with important toxicology principles.

For exposure, the best standards and methods of evaluation are those promulgated by the American Conference of Governmental Industrial Hygienists (http://www.acgih.org). In particular, the group's biological exposure indices and threshold limit values are more frequently evaluated and updated than data from the Agency for Toxic Substances and Disease Registry, the Environmental Protection Agency, the Centers for Disease Control and Prevention Third National Report on Human Exposure to Environmental Chemicals,[5] and the permissible exposure limits defined by NIOSH. Biologic monitoring of these exposures requires a clear understanding of the underlying principles.[6]

For workplace risk assessment, the *NIOSH Pocket Guide to Chemical Hazards*[7] provides a concise summary of toxicologic information. In particular, respirable particles must be smaller than 5 μm to enter the lungs, with 2- to 5-μm particles able to reach the trachea and bronchi and particles smaller than 2 μm able to reach terminal respiratory units.[8] Of importance in evaluation of respirable exposures is the distance of the worker from the source; the area tested should usually be within 2 ft of the worker's area.[9]

The greatest threat to personal lung health is from tobacco inhalation.[10,11] Although it is customary to quantitate tobacco use in terms of pack-years, the variation in cigarette type and inhalational habits does not permit more than an approximation for potential lung injury.[12] Data show that smoking is associated with decreased worker productivity.[13] Of growing recognition and concern are the pulmonary effects of air pollution on all people and in all countries.[14-17] People seem to have genetic susceptibility to the effects of air pollution.[18] The majority of the US population is skin-test-positive to at least one environmental allergen.[19] This fact increases the difficulty in determining the relative contribution of work-related and non–work-related factors to the genesis of symptoms in people with multiple risk factors or exposures.

Occupational Pulmonary Diseases

The common categories of occupational pulmonary diseases include occupational asthma with latency, occupational asthma without latency (also called Irritant asthma or RADS), hypersensitivity pneumonitis, inhalational fever, and fibrotic lung disorders (pneumoconiosis). Certain cancers (such as mesothelioma and bronchogenic lung carcinoma) and chronic obstructive pulmonary disease (COPD) can also be caused by occupational exposures.

General Considerations for Asthma

Also known as reactive airways disease, bronchospasm, and irritable airways disease, asthma is currently viewed as a growing epidemic.[20,21] Although occupational and environmental factors can clearly be causal, literature and clinical experience identify genetic risk in asthma.[22,23] The development of asthma in children as a consequence of exposure to air pollution is a sentinel warning of a growing epidemic because many will carry this diagnosis into adulthood.[24] In addition, indoor home exposures are also strongly linked to asthma,[25] as is obesity.[26] Athletes have an increased prevalence of asthma because increased ventilation during performance of their sport can enhance inhalation of allergens and irritants,[27] and exercise-induced asthma is well described.[28]

The terms *sick building syndrome* and *building-related illness* have come to be associated with asthma symptoms related to indoor air quality. One must have a careful study of the indoor air because certain temperature, humidity, and respirable gas levels can result in patient reports of symptoms.[29] The degree to which subsequent symptoms represent a demonstrable physiologic response to exposure as opposed to a conditioned response to a particular olfactory or physical stimulus remains unclear.

An area of more intense interest is the relationship of molds to asthma.[30-32] Certain molds are clearly associated with an increase in asthma symptoms, although resolution of symptoms is the rule once exposure is eliminated. Mold remediation efforts require a thorough process that involves identification of the source and worker protection.[33,34] Therefore, PFTs are mandatory to help support the diagnosis of respiratory complaints.

Occupational Asthma

Occupational asthma is caused or exacerbated by environmental agents in the workplace. The signs or symptoms of occupational asthma can be due to abnormal concentrations of an environmental agent or an exaggerated response in a worker. Occupational asthma is known as RADS when it develops after a single (usually) or several (occasionally) exposure(s) to a gaseous substance that is highly irritating or caustic, leads to an immediate bronchoconstrictive reaction, and recurs when the person is challenged with the substance (or other substances) subsequently. Modifications of the clinical criteria for RADS as initially described are as follows[35]:

1. Documented absence of preceding respiratory complaints (if possible)
2. Onset of symptoms after a single (usually) specific exposure
3. Exposure to a gas, smoke, fume, or vapor that was present in high concentrations and had irritant qualities
4. Onset of symptoms within 24 hours of exposure
5. Symptoms simulate asthma, with cough, wheezing, and dyspnea predominating
6. Possible demonstration of airflow obstruction by PFTs
7. Positive results of methacholine challenge testing, if performed (not mandated)
8. Other types of pulmonary disease ruled out

Reactive airways dysfunction syndrome is only one type of occupational asthma. The history of irritant causation is usually straightforward when the response is immediate, occurs after a known inhalational exposure of an aerosol at high levels,[36] and is manifested by a response that can range from inhalational fever due to a nonallergic inflammation to asphyxiation.[37] The hallmark of irritant lung disease is that it does not usually cause persistent reactive airway disease as classically seen in asthma.[38] Many studies have identified the incidence and prevalence of this condition.[39-41] Good reviews are available to examine the types of exposures and known causes.[42]

Occupational asthma can also be precipitated by exposure, over time, to high- and low-molecular-weight compounds. Asthma resulting from high-molecular-weight compounds is usually allergic. The response can be immediate (occupational asthma without latency) or delayed (occupational asthma with latency). Occupational asthma without latency is characterized by asthmatic reactions that occur from one to several hours after exposure. Many studies have identified the incidence, prevalence, and disability of this condition.[43-45] As opposed to mold exposure, complete resolution is usually not seen in the various occupational exposures, although the degree of resolution depends on the agent and the duration of exposure.[43] There are many reviews and chapters on this subject.[4, 44-46] A high index of suspicion is the first step toward addressing this entity. Making a definitive diagnosis is based on the timing of symptoms, the degree to which symptoms resolve when the affected person is away from work and recur with subsequent workplace and later environmental exposures, and objective testing results.

Standard pulmonary function testing for asthma requires performance of baseline spirometry and repeated testing after administration of bronchodilators. A 15% improvement in the FEV_1 or FVC or a 30% improvement in the $FEF_{25\%-75\%}$ is required for a diagnosis of asthma. An alternative to standard testing is bronchocoprovocation testing, with a positive response manifested by decreases in FEV_1 of at least 20%, FVC of at least 10%, peak expiratory flow of at least 25%, and $FEF_{25\%-75\%}$ of at least 25%.[47] The peak flow rate can be assessed at the workplace in the context of exposure using readily available handheld devices. Submaximal effort and the presence of other anatomic factors that affect peak flow limit the usefulness of this testing.

Occupational asthma with latency is an allergic disease. The latency period reflects the time required to develop sensitization following initial exposure to the relevant antigen. This period can range from months to years, with high-molecular-weight allergens, such as flour and grain dust, and latex typically provoking an IgE-mediated immunologic response in susceptible people. Skin testing and *in vitro* laboratory tests (e.g., radioallergosorbent testing) can be performed to determine the antigen-specific IgE concentration in serum. However, they must be correctly interpreted and correlated with the patient's history and examination findings because although the demonstration of IgE antibodies to an allergen demonstrates prior exposure, it does not necessarily prove that the patient's allergic symptoms are related to that specific allergen.

Many reviews list agents and occupations at risk for work-related asthma.[47-49] Potential high-molecular-weight causative factors consist of animal and plant proteins and enzymes; fumes, drugs, diisocyanates, anhydrides, dyes, wood dust, and a number of other miscellaneous chemicals are classified as low-molecular-weight compounds. Some examples of high- and low-molecular-weight compounds are as listed in Tables 13-1 and 13-2.[50] A more extensive list of compounds is available at the Haz-Map web site (http://hazmap.nlm.nih.gov/cgi-bin/hazmap_adveff?form=adveff&Ag_Asthma=1).

TABLE 13-1	High-Molecular-Weight Agents*

Agent

Animals

 Cow dander/hair allergen

 Crab

 Laboratory animal allergens

 Salmon

Baking allergens

 Baking allergens

 Fungal amylase

Biological enzyme

 Detergent enzyme

 Phytase

Mold

 Aspergillus niger

 Plants

 Grain

 Latex

 Wheat, buckwheat

* Adapted from NIOSH[50]
NOTE: This is only a partial list.

TABLE 13-2   Low-Molecular-Weight Agents*

Anhydrides

Hexahydro-phthalic anhydride (HHPA)

Maleic anhydride

Methyltetrahydrophthalic anhydride (MTHPA)

Phthalic anhydride

Pyromellitic dianhydride (PMDA)

Tetracholaphthalic anhydride (TCPA)

Trimellitic anhydride (TMA)

Other Chemicals

Persulfate salts

Diisocyanates

Diphenylmethane diisocyanate (MDI)

Hexamethylene diisocyanate (HDI)

Isocyanates (unspecified)

Napthylene diisocyanate (NDI)

Toluene diisocyanate (TDI)

Fluxes

Colophony

Metals

Aluminum

Chromium

Cobalt

Platinum

Wood dust or bark

Red cedar (western)

* Adapted from NIOSH.[50]
NOTE: This is only a partial list.

Review of the Material Safety Data Sheets can help establish all the primary chemical agents to which a worker has been exposed when symptoms occur after inhalation of a compound with multiple components. A recent example of novel occupational exposures causing reactive airway disease was seen in the World Trade Center experience.[51]

Hypersensitivity Pneumonitis

The classic example of hypersensitivity pneumonitis was the development of a flulike illness in patients exposed to high levels of an antigen (Farmer's lung), with chronic conditions of exposure leading to fibrotic changes. Hypersensitivity pneumonitis is defined as "a granulomatous interstitial lung disorder resulting from a reaction to repeated inhalation of and sensitization to organic dusts of 1 to 5 µg in size occurring in a predisposed host."[52] Workers in occupations that involve exposure to animal and/or plant proteins, such as bird breeders, cheese washers, and sugar cane workers (the disease is bagassosis), and workers exposed to wood dusts and pulps, hot tubs, humidifiers, compost, metal working fluids, mollusk shells, and peat moss are at risk of developing this disorder. Agents that can lead to the development of hypersensitivity pneumonitis are as listed in Table 13-3.

TABLE 13-3   Agents Associated With Hypersensitivity Pneumonitis*

Micropolyspora faeni

Thermoactinomyces vulgaris

Thermoactinomyces sacchari

Penicillium casei or *Penicillium roqueforti*

Penicillium frequentans

Aspergillus clavatus

Cryptostroma corticale

Alternaria species

Graphium species

Aureobasidium pullulans

Merulius lacrymans

Trichosporon cutaneum

* Adapted from Haz-Map.[53]
NOTE: This is only a partial list.

CHAPTER 13

The disease is a consequence of immunologically mediated inflammation and differs from occupational asthma because it is infiltrative and interstitial rather than bronchospastic. The degree to which disease develops after a given exposure differs among affected people, ie, genetic and baseline immunologic factors have a role[52] in affecting the pulmonary interstitium. The results of PFTs reveal decreases in FVC, FEV_1, and D_{LCO}, which reflect the restriction, stiffness, and alveolar membrane thickening that result from this disorder.

Criteria for the diagnosis of hypersensitivity pneumonitis are as follows[52]:
1. History of exposure to a known causative antigen or clearly sufficient amounts of a putative antigen
2. Symptoms of cough, fever, and dyspnea
3. Abnormal chest X-ray and PFT results
4. Evidence of immunologic sensitization based on the results of testing for precipitating antibodies to the suspected organic antigen or skin testing (The finding of lymphocytosis with CD8 predominance, IgM and IgG antibodies, and increased total protein in fluid obtained through bronchoalveolar lavage is an alternative.)
5. Findings consistent with the disorder if pulmonary biopsy performed

Fibrotic Lung Disorders (Pneumoconiosis)

The classic inorganic dusts associated with this condition are silicon-containing materials, coal dust,[54] and asbestos.[55] The effects of exposure to beryllium dust or fumes will be discussed, even though the disorder is primarily considered to represent hypersensitivity,[56] as will deliberations regarding the association between inhalation of manufactured vitreous fibers and pneumoconiosis. Exposures to compounds containing talc,[57] chromium,[58] attapulgite,[59] zirconium,[60] carbon black,[61] vinyl chloride,[62] aluminum,[63] nickel,[64] hematite,[65] and molybdenum[66] have also been implicated in the development of symptomatic pneumoconiosis. There is usually a latency period between exposure and the development of symptoms; this period is based on the dose and duration of exposure and the physical and chemical properties of the dust inhaled.

When radiologic abnormalities consistent with pneumoconiosis are not accompanied by respiratory symptoms of consequence, the pneumoconiosis is considered benign. Barium sulfate inhalation occurring in association with mining, grinding, or bagging barite may lead to its deposition in the lung in sufficient quantities to produce baritosis, one of the classic, benign pneumoconioses.[67] Benign pneumoconioses are also caused by tin oxide (stannosis), gypsum, iron oxide (siderosis),[68] elemental antimony[69] and its oxides,[70] mica dust (unless heavily contaminated with silica),[71] kaolin,[72] nickel oxide,[73] and others.

Silica occurs in crystalline and amorphous forms. Crystalline forms are responsible for most cases of silicosis. Although quartz is the most common of the crystalline forms, cristobalite and tridymite are more potent forms of crystalline silica. Workers who blast, drill, remove, crush, grind, or cut silica-containing rock, brick, stone, tiles, or terrazzo or load, dump, or are otherwise exposed to silica powder or dust are at risk of disease development. Although usually characterized by a long latency, acute and accelerated forms of silicosis have been described. *Extrapulmonary silicosis,* a term encompassing the spread of lesions to the liver, spleen, kidneys, bone marrow, and extrathoracic lymph nodes, may also occur.[74]

Anthracite coal dust, bituminous coal dust, and lignite coal dust exposures have been established as causes of bronchitis and pneumoconiosis. Although the heaviest exposures occur in underground mines, exposures also occur in handling and transporting coal. Simple coal workers' pneumoconiosis is defined by the presence of small lung opacities that develop after at least 10 years of exposure to coal dust, but it is rarely seen in miners who have spent fewer than 20 years working underground.[75]

Asbestos fibers belong to one of two mineral groups, serpentines and amphiboles. Although the serpentine group contains only chrysotile asbestos, there are five varieties of amphiboles: anthophyllite asbestos, grunerite asbestos (amosite), riebeckite asbestos (crocidolite), tremolite, and actinolite asbestos. Commercial products may contain one or more forms of asbestos; however, chrysotile asbestos is most commonly found in industry (95% of world production) and, even though considered less toxic than other forms of asbestos, is, nevertheless, the form most frequently associated with disease.[76] Asbestos may also contaminate talc and vermiculite. Effects of asbestos are dose-related,[77] with the diagnosis of asbestosis dependent on a history of exposure to asbestos dust. Latency between exposure and disease onset is at least 10 years (usually 25 years or more), with early signs of disease objectively manifested by diffuse fibrosis and pleural plaques by chest X-ray or computed tomographic scan, and, later, a restrictive pattern on pulmonary function testing.[78]

Exposure to relatively high concentrations of *beryllium* (100 µg/m^3) can lead to acute *berylliosis,* a chemical pneumonitis characterized by edema, inflammation, and necrosis due to a direct toxic effect on the mucosa of the tracheobronchial tree. Chronic berylliosis is characterized by radiographic evidence of granulomatous inflammation similar to what is seen in pneumoconiosis or sarcoidosis but is actually a hypersensitivity disorder characterized by the accumulation of beryllium-specific CD4$^+$ T cells in the lung. This disorder occurs in 2% to 16% of exposed workers, depending on genetic susceptibility and the nature of the exposure.[79-82]

CHAPTER 13

Manufactured vitreous fibers such as fibrous glass (glass wool and fibers), continuous filament, mineral wool (slag and rock), and ceramic fiber have been considered potential causes of fibrous lung disorders; however, their precise role is still under investigation.[83,84] They differ from asbestos *fibers* in several ways that decrease initial deposition in the lungs and increase elimination of fibers that have been deposited.[85,86] Thus, at long-term exposure levels less than the currently recommended occupational exposure limits of 1 fiber per cubic centimeter, elevated risks for developing respiratory disease are not expected.[87]

Chronic Obstructive Pulmonary Disease

Chronic obstructive pulmonary disease is characterized by mildly reversible, progressive pulmonary changes with underlying inflammatory components.[88] Many cases of this condition are undiagnosed.[89] Smoking accounts for approximately 85% to 90% of cases, with a certain additional percentage attributed to secondhand smoke (also know as ETS, or environmental tobacco smoke).[90,91] Genetic susceptibility due to alpha$_1$-antitrypsin deficiency accounts for approximately 5% of cases and is suggested by a positive family history.[92] As opposed to asthma, lower body weight is more often associated with COPD.[93] Air pollution is causative in COPD.[94] Occupational risk is less extensive than with the respiratory conditions previously reviewed in this chapter. Increased occupational risk is noted in the polymer industry, in particular with toluene diisocyanate, in tire workers,[95] and in workers exposed to inorganic dusts.[96] Although many jurisdictions presumptively accept COPD as an occupational disease in firefighters, only firefighters with certain genetic predispositions may actually be at increased risk.[97]

Lung Cancer

Epidemiologic studies have shown an increased risk of lung cancer for workers exposed to silica, but confounding factors include tobacco smoking and radon exposure. Quartz and cristobalite crystalline silica are classified as known carcinogens, whereas tridymite and tripoli are classified as probable human carcinogens by the International Agency for Research on Cancer (IARC).[98]

There is an extensive body of literature documenting the relationship between mesothelioma and asbestos exposure. Although asbestos exposure may come through work, contact with the clothing or other belongings of asbestos-exposed workers may be causative.[99] However, mesothelioma may develop as a result of environmental asbestos sources[100-102] or in the absence of exposure to asbestos.[103] Genetic factors have a role in whether it develops in the context of a given exposure.[104,105] Although initially mesothelioma was thought to be caused only by various forms of amphibole asbestos (crocidolite, tremolite, amosite), more recent studies have established chrysotile, which is 95% of the world production of asbestos and was presumed safer, as similar in potency to amphibole asbestos.[106-108] Enzyme-linked immunosorbent assay testing for asbestos-related mesothelioma has recently been developed.[109] Monitoring of serum osteopontin levels has been suggested as a means of assessing whether mesothelioma is present in asbestos-exposed people.[110] When there has been exposure to asbestos from multiple sources, use of the mesothelioma risk model is recommended to achieve apportionment.[111]

Beryllium is a suspected human carcinogen, based on results of studies of animals. Epidemiologic evidence relating beryllium exposure to cancer in humans is inadequate to demonstrate or refute that beryllium is carcinogenic in humans, and the IARC lists the evidence for beryllium-induced carcinogenicity in humans as limited.[64] As noted previously, although possible health hazards from long-term exposure to manufactured vitreous fibers such as airborne fibrous glass, rock wool, and slag wool include effects associated with occupational exposure to asbestos (lung scarring, lung cancer, and mesothelioma), epidemiologic studies of fibrous glass, rock wool, and slag wool workers provide no consistent evidence for increased risks of mortality from nonmalignant respiratory disease, lung cancer, or pleural mesothelioma. Results from recent animal research suggest that glass wool, rock wool, and slag wool are less potent than asbestos in producing tissue scarring and tumors owing, at least in part, to their relatively rapid rates of dissolution in lung tissue. The IARC has most recently concluded (in 2001) that insulation glass wool, rock (stone) wool, and slag wool, as well as continuous filament glass, are *not classifiable* as to carcinogenicity in humans because of the inadequate evidence of carcinogenicity in humans and the relatively low biopersistence of these materials, although the data from studies of animals exposed to glass wool are suggestive. The American Conference of Governmental Industrial Hygienists in 2001 recommended threshold limit values–time-weighted averages as 1 fiber per cubic centimeter for continuous filament glass fibers, with an A4, *not classifiable as a human carcinogen*, designation, and 1 fiber per cubic centimeter for glass wool, rock wool, slag wool, and special-purpose glass fibers, with an A3, *confirmed animal carcinogen with unknown relevance to humans*, designation.[112] Thus, in the absence of ongoing continuous exposure to high levels of long fibers, the risk for lung cancer and mesothelioma from exposure to conventional glass fiber is extremely small. The IARC Web site (http://www.iarc.fr/index.html) permits research of the most current literature about the link between exposures to specific agents and lung cancer.

CHAPTER 13

Obstructive Sleep Apnea

Sleep disorders, particularly obstructive sleep apnea (OSA), have garnered greatly increased attention in recent years.[113-115] Portable monitoring makes detection more readily achievable. Sleep-disordered breathing has been associated with novel inflammatory markers that may aid in diagnostic detection or, possibly, in predicting response to treatment.[116-118] Obstructive sleep apnea and sleep-disordered breathing have been identified as contributing to diabetes,[119,120] hypertension,[121] metabolic syndrome,[122] stroke,[123] and heart disease.[124] Altered sleep as seen in OSA is overwhelmingly due to obesity[125]; although the weight effect may diminish with age,[126] weight change directly affects the level of altered breathing.[127] Treatment of the OSA condition, with weight loss or continuous positive airway pressure therapy, improves the aforementioned conditions to which OSA contributes.[128-130] Obstructive sleep apnea is seen more commonly in middle-aged men with familial predilection and in patients with craniofacial or upper airway abnormalities.[131] The effects on the work environment are significant and measurable.[132,133]

Bronchiolitis Obliterans

Bronchiolitis obliterans, a respiratory illness producing fibrosis and obstruction of the small airways, is the term commonly used to describe a number of unrelated conditions with a common end point. In May 2000, eight persons who had formerly worked at a microwave-popcorn production plant were reported to have severe bronchiolitis obliterans. Analysis of data for the affected people indicated an association between the development of this disorder and their cumulative exposure to diacetyl, the predominant ketone in artificial butter flavoring.[134] Other common conditions associated with bronchiolitis obliterans are listed in Table 13-4.

TABLE 13-4	Conditions Associated With Bronchiolitis Obliterans

Toxic fume inhalation

Mineral dust exposure

Infection (viral, *Mycoplasma* species, *Legionella* species)

Bone marrow transplantation

Lung and heart-lung transplantation

Rheumatoid arthritis

Penicillamine use

Systemic lupus erythematosus

Dermatomyositis, polymyositis

Hypersensitivity pneumonitis

Assessing the Contribution of Occupational Risk Factors to Pulmonary Disease

In assessing the relationship between pulmonary disease and a given work-related factor, one needs to address the following questions:

1. Is there documented pulmonary disease (using spirometry, imaging, and, if relevant, the presence of specific biological markers)?
2. What were the relevant exposures, occupational and environmental?
3. Are there genetic factors that could account for, or contribute to, the disease?
4. Is there a plausible mechanism linking the occupational exposure to the disease under investigation? Was the dose sufficient?
5. Does the medical literature support a causal relationship between the two?

If there has been a documented exposure of sufficient magnitude to lead to the pulmonary condition under investigation, and there is appropriate supportive literature, it is reasonable to state the condition is causally linked to the occupational exposure.

References

1. Hyman MH. Working with common cardiopulmonary problems. In: Talmage JB, Melhom JM, eds. *A Physician's Guide to Return to Work*. Chicago, IL: AMA Press; 2005:233-266.
2. Pratter MR, Brightling CE, Boulet LP, et al. An empiric integrative approach to the management of cough: ACCP evidence-based clinical practice guidelines. *Chest*. 2006;129(1 suppl):222S-231S.
3. Grayson MH, Holtzman MJ. Asthma. In: Dale DC, Federman DD, eds. *ACP Medicine*. 3rd ed. Philadelphia, PA: American College of Physicians; 2005.
4. Friesen MC, Davies HW, Teschke K. Impact of the specificity of the exposure metric on exposure-response relationships. *Epidemiology*. 2007:18:88-94.
5. Centers for Disease Control and Prevention. Third National Report on Human Exposure to Environmental Chemicals. Atlanta, GA: CDC; 2005. http://www.cdc.gov/exposurereport/3rd/report.htm. Accessed December 24, 2006.
6. Jakubowski M, Trzcinka-Ochoka M. Biological monitoring of exposure: trends and key developments. *J Occup Health*. 2005:47:22-48.
7. National Institute for Occupational Safety and Health. *NIOSH Pocket Guide to Chemical Hazards*. NIOSH publication 2005-149. http://www.cdc.gov/niosh/npg/. Accessed December 24, 2006.
8. Mason RJ, Murray JF, Broaddus VC, et al, eds. *Murray & Nadel's Textbook of Respiratory Medicine*. 4th ed. Philadelphia, PA: Saunders; 2005.
9. Phillips S. Medical surveillance and monitoring. In: American College of Occupational and Environmental Medicine Basic Curriculum. Elk Grove, IL: American College of Occupational and Environmental Medicine; 2006.
10. NIH State-of-the-Science Panel. National Institutes of Health State-of-the-Science Conference Statement: Tobacco Use: Prevention, Cessation, and Control. *Ann Intern Med*. 2006:145:839-844.
11. Surgeon General 2004 Report: Health Consequences of Smoking on the Human Body. http://www.cdc.gov/tobacco/sgr/sqr 2004/sgranimation/home effects.html. Accessed December 24, 2006.
12. Fitzgerald FT, Murray JF. History and physical examinations. In: Mason RJ, Murray JF, Broaddus VC, et al, eds. *Murray & Nadel's Textbook of Respiratory Medicine*. 4th ed. Philadelphia, PA: Saunders; 2005: chap 18.
13. Bunn WB, Stave GM, Downs KE, et al. Effect of smoking status on productivity loss. *J Occup Environ Med*. 2006:48:1099-1108.
14. Delfino RJ. Epidemiologic evidence for asthma and exposure to air toxics: linkages between occupational, indoor, and community air pollution research. *Environ Health Perspect*. 2002;110(suppl 4):573-589.
15. Leikauf GD. Hazardous air pollutants and asthma. *Environ Health Perspect*. 2002;110(suppl 4):505-526.
16. Lugogo NL, Kraft M. Epidemiology of asthma. *Clin Chest Med*. 2006;27:1-15.
17. Dorsey TF, Lafleur AL, Kumata H, et al. Correlations of asthma mortality with traffic-related factors: use of catalytic converters and radial tires. *J Occup Environ Med*. 2006;48:1321-1327.
18. McCunney RJ. Asthma, genes, and air pollution. *J Occup Environ Med*. 2005;47:1285-1291.

19. Arbes SJ, Gergen PJ, Elliott L, Zeldin DC. Prevalences of positive skin test responses to 10 common allergens in the US population: results from the Third National Health and Nutrition Examination Survey. *J Allergy Clin Immunol.* 2005;116:377-383.

20. Flattery J, Davis L, Rosenman KD, et al. The proportion of self-reported asthma associated with work in three states: California, Massachusetts, and Michigan, 2001. *J Asthma.* 2006;43:213-218.

21. Eder W, Ege MJ, von Mutius E. The asthma epidemic. *N Engl J Med.* 2006;355:2226-2235.

22. Haland G, Carlsen KCL, Sandvik L, et al. Reduced lung function at birth and the risk of asthma at 10 years of age. *N Engl J Med.* 2006;355:1682-1689.

23. Ober C. Perspectives on the past decade of asthma genetics. *J Allergy Clin Immunol.* 2005;116:274-278.

24. Gauderman WJ. Air pollution and children: an unhealthy mix [editorial]. *N Engl J Med.* 2006;355:78-79.

25. Blanc PD, Eisner MD, Katz PP, et al. Impact of the home indoor environment on adult asthma and rhinitis. *J Occup Environ Med.* 2005;47:362-372.

26. Camargo CA, Weiss ST, Zhang S, et al. Prospective study of body mass index, weight change, and risk of adult-onset asthma in women. *Arch Intern Med.* 1999;159:2582-2588.

27. Randolph CC. Allergic rhinitis and asthma in the athlete. *Allergy Asthma Proc.* 2006;27:104-109.

28. Cummiskey J. Exercise-induced asthma: an overview. *Am J Med Sci.* 2001;322:200-203.

29. ASHRAE 1999. American Society of Heating, Refrigeration and Air-Conditioning Engineers. Ventilation for acceptable indoor air quality standards. 62-1999. http://www.ashrae.org. Accessed Sept. 18, 2007.

30. American College of Environmental and Occupational Medicine. Adverse human health effects associated with molds in the indoor environment. *J Occup Environ Med.* 2003;45:470-478.

31. Board on Health Promotion and Disease Prevention, Institute of Medicine. *Damp Indoor Spaces and Health.* Washigton, DC: National Academies Press; 2004.

32. Bush RK, Portnoy JM, Saxon A, et al. The medical effects of mold exposure. *J Allergy Clin Immunol.* 2006;117:326-333.

33. New York City Department of Health and Mental Hygiene, Bureau of Environmental and Occupational Disease Epidemiology. Guidelines on assessment and remediation of fungi in indoor environments. http://www.nyc.gov/html/doh/html/epi/moldrpt1.shtml. Accessed December 25, 2006.

34. Mitchell CS, Hodgson MJ. Respiratory protection for mold remediation. *J Occup Environ Med.* 2004;46:1099-1100.

35. Brooks SM. Weiss MA, Bernstein IL, et al. Reactive airways dysfunction syndrome (RADS): persistent asthma syndrome after high level irritant exposures. *Chest.* 1985;88:376-384.

36. Youakim S. Work-related asthma. Am Fam Phys.2001; 64:1839-1848.

37. Glazer CS. Acute inhalational injury. In: Hanley ME, Welsh CH, eds. *Current Diagnosis and Treatment in Pulmonary Medicine.* New York, NY: McGraw-Hill; 2006: chap 35.

CHAPTER 13

38. Bardana EJ. Occupational asthma and related respiratory disorders. *Dis Mon.* 1995;61:144-199.

39. Vollmer WM, Heumann MA, Breen VR, et al. Incidence of work-related asthma in members of a health maintenance organization. *J Occup Environ Med.* 2005;47:1292-1297.

40. Berger Z, Rom WN, Reibman J, et al. Prevalence of workplace exacerbation of asthma symptoms in an urban working population of asthmatics. *J Occup Environ Med.* 2006;48:833-839.

41. Eisner MD, Yelin EH, Katz PP, et al. Risk factors for work disability in severe adult asthma. *Am J Med.* 2006;119:884-891.

42. Miller K, Chang A. Acute inhalation injury. *Emerg Med Clin North Am.* 2003;21:533-557.

43. Labrecque M, Khemici E, Cartier A, et al. Impairment in workers with isocyanate-induced occupational asthma and removed from exposure in the province of Quebec between 1985 and 2002. *J Occup Environ Med.* 2006;48:1093-1098.

44. Balmes J, Becklake M, Blanc P, et al. American Thoracic Society Statement: Occupational contribution to the burden of airway disease. *Am J Respir Crit Care Med.* 2003;167:787-797.

45. Chan-Yeung M. Assessment of asthma in the workplace. ACCP Consensus Statement. American College of Chest Physicians. *Chest.*1995;108:1084-1117.

46. Tarlo SM, Boulet LP, Cartier A, et al. Canadian Thoracic Society guidelines for occupational asthma. *Can Respir J.*1998;5:289-300.

47. Demeter SL, Corasco EM. Occupational asthma. In Zenz C, Dickerson OB, Horvath EP, eds. *Occupational Medicine.* 3rd ed. St Louis, MO: Mosby-Year Book; 1994:213-228.

48. Zacharisen MC. Occupational asthma. *Med Clin North Am.* 2002;86:951-971.

49. Beach J, Rowe BH, Blitz S, et al. *Diagnosis and Management of Work-related Asthma.* Rockville, MD: Agency for Healthcare Research and Quality; October 2005. Summary Evidence Report/Technology Assessment 129. AHRQ publication 06-E003-1.

50. NIOSH Health and Safety Topic: Asthma and Allergens: Prevention of Occupational Asthma. http://www.cdc.gov/niosh/topics/asthma/OccAsthmaPrevention.html. Accessed Sep. 18, 2007.

51. Prezant DJ, Welden M, Banauch GI, et al. Cough and bronchial responsiveness in the World Trade Center site. *N Engl J Med.* 2002;347:806-815.

52. Fink JN, Lindesmith LA, Horvath EP. Hypersensitivity pneumonitis. In: Zenz C, Dickerson OB, Horvath EP, eds. *Occupational Medicine.* 3rd ed. St Louis, MO: Mosby-Year Book; 1994: 205-212.

53. Hypersensitivity pneumonitis in Haz-Map: Occupational Exposure to Hazardous Agents. http://hazmap.nlm.nih.gov/cgi-bin/hazmap_generic?tbl=TblDiseases&id=425. Accessed Sept. 18, 2007.

54. Schlueter DP. Silicosis and coal worker's pnuemoconiosis. In: Zenz C, Dickerson OB, Horvath EP, eds. *Occupational Medicine.* 3rd ed. St Louis, MO: Mosby-Year Book; 1994: 171-178.

55. Carrier DD, Newman LS. Pneumoconiosis. In: Hanley ME, Welsh CH, eds. *Current Diagnosis and Treatment in Pulmonary Medicine.* New York, NY: McGraw-Hill; 2006: chap 31.

56. Aronchick JM. Chronic beryllium disease. *Radiol Clin North Am.* 1992; 30 :1209-1217.

57. NTP Toxicology and Carcinogenesis Studies of Talc (CAS No. 14807-96-6) (Non-Asbestiform) in F344/N Rats and B6C3F1 Mice (Inhalation Studies); Natl Toxicol Program Tech Rep Ser 1993; 421 1 287.

58. Hazardous Substance Data Bank. Chromium compounds. : http://toxnet.nlm.nih.gov/cgi-bin/sis/search/f?./temp/~2Bf19s:12. Accessed Sept. 18, 2007.

59. Hazardous Substance Data Bank. Attapulgite: CASRN 12174-11-7. http://toxnet.nlm.nih.gov/cgi-bin/sis/search/f?./temp/~2Bf19s:16. Accessed Sept. 18, 2007.

60. Hazardous Substance Data Bank. Zirconium compounds. http://toxnet.nlm.nih.gov/cgi-bin/sis/search/f?./temp/~2Bf19s:17. Accessed Sept. 18, 2007.

61. Hazardous Substance Data Bank. Carbon black: CASRN 1333-86-4. http://toxnet.nlm.nih.gov/cgi-bin/sis/search/f?./temp/~2Bf19s:22. Accessed Sept. 18, 2007.

62. Hazardous Substance Data Bank. Vinyl chloride: CASRN 75-01-4. http://toxnet.nlm.nih.gov/cgi-bin/sis/search/f?./temp/~2Bf19s:23. Accessed Sept. 18, 2007.

63. Hazardous Substance Data Bank. Aluminum compounds (general). http://toxnet.nlm.nih.gov/cgi-bin/sis/search/f?./temp/~2Bf19s:15. Accessed Sept. 18, 2007.

64. Hazardous Substance Data Bank. Nickel compounds. http://toxnet.nlm.nih.gov/cgi-bin/sis/search/f?./temp/~2Bf19s:25. Accessed Sept. 18, 2007.

65. Hazardous Substance Data Bank. Hematite: CAS-RN 1317-60-8. http://toxnet.nlm.nih.gov/cgibin/sis/search/f?./temp/~2Bf19s:31. Accessed Sept. 18, 2007.

66. Hazardous Substance Data Bank. Molybedenum: CASRN 7439-98-7. http://toxnet.nlm.nih.gov/cgi-bin/sis/search/f?./temp/~2Bf19s:37. Accessed Sept. 18, 2007.

67. Hazardous Substance Data Bank. Barium sulfate: CASRN 7727-43-7. http://toxnet.nlm.nih.gov/cgibin/sis/search/r?dbs+hsdb:@term+@rn+7727-43-7. Accessed Sept. 18, 2007.

68. Hazardous Substance Data Bank. Elemental iron: CASRN 7439-89-6. http://toxnet.nlm.nih.gov/cgi-bin/sis/search/f?./temp/~gG9Tj3:3. Accessed Sept. 18, 2007.

69. Hazardous Substance Data Bank. Antimony, elemental: CAS-RN:7440-36-0. http://toxnet.nlm.nih.gov/cgi-bin/sis/search/f?./temp/~iktW8g:1. Accessed Sept. 18, 2007.

70. Pneumoconioses, benign. http://hazmap.nlm.nih.gov/cgi-bin/hazmap_generic?tbl=TblDisease&id=235. Accessed Sept. 18, 2007.

71. Hazardous Substance Data Bank. Mica: CASRN 12001-26-2. http://toxnet.nlm.nih.gov/cgi-bin/sis/search/f?./temp/~2Bf19s:2. Accessed Sept. 18, 2007.

72. Hazardous Substance Data Bank. Kaolin: CASRN 1332-58-7. http://toxnet.nlm.nih.gov/cgi-bin/sis/search/f?./temp/~2Bf19s:3. Accessed Sept. 18, 2007.

73. Hazardous Substance Data Bank. Nickel oxide: CASRN 1313-99-1. http://toxnet.nlm.nih.gov/cgi-in/sis/search/f?./temp/~2Bf19s:11. Accessed Sept. 18, 2007.

74. Hazardous Substance Data Bank. Crystalline silica. http://toxnet.nlm.nih.gov/cgi-bin/sis/search/f?./temp/~XltHJ0:1. Accessed Sept. 18, 2007.

75. Coal workers, pneumoconiosis of. http://hazmap.nlm.nih.gov/cgi-bin/hazmap_generic?tbl=TblDiseases&id=117. Accessed Sept. 18, 2007.

76. Hein MJ, Stayner L, Lehman E, Dements JM. Follow-up study of chrysotile textile workers: cohort mortality and exposure-response. *Occup Environ Med.* 2007;64:616-625.

CHAPTER 13

77. Asbestos. http://hazmap.nlm.nih.gov/cgibin/hazmap_generic?tbl=TblAgents&id=1. Accessed Sept. 18, 2007.

78. Levy SA. Asbestosis. In: Zenz C, Dickerson OB, Horvath EP, eds. *Occupational Medicine.* 3rd ed. St Louis, MO: Mosby-Year Book; 1994.

79. Kreiss K, Mroz MM, Zhen B, Martyny JW, Newman LS. Epidemiology of beryllium sensitization and disease in nuclear workers. *Am Rev Respir Dis.* 1993;148(4 pt 1):985-991.

80. Fontenot AP, Maier LA. Genetic susceptibility and immune-mediated destruction in beryllium-induced disease. *Trends Immunol.* 2005;26:543-549.

81. Maier LA. Genetic and exposure risks for chronic beryllium disease. *Clin Chest Med.* 2002;23:827-839.

82. Hazardous Substance Data Bank. Beryllium. http://toxnet.nlm.nih.gov/cgibin/sis/search/f?./temp/~WqOG3l:1. Accessed Sept. 18, 2007.

83. Mast RW, Utell MJ. Man-made vitreous fibers. In: Zenz C, Dickerson OB, Horvath EP, eds. *Occupational Medicine.* 3rd ed. St Louis, MO: Mosby-Year Book; 1994: 185-193.

84. LeMasters GK, Lockey JE, Ylin JH, Hilberts TJ, Levin LS, Rice CH. Mortality of workers occupationally exposed to refractory ceramic fibers. *J Occup Environ Med.* 2003;45:440-450.

85. Hazardous Substance Data Bank. Synthetic vitreous fibers. http://toxnet.nlm.nih.gov/cgi-bin/sis/search/f?./temp/~u6YLjV:1. Accessed Sept. 18, 2007.

86. Agency for Toxic Substances and Disease Registry. *Toxicological Profile for Synthetic Vitreous Fibers.* Atlanta, GA: US Department of Health and Human Services, Public Health Service; 2004.

87. Agency for Toxic Substances and Disease Registry. Report on the Health Effects of Asbestos and Synthetic Vitreous Fibers: The Influence of Fiber Length. March 17, 2003. http://www.atsdr.cdc.gov/HAC/asbestospanel/. Accessed Sept. 18, 2007.

88. Dewar M, Curry RW. Chronic obstructive pulmonary disease: diagnostic considerations. *Am Fam Physician.* 2006;73:669-676.

89. Coultas DB, Mapel D, Gagnon R, et al. The health impact of undiagnosed airflow obstruction in a national sample of United States adults. *Am J Respir Crit Care Med.* 2001;164:372-377.

90. Report of the Surgeon General. The Health Consequences of Involuntary Exposure to Tobacco Smoke: 6 Major Conclusions of the Surgeon General Report. Washington, DC: US Department of Health and Human Services; 2006. http://www.surgeongeneral.gov/library/secondhandsmoke/factsheets/factsheet6.html. Accessed December 25, 2006.

91. Petty TL. Chronic obstructive pulmonary disease. In: Hanley ME, Welsh CH. *Current Diagnosis and Treatment in Pulmonary Medicine.* New York, NY: McGraw-Hill; 2006: chap 7.

92. Higgins M. Risk factors associated with chronic obstructive lung disease. *Ann N Y Acad Sci.*1991;624:7-17.

93. Harik-Khan RI, Fleg JL, Wise RA. Body mass index and the risk of COPD. *Chest.* 2002;121:370-376.

94. Viegi G, Maio S, Pistelli F, Balducci S, Carrozzi L. Epidemiology of chronic obstructive pulmonary disease: health effects of air pollution. *Respirology.* 2006;11:523-532.

95. Holmberg B, Zenz C, Dodson VN. The polymer industry. In: Zenz C, Dickerson OB, Horvath EP. *Occupational Medicine.* 3rd ed. St Louis, MO: Mosby-Year Book; 1994:719-749.
96. Viegi G, Di Pede C. Chronic obstructive lung diseases and occupational exposure. *Curr Opin Allergy Clin Immunol.* 2002;2:115-121.
97. Burgess JL, Fierro M, Lantz RC, et al. Longitudinal decline in lung function: evaluation of interleukin-10 genetic polymorphisms in firefighters. *J Occup Environ Med.* 2004;46:1013-1022.
98. Silica, crystalline. http://hazmap.nlm.nih.gov/cgi-bin/hazmap_generic?tbl=TblAgents&id=427. Accessed 9/18/07.
99. Miller A. Mesothelioma in household members of asbestos-exposed workers: 32 United States cases since 1990. *Am J Ind Med.* 2005;47:458-462.
100. Pan XL, Day HW, Wang W, Beckett LA, Shenker MB. Residential proximity to naturally occurring asbestos and mesothelioma risk in California. *Am J Respir Crit Care Med.* 2005;172:1019-1025.
101. Metintas M, Ozdemir N, Hillerdal G, et al. Environmental asbestos exposure and malignant pleural mesothelioma. *Respir Med.* 1999;93:349-355.
102. Bourdès V, Boffetta P, Pisani P. Environmental exposure to asbestos and risk of pleural mesothelioma: review and meta-analysis. *Eur J Epidemiol.* 2000; 16:411-417.
103. Marchevsky AM, Harber P, Crawford L, Wick MR. Mesothelioma in patients with nonoccupational asbestos exposure: an evidence-based approach to causation assessment. *Ann Diagn Pathol.* 2006;10:241-250.
104. Neri M, Taioli E, Filiberti R, et al. Metabolic genotypes as modulators of asbestos-related pleural malignant mesothelioma risk: a comparison of Finnish and Italian populations. *Int J Hyg Environ Health.* 2006;209:393-398.
105. Neri M, Filiberti R, Taioli E, et al. Pleural malignant mesothelioma, genetic susceptibility and asbestos exposure. *Mutat Res.* 2005;592:36-44.
106. Lemen RA. Chrysotile asbestos as a cause of mesothelioma: application of the Hill causation model. *Int J Occup Environ Health.* 2004;10:233-239.
107. Smith AH, Wright CC. Chrysotile asbestos is the main cause of pleural mesothelioma. *Am J Ind Med.* 1996;30:252-266.
108. Li L, Sun TD, Zhang X, et al. Cohort studies on cancer mortality among workers exposed only to chrysotile asbestos: a meta-analysis. *Biomed Environ Sci.* 2004;17:459-468.
109. Maeda M, Hino O Blood tests for asbestos-related mesothelioma. *Oncology.* 2006;71:26-31.
110. Pass HI, Lott D, Lonardo F, et al. Asbestos exposure, pleural mesothelioma, and serum osteopontin levels. *N Engl J Med.* 2005;353:1564-1573.
111. Price B, Ware A Mesothelioma: risk apportionment among asbestos exposure sources. *Risk Anal.* 2005;25:937-943.
112. Department of Health and Human Services, Public Health Service, Agency for Toxic Substances and Disease Registry. Technical Briefing Paper: Health Effects From Exposure to Fibrous Glass, Rock Wool, or Slag Wool. Washington, DC: Dept of Health and Human Services, Public Health Service, Agency for Toxic Substances and Disease Registry. June 14 2002.
113. Zee PC, Turek FW. Sleep and health. *Arch Intern Med.* 2006;166:1686-1688.

CHAPTER 13

114. Caples SM, Gami AS, Somers VK. Obstructive sleep apnea. *Ann Intern Med.* 2005;142:187-197.
115. Shamsuzzaman AS, Gersh BJ, Somers VK. Obstructive sleep apnea: implications for cardiac and vascular disease. *JAMA.* 2003;290:1906-1914.
116. Lange T, Dimitrov S, Fehm HL, et al. Shift of monocyte function toward cellular immunity during sleep. *Arch Intern Med.* 2006;166:1695-1700.
117. Mehra R, Storfer-Isser A, Kirchner L, et al. Soluble interleukin 6 receptor. *Arch Intern Med.* 2006;166:1725-1731.
118. Himmerich H, Beitinger PA, Fulda S, et al. Plasma levels of tumor necrosis factor alpha and soluble tumor necrosis factor receptors in patients with narcolepsy. *Arch Intern Med.* 2006;166:1739-1743.
119. Knutson KL, Ryden AM, Mander BA, et al. Role of sleep duration and quality in the risk and severity of type 2 diabetes mellitus. *Arch Intern Med.* 2006;166:1768-1774.
120. Reichmuth KJ, Austin D, Skatrud, JB, et al. Association of sleep apnea and type II diabetes: a population based study. *Am J Respir Crit Care Med.* 2005;172:1590-1595.
121. Bixler EO, Vgontzas AN, Lin HM, et al. Association of hypertension and sleep-disordered breathing. *Arch Intern Med.* 2000;160:2289-2295.
122. Coughlin SR, Mawdsley L, Murgaza JA, et al. Obstructive sleep apnea is independently associated with an increased prevalence of the metabolic syndrome. *Eur Heart J.* 2004;25:735-741.
123. Yaggi HK, Concato J, Kernan WN, et al. Obstructive sleep apnea as a risk factor for stroke and death. *N Engl J Med.* 2005;353:2034-2041.
124. Bradley TD, Logan AG, Kimoff RJ, et al. Continuous positive airway pressure for central sleep apnea and heart failure. *N Engl J Med.* 2005;353:2025-2033.
125. Kohatsu ND, Tsai R, Young T, et al. Sleep duration and body mass index in a rural population. *Arch Intern Med.* 2006;166:1701-1705.
126. Tishler PV, Larkin EK, Schluchter MD, et al. Incidence of sleep-disordered breathing in an urban adult population. *JAMA.* 2003;289:2230-2237.
127. Newman AB, Foster G, Givelber R, et al. Progression of sleep-disordered breathing with changes in weight. *Arch Intern Med.* 2005;165:2408-2413.
128. Babu AR, Herdegen J, Fogelfeld L, et al. Type 2 diabetes, glycemic control, and continuous positive airway pressure in obstructive sleep apnea. *Arch Intern Med.* 2005;165:447-452.
129. Silverberg DS, Iaina A. Treating obstructive sleep apnea improves essential hypertension and quality of life. *Am Fam Physician.* 2002;65:229-236.
130. Faccenda JF, Mackay TW, Boon NA, et al. Continuous positive airway pressure reduces blood pressure. *Am J Respir Crit Care Med.* 2001;163:344-348.
131. Young T, Skatrud J, Peppard PE. Risk factors for obstructive sleep apnea in adults. *JAMA.* 2004;291:2013-2016.
132. Wittman V, Rodenstein DO. Health care costs and the sleep apnea syndrome. *Sleep Med Rev.* 2004;8:269-279.

CHAPTER 13

133. Hartenbaum N, Collop N, Rosen IM, et al. Sleep apnea and commercial motor vehicle operators: statement from the Joint Task Force of the American College of Chest Physicians, American College of Occupational and Environmental Medicine, and the National Sleep Foundation. *J Occup Environ Med.* 2006; 48(9 suppl):S4-S37.

134. Kreiss K, Gomaa A, Kullman G, Fedan K, Simoes EJ, Enright PL. Clinical bronchiolitis obliterans in workers at a microwave-popcorn plant. *N Engl J Med.* 2002;347:330-338.

CHAPTER 14

Neurological Disorders

Brian Cicuto, DO, and Albert Carvelli, MD

Neurological disorders that affect the central nervous system (CNS) and peripheral nervous system (PNS) often require extensive diagnostic testing and treatment. Work exposure to environmental factors and caustic agents has led to speculation that certain jobs and occupations may cause neurological injury and disease. Conditions implicated in this discussion are considered in this chapter.

Central Nervous System

Parkinson Disease

Parkinson disease (PD) is a movement disorder characterized by tremor at rest, rigidity, and bradykinesia and accompanied by a flexed posture of the torso and limbs. This chronic disease is progressive in nature and can lead to akinesia and dementia. Parkinsonism describes the common motor symptoms of PD. The causes of PD are categorized as primary (idiopathic), which is most common, and secondary. Common causes of parkinsonism include head trauma, drugs, and hereditary factors. Toxins identified as causes of PD include manganese, MPTP (1-methyl-4-phenyl-1, 2, 3, 6-tetrahydropyridine), pesticides, fungicides, and paraquat.

Risk Factors

Occupations associated with PD include farming, welding, and occupations that expose workers to heavy metals, including electrical and laboratory occupations. A uniform hypothesis is lacking, but theories include the long-term exposure to manganese inhaled in welding fumes and the routine contact with pesticides, herbicides, and insecticides in farming as possibly leading to neurotoxic effects at the basal ganglia.[1-14]

Welding and PD

Welding is a process that joins materials, usually metals, in fabricating that requires a filler material called a *consumable*. This process of melting the consumable with the native metals results in the production of fumes and gases.[15,16] The fumes produce many elements, including fluorine, manganese, zinc, lead, arsenic, calcium, sulfur, chromium, and nickel.[15,16] In addition, gases are released, including carbon monoxide, carbon dioxide, fluoride, and hydrogen fluoride.

Manganese is a naturally occurring metal that is highly reactive and is often added to carbon steel to increase hardness and strength. It is also a necessary element required in many enzymatic reactions in the body. Manganese is ubiquitous in nature, found in air and water.

Manganism is manganese toxicity and has predominantly extrapyramidal manifestations. It was described in Moroccan manganese miners and in manganese smelting plant and steelworkers with parkinsonism and neuropsychiatric changes.[17-22]

Manganese-induced parkinsonism can be distinguished from PD by clinical manifestations, imaging by magnetic resonance imaging and positron emission tomography scan, and pathologic features secondary to the preferential accumulation of manganese in and damage to the pallidum and striatum rather than the nigrostriatal system.[23-29] Olanow[23] discussed the differences in response to levodopa due to the degeneration of dopaminergic receptors in the nigra, but preservation of the striatal neurons is noted. This observation may explain the improvement in the condition of patients with PD with levodopa therapy but the lack of response in people with manganese toxicity. In manganese-induced parkinsonism, the damage occurs later in the circuitry and accounts for the poor response to levodopa.[23] Animal models of manganese toxicity and manganese-induced parkinsonism in patients with liver failure have further clarified the differences in anatomic and clinical manifestations between the two entities.[30-35]

Farming and PD

Farming and related occupations and well water and rural living have been suggested as causes of PD.[1,3,6,7,11,36] At least three studies found no significant relationship with rural living or well-water consumption.[11,31,37] Exposure to common herbicides and insecticides is associated with acute toxicity.[11,38,39] The proposed mechanism of injury is oxidative stress, which induces a biochemical defect in the nigra by interfering with the complex cascade of events that occurs during oxidative phosphorylation. Depletion of glutathione in the cells and the loss of ability to scavenge free radicals result.

Several studies have reported an increased risk of PD from exposure to insecticides and herbicides, although no specific pesticide was determined to be the cause.[3,4,11,31,37,40] Inconsistent results have been reported, even within the same investigation, regarding paraquat; some studies have shown no association.[41-43] Although exposure to pesticides is suspected as a cause of PD, a link between exposure to specific pesticides used in farming and related industries cannot be established at this time. Difficulties encountered in interpreting results of the studies involving the pesticides include length of exposure, class of pesticide used, and the definition of the job title.

CHAPTER 14

Multiple Sclerosis

Multiple sclerosis (MS) is a severe, chronic neurological disease that results in the destruction of myelin and, eventually, the loss of the axons and cell bodies in the CNS. The characteristic lesion is the plaque noted by magnetic resonance imaging of the CNS, which is a zone of demyelinization. These plaques may occur anywhere in the CNS and in the optic nerves but are most frequently found in the spinal cord, particularly the dorsal columns, in the brain stem, and periventricularly in the forebrain. Multiple sclerosis can result in severe disability and chronic pain. The two major forms are the slowly progressive and remitting-relapsing forms.[44]

The cause of MS is generally thought to be a complex interplay between genetic and environmental factors.[45-48] Only a few work-related factors have been shown to be associated with an increased risk of developing MS. Occupational exposure to organic solvents and ionizing radiation are the two occupational factors most commonly reported in the literature as potential risk factors for the development of MS.[48]

In regard to solvents, there have been several case-control and cohort studies that have looked particularly at exposure to volatile anesthetic agents.[48-51] There is a suggestion in the European literature that nurse anesthetists have a higher risk of developing MS. However, there is conflicting evidence in regard to causality, with some studies showing no difference in the rates of MS among nurse anesthetists[50] and others showing a twofold increased risk.[48] Overall, there seems to be some support for volatile anesthetics having a potential role in the complex interplay of factors that leads to the development of MS, but at this point, there does not seem to be definitive evidence linking the two.

There have been multiple studies published in the literature concerning the exposure to other organic solvents and the risks of developing MS. Several occupations have been studied specifically because of their inherent exposure to organic solvents, including painting, carpentry, printing, construction, and food processing. The majority of the literature involves case-control studies. Again, there is conflicting evidence, with several studies reporting no association between occupational exposure to organic solvents and MS,[52,53] and several showing organic solvents as potential risk factors.[54,55] One of these investigations was a cohort study from Norway showing the relative risk as 2.0 for painters receiving disability pension because of MS compared with workers not exposed to organic solvents.[55]

Radiologic work has also been studied as a potential risk factor for the development of MS. Some investigators have observed an increased frequency of radiologic work and X-ray examinations among patients with MS.[56,57]

The available literature seems to indicate, in general, that occupational exposures are possible risk factors for the development of MS. However, the exact cause of MS itself remains elusive, and several other environmental exposures, including viral infections and smoking, have been identified as risk factors as well.[58,59] Thus, it is our opinion that the present literature basis is inadequate to make a definitive association between occupational exposure and the development of MS. This conclusion is based on the conflicting findings in the available body of literature, in which the majority of studies are case-control studies.

Peripheral Nervous System

Brachial Plexopathy

The brachial plexus is a network of nerves that supply the shoulder and upper extremity. It has well-defined borders described by the position of the plexus along its route from the cervical spine to the hand. Classically, it is discussed as having roots, trunks, divisions, cords, and peripheral nerves.[60] The anatomy of the cervical spine and shoulder is responsible for the vulnerability of the structure to mechanical forces such as pressure and traction and to exposure to caustic agents and radiation.[60,61]

Injuries to the plexus result in complaints characterized by neuropathic symptoms, including pain with associated paresthesias and motor signs of weakness and tremors. Location of injury along the course of the plexus determines which structure is involved and aids in predicting the extent of injury. The injuries located above the clavicle are most commonly known as supraclavicular injuries.

Thoracic Outlet Syndrome

Thoracic outlet syndrome (TOS) is a condition considered a supraclavicular plexopathy that involves the lower trunk, specifically the C8 and T1 fibers. The anatomy consists of the brachial plexus and subclavian vessels that traverse the base of the neck and axilla.[63] This space between the first rib and clavicle is commonly referred to as the *thoracic outlet*. Owing to the controversy of the diagnosis, it is further subdivided into true neurogenic, vascular, and disputed or "symptomatic" TOS.[62]

Neurogenic TOS is also known as cervical rib and band syndrome because the affected C8 and T1 fibers are stretched or compressed by a cervical rib or an

CHAPTER 14

elongated C7 transverse process. Vascular TOS develops after thrombus formation or trauma to the arterial or venous subclavian vessels.[63]

Disputed, or symptomatic, TOS often occurs in the workplace, where its existence is questioned. It is more common than the other types and is often described as a symptom complex rather than a true anatomic pathologic process.[64-71] The physical examination reveals normal neurological and vascular findings.

Diagnostic Criteria

Criteria for neurogenic TOS include subjective complaints of pain, and numbness and tingling in the ulnar distribution. In addition, all three of the following electrodiagnostic abnormalities must be found: (1) reduced-amplitude median nerve motor response, (2) reduced-amplitude ulnar sensory response, and (3) denervation in the muscles innervated by the lower trunk of the brachial plexus.[72-76]

Criteria for vascular TOS include subjective symptoms of pain heaviness, swelling, or color changes coupled with an abnormal results of venous or arterial vascular imaging testing.[73]

Peripheral Neuropathies

Peripheral nerves can be affected by a variety of diseases and toxins. Several unique features of the PNS make it particularly susceptible to trauma and metabolic derangements. The peripheral neuropathies involving smaller afferent fibers are usually painful. Those affecting large-diameter afferent fibers and Schwann cells are generally painless. The pain of a peripheral neuropathy is usually not distinctive, and the diagnosis must, therefore, be based on other criteria.[77] Regardless of their causes, peripheral neuropathies have several characteristics: paresthesias and dysethesias, sensory loss, loss or diminution of tendon reflexes, and impaired motor function. Tremors and disorders of autonomic function also may be seen with peripheral neuropathies. Useful diagnostic laboratory tests include nerve conduction studies, nerve biopsies, and cerebrospinal fluid examination.[77]

The development of peripheral neuropathies has been attributed to a wide range of environmental factors. The majority of available literature linking peripheral neuropathy to occupational exposures focuses primarily on the following: (1) organic solvents, (2) organophosphates, (3) arsenic, (4) mercury, (5) lead, and (6) thallium. Of the studies, most examine the relationship between exposure to organic solvents in the workplace and the development of peripheral neuropathy.

Organic solvents are chemically different compounds with one common feature: they dissolve fats, oils, resins, cellulose acetate, and cellulose nitrate, which makes them widely used in industry.[78] Most of the studies done on organic solvents are case reports and case-control studies; however, they have the advantage of using nerve conduction studies as an objective end point to show differences between the cases and controls.[78-82] Solvents, glues, spray paints, coatings, silicones, and other products contain n-hexane, a petroleum distillate and simple alkane hydrocarbon. n-Hexane is an isomer of hexane and was identified as a peripheral neurotoxin in 1964.[80] Since then, many cases of n-hexane-related neurotoxicity have occurred in printing plants and in furniture factories in Asia, Europe, and the United States.[80] Long-term exposure to n-hexane can result in n-hexane intoxication.[82] The main lesion of the disease is multiple peripheral neuropathy. A diagnosis can be made according to a history of exposure, the typical clinical manifestations of peripheral neuropathy, and changes shown by electromyography and nerve conduction testing.[82]

Organophosphorus esters (OP) are commercially available as insecticides and have the potential to cause several neurotoxic disorders in humans: cholinergic syndrome, intermediate syndrome, and organophosphate-induced delayed polyneuropathy (OPIDP).[83] Organophosphate pesticides are designed to be effective inhibitors of acetylcholinesterase. However, they are a toxicologically disparate group, ranging from very hazardous nerve agents to those with virtually no toxic potential in humans.[84]

The most common and best understood form of OP-induced neurotoxicity results from inhibition of acetylcholinesterase, accumulation of acetylcholine at cholinergic synapses, and overstimulation of the post-synaptic terminal.[85] Organophosphate-induced delayed polyneuropathy is a rare toxicity resulting from exposure to certain organophosphorus esters. It is characterized by distal degeneration of some axons of the PNS and CNS occurring 1 to 4 weeks after a single or short-term exposure. Cramping muscle pain in the lower limbs, distal numbness, and paresthesias occur, followed by progressive weakness and depression of deep tendon reflexes in the lower limbs and, in severe cases, in the upper limbs. Signs include high-stepping gait associated with bilateral footdrop and, in severe cases, quadriplegia with footdrop and wristdrop and pyramidal signs.[86] Pre-marketing toxicity-testing in animals used OP insecticides with cholinergic toxicity potential that is much higher than that of these listed agents to result in OPIDP. Therefore, OPIDP may develop only after very large exposures to insecticides causing severe cholinergic toxicity. However, this was not the case with certain triaryl phosphates that were not used as insecticides but as hydraulic fluids, lubricants, and plasticizers which did not result in cholinergic toxicity. Several thousand cases of OPIDP as a result of exposure to triorthocresyl phosphate have been reported, whereas the number of cases of OPIDP as a result of OP pesticide poisoning is much lower.[86]

There has been the suggestion in the literature that long-term, low-level exposure to some organophosphate esters used for pesticides in doses too low to produce cholinergic signs may result in peripheral neuropathy in humans. However, a single pattern of subclinical disturbances that relates low-level OP exposure to human peripheral neuropathy has not been identified.[83]

Arsenic is found in the earth's crust and is a contaminant in a wide variety of metal ores.[87,88] It is extracted in the smelting of copper, gold, lead, and zinc.[87-89] It is used in metallurgy for hardening alloys of copper and lead, as a dopant in semiconductor production, in the manufacturing of pigments and glass, and in organic rodenticides, pesticides, and fungicides.[88,89] In Swedish copper smelter workers, subclinical nerve injuries were associated with long-term occupational exposure to arsenic trioxide.[88,90] A recent study looking at a history of drinking well water containing arsenic found that this exposure might induce peripheral neuropathy.[91] Chromated copper arsenate has been used to treat wood used to make children's playground equipment and decks. However, only the burning of chromated copper arsenate-treated wood in fireplaces has very rarely resulted in chronic arsenic toxicity.[88]

Mercury poisoning has been reported to cause residual peripheral neuropathy after industrial exposure.[93] Acute mercury vapor poisoning was reported to result in residual peripheral neuropathy in shipyard workers after an industrial accident as well.[94] These cases are rare.

Sensory abnormalities had not been a noted feature of poisoning with lead, unlike poisoning with other heavy metals. However, long-term exposure to lead occurred in industrial workers in Latvia until the end of the 1990s; in a large cohort of the workers with increased lead concentrations who were followed up, nearly a third complained of neuropathic symptoms.[95,96]

Thallium is a neurotoxic metal that has been used in the manufacturing of optical lenses, semiconductors, scintillation counters, some fireworks, insecticides, and rodenticides.[97,98] Thallium causes a predominantly small-fiber neuropathy, with painful dysethesias in the distal lower extremities. Dysautonomia often is present and may precede neuropathy.[97,99]

Complex Regional Pain Syndrome

The complex regional pain syndrome (CRPS) is a controversial diagnosis associated with a range of injury and trauma from catastrophic to minor. It was formerly called *reflex sympathetic dystrophy*. The nomenclature changed in 1993 when, despite significant efforts to implicate the sympathetic nervous system in the pain and distress exhibited by patients with a spectrum of serious and at other times insignificant-appearing injuries, no connection could be established. The syndrome is not a disease, but rather a constellation of symptoms that has no known cause or established pathophysiology and no cure. The International Association for the Study of Pain (IASP) has suggested guidelines for the clinical diagnosis of CRPS.[100] However, confusion and misdiagnosis of the entity are not unusual, particularly in the litigious environment that exists with work injuries and the associated compensation systems. The symptom complex occurs predominantly in the extremities and consists of burning pain accompanied by edema and color changes.

Complex regional pain syndrome has been divided into CRPS-I, in which no peripheral nerve injury exists, and CRPS-II, also known as *causalgia,* in which there is evidence of nerve injury but the pain is beyond the anatomic distribution of that nerve.

The syndrome is considered a neuropathic pain syndrome, and proposed mechanisms of pain generation include PNS and CNS sensitization[100,101] coupled with regional inflammation.[102,103]

No occupations or job classifications have been demonstrated to cause CRPS.

Risk Factors

There are no known risk factors for the development of CRPS. Authors have attributed certain personality types, lifestyle habits, specific injuries, such as repetitive work, as precursors to the development of CRPS, but, to date, none have been proven as causes.[101,103] Immobilization has been suggested as a contributing factor in the development of CRPS, and immobilization has been demonstrated to produce the symptoms and signs found at the time of diagnosis.[101,104]

Diagnosis

There are no "gold standard" diagnostic tests available to accurately confirm or eliminate the diagnosis of CRPS. Many diagnostic tests and procedures have been suggested and performed, but, to date, no studies have been shown to be definitive.[105-107] The clinical diagnosis requires the following: (1) the presence of an initiating noxious event or cause of immobilization that leads to the development of the syndrome; (2) continuing pain, allodynia, or hyperalgesia that is disproportionate to the inciting event and/or spontaneous pain in the absence of external stimuli; (3) evidence at some time of edema, changes in blood flow, or abnormal sweating activity in the region of the pain; and (4) exclusion of conditions that would otherwise account for the degree of pain or dysfunction.[99]

Criteria 2 through 4 must be present to support the diagnosis. It is essential to determine that other conditions in the differential diagnosis of extremity pain be excluded before the diagnosis of CRPS is made. Examples include sprains, fractures, peripheral neuropathies, inflammatory and rheumatologic disorders, and factious disorder.[108]

External validation of the IASP criteria has determined that the guidelines established for the diagnosis of CRPS have inadequate specificity and may lead to overdiagnosis of this condition.[110] At least two states have further clarified the criteria necessary to establish the diagnosis of CRPS in workers' compensation injuries.[104,110] Widespread pain in an extremity without an obvious anatomic pattern alone is insufficient to make the diagnosis of CRPS and is best described as "regional pain of undetermined origin."[104]

Treatment

With no discernable cause or known mechanism of pain generation, treatment is largely empirical.[111] Intravenous administration of guanethidine has been shown to be no more effective than administration of saline.[112] Sympathetic nerve blocks (injections) have resulted in mixed results,[113] and permanent sympathectomies have been demonstrated to be risky with no demonstrable reduction in pain or improvement in function.[114] Spinal cord stimulation has been promoted as an effective treatment for intractable cases of CRPS; however, there is limited evidence to support this claim.[115-119] Evidence supports as helpful a progressive, active exercise program, including a monitored home exercise program, that requires desensitization and weight bearing of the extremity.[120,121] Return to work is considered therapeutic, and efforts should be made to include this in the treatment strategy from the onset.[122-124]

References

1. Tanner CM, Goldman SM, Quinlan P, et al. Occupation and risk of Parkinson's disease (PD): a preliminary investigation of standard occupational codes (SOC) in twins discordant for disease. Abstract. *Neurology.* 2003;60(suppl 1):A415.

2. Goldman SM, Tanner CM, Olanow CW, Wattes RL, Field RD, Langston JW. Occupation and Parkinsonism in three movement disorders clinics. *Neurology.* 2005;65:1430-1435.

3. Gorell JM, Johnson CC, Rybicki BA, Peterson EL, Richardson RJ. The risk of Parkinson's disease with the exposure to pesticides, farming, well water and rural living. *Neurology.* 1998;50:1346-1350.

4. Ho SC, Woo J, Lee CM. Epidemiologic study of Parkinson's disease in Hong Kong. *Neurology.* 1989;39:1314-1318.

5. Schulte PA, Burnett CA, Boeniger MF, Johnson J. Neurodegenerative diseases: occupational occurrence and potential risk factors, 1982 though 1991. *Am J Public Health.* 1996;86:1281-1288.

6. Tuchsen F, Jensen AA. Agricultural work and risk of Parkinson's disease in Denmark, 1981-1993. *Scand J Work Environ Health.* 2000;26:359-362.

7. Lee E, Burnett CA, Lalich N, Cameron LL, Sestito JP. Proportionate mortality of crop and livestock farmers in the United States, 1984 1993. *Am J Ind Med.* 2002;42:410-420.

8. Tanner C, Grabler P, Goetz C. Occupation and risk of Parkinson's disease: a case-control study in young onset patients. Abstract. *Neurology.* 1990; 40(suppl 1):A415.

9. Rocca WA, Anderson DW, Meneghini F, et al. Occupation, education, and Parkinson's disease: a case-control study in an Italian population. *Mov Disord.* 1996;11:201-206.

10. Racette BA, McGee-Minnich L, Moerlein SM, Mink JW, Videen TO, Perlmutter JS. Welding-related parkinsonism: clinical features, treatment, and pathophysiology. *Neurology.* 2001;56:8-13.

11. Seidler A, Hallenbrand W, Rulera BP, et al. Possible environmental, occupational and other etiologic factors for Parkinson's disease: a case-control study in Germany. *Neurology.* 1996;46:1275-1284.

12. Kirkey KL, Johnson CC, Rybicki BA, Peterson EL, Kortsha GX, Gorell JM. Occupational categories at risk for Parkinson's disease. *Am J Ind Med.* 2001;39:564-571.

13. Goldman SM, Smith A, Comyns K, et al. Welding and risk of Parkinson's disease. Abstract. *Neuroepidemiology.* 2004;23:154.

14. Racette BA, Tabbal SD, Jennings D, Good JS, Perlmutter JS. Prevalence of parkinsonism in a large cohort of welders. [Abstract 5186]. *Mov Disord.* 2004;19(suppl 9):521.

15. National Institute of Occupational Safety and Health. Criteria for a Recommended Standard: Occupational Exposure to Welding, Brazing, and Thermal Cutting. Cincinnati, OH: US Dept of Health and Human Services, Public Health Service, Centers for Disease Control, National Institute for Occupational Health; 1988.

CHAPTER 14

16. American Welding Society Safety and Health Committee. *Effects of Welding on Health VIII*. Miami, FL: American Welding Society Safety and Health Committee; 1993.

17. Rodier J. Manganese poisoning in Moroccan mines. *Br J Ind Med*. 1995;12:21-35.

18. Wang JD, Hwang CC, Hwang YH, et al. Manganese induced parkinsonism: and outbreak due to an unrepaired ventilation control system in a ferromanganese smelter. *Br J Ind Med*. 1989;46:856-859.

19. Calne DB, Chu NS, Huang CC, Lu CS, Olanow W. Manganese and idiopathic parkinsonism; similarities and differences. *Neurology*. 1994;44:1583-1586.

20. Mena I, Marin O, Fuenzalida S, Cotzias GC. Chronic manganese poisoning: clinical picture and manganese turnover. *Neurology*. 1967;17:128-136.

21. Huang CC, Chu NS, Lu CS, et al. Chronic manganese intoxication. *Arch Neurol*. 1989;46:1104-1106.

22. Huang CC, Lu CS, Chu NS, et al. Progression after chronic manganese exposure. *Neurology*. 1993;43:1479-1483.

23. Olanow CW. Manganese-induced parkinsonism and Parkinson's disease. *Ann N Y Acad Sci*. 2004;1012:204-223.

24. Forno, LS. Neuropathy of Parkinson's disease. *J Neuropathol Exp Neurol*. 1996;55:259-272.

25. Olanow CW, Alberts M, Djang W, Stajicj J. MR imaging of putamenal iron predicts response to dopaminergic therapy in parkinsonian patients. In: *Early Markers in Parkinson's and Alzheimer's Disease*. Berlin, Germany: Springer-Verlag;1990: 99-109.

26. Brooks DJ, The early diagnosis of Parkinson's disease. Ann *Neurol*. 1998;44 (suppl 1):10-18.

27. Leenders KL, Salmon EP, Tyrrell P, et al. The nigrostriatal dopaminergic system assessed in vivo by positron emission tomography in healthy volunteer subjects and patients with Parkinson's disease. *Arch Neurol*. 1990;47:1290-1298.

28. Wolters ECH, Huang CC, Clark C, et al. Positron emission tomography in manganese intoxication. *Ann Neurol*. 1989;26:647-651.

29. Shinotoh H, Snow BJ, Chu NS, et al. Presynaptic and postsynaptic striatal dopaminergic function in patients with manganese intoxication: a positron emission tomography study. *Neurology*. 1997;48:1053-1056.

30. Semchuk KM, Love EJ, Lee RG. Parkinson's disease and exposure to rural environment factors: a population-based case-control study. *Can J Neurol Sci*. 1991;18:279-286.

31. Gerlach M, Ben-Shachar D, Riederer P, Youdim MB. Altered brain metabolism of iron as a cause of neurodegenerative diseases? *J Neurochem*. 1994;63:793-807.

32. Corbett JR. Pesticides interfering with respiration. In: Corbett JR, Wright K, bailee AC, eds. *The Biochemical Mode of Action of Pesticides*. 2nd ed. London, England: Academic Press; 1984:1-49.

33. Jewess PJ. Insecticides and acaroids which act at the rotenone-binding site of mitochondrial NAOH: ubiquinone oxidoreductase: competitive displacement studies using a 3H-labeled rotenone analogue. *Biochem Soc Trans*. 1994; 22:247-251.

34. Mella H. The experimental production of basal ganglion symptomatology in Macacus rhesus. *Arch Neurol Psychiatry*. 1924;11:405-417.

35. Olanow CW, Good PF, Shinotoh H, et al. Manganese intoxication in the rhesus monkey: a clinical, imaging, pathologic, and biochemical study. *Neurology.* 1996;46:492-498.
36. Semchuk KM, Love EJ, Lee RG. Parkinson's disease and exposure to agricultural work and pesticide chemicals. *Neurology.* 1992;42:1328-1335.
37. Engel LS, Checkoway H, Kiefer MC, et al. Parkinsonism and occupational exposure to pesticides 2001. *Occup Environ Med.* 2001;58:582-589.
38. Ecobichon DJ. Toxic effects of pesticides. In: Klaasen CD, ed. *Casarett and Dowll's Toxicology: The Basic Science of Poisons.* 5th ed. New York, NY: McGraw-Hill; 1996:643-689.
39. Hayes WJ, Laws ER. *Handbook of Pesticides Toxicology.* San Diego, CA: Academic Press; 1991.
40. Semchuk KM, Love EJ, Lee RG. Parkinson's disease: a test of the multifactorial etiologic hypothesis. *Neurology.* 1993;42:1173-1180.
41. Hertzman C, Weins M, Bowering D, Snow B, Caine D. Parkinson's disease: a case-control study of occupational and environmental risk factors. *Am J Ind Med.* 1990;17:349-355.
42. Hertzman C, Weins M, Snow B, et al. A case-control study of Parkinson's disease in a horticultural region of British Columbia. *Mov Disord.* 1994;9:69-75.
43. Rajput AH, Uitti RJ, Stern W, et al. Geography, drinking water chemistry, pesticides and herbicides and the etiology of Parkinson's disease. *Can J Neurol Sci.* 1987;14:414-418.
44. McMahon S, Koltzenburg M. Central pain. In: McMahon S, Koltzenburg M. *Wall and Melzack's Textbook of Pain.* 5th ed. New York, NY: Elsevier Ltd; 2006:1070-1071.
45. Compston DAS, Ebers G, Lassmann H, McDonald I, Matthews B, Wekerle H. Exogenous factors and multiple sclerosis. In: *McAlpine's Multiple Sclerosis.* 3rd ed. London, England: Churchill-Livingstone; 1998:94-100.
46. Jersild C, Fog T, Hansen GS, et al. Histocompatibility determinants in multiple sclerosis, with special reference to clinical cause. *Lancet.* 1973;2:1221-1225.
47. Detels R. Case control studies of multiple sclerosis. *Neuroepidemiology.* 1982;1:117.
48. Landtblom A-M, Tondel M, Hjalmarsson P, Flodin U, Axelson O. The risk for multiple sclerosis in female nurse anaesthetists: a register based study. *Occup Environ Med.* 2006;63:387-389.
49. Flodin U, Landtblom AM, Axelson O. Multiple sclerosis in nurse anesthetists. *Occup Environ Med.* 2003;60:66-68.
50. Stenager E, Bronnum-Hansen H, Koch-Henriksen N. Risk of multiple sclerosis in nurses: a population-based epidemiological study. *Multiple Sclerosis.* 2003;9:299-301.
51. Stenager E, Bronnum-Hansen, Koch-Henriksen N. Risk of multiple sclerosis in nurse anesthetists. *Multiple Sclerosis.* 2003;9:427-428.
52. Mortensen JT, Bronnum-Hansen H, Rasmussen K. Multiple sclerosis and organic solvents. *Epidemiology.* 1998;9:168-171.
53. Gronnin M, Albrektsen G, Kvale G, et al. Organic solvents and multiple sclerosis: a case-control study. *Acta Neurol Scand.* 1993;88:247-250.

CHAPTER 14

54. Landtblom AM, Flodin U, Karlson M, et al. Multiple sclerosis and exposure to solvents, ionizing radiation and animals. *Scand J Work Environ Health.* 1993;19:399-404.

55. Riise T, Moen BE, Kyvik KR. Organic solvents and the risk of multiple sclerosis. *Epidemiology.* 2002;13:718-720.

56. Riise T. Can we contract multiple sclerosis from our working environment [editorial]? *Multiple Sclerosis.* 2003;9:217-218.

57. Axelson O, Landtblom AM, Flodin U. Multiple sclerosis and ionizing radiation. *Neuroepidemiology.* 2001;20:175-178.

58. Riise T, Norvedt MW, Ascherio A. Smoking is a risk factor for multiple sclerosis. *Neurology.* 2003;61:1122-1124.

59. Haahr S, Koch-Henriksen N, Moller-Larsen A, et al. Increased risk after late Epstein-Barr virus infection: a historical prospective study. *Multiple Sclerosis.* 1995;1:73-77.

60. Hollinshead WH. *The Back and Limbs.* 3rd ed. Philadelphia, PA: Harper and Row; 1982880. *Anatomy for Surgeons*; vol 3.

61. Hoppenfeld S. *Physical Examination of the Spine and Extremities.* Appleton-Century-Crofts New York; 1976:118-119.

62. Pasquina P. Thoracic outlet syndrome. In: Frontera W, Silver J, eds. *Essentials of Physical Medicine and Rehabilitation.* Philadelphia, PA: Hanley and Belfus, Inc; 2002.

63. Roos DB. Thoracic outlet nerve compression. In: Rutherford RB, ed. *Vascular Surgery.* Philadelphia, PA: WB Saunders; 1989:858-875.

64. Rosenman KD, Gardiner JC, Wang J, et al. Why most workers with occupational repetitive trauma do not file for workers' compensation. *J Occup Environ Med.* 2000;42:25-34.

65. Sucher BM, Heath DM. Thoracic outlet syndrome: a myofascial variant, part 3: structural and postural considerations. *J Am Osteopath Assoc.* 1993;93:334-345.

66. Hadler NM. Repetitive upper-extremity motions in the workplace are not hazardous. *J Hand Surg Am.* 1997;22:19-29.

67. Sucher BM. Thoracic outlet syndrome: a myofascial variant, part 2: treatment. *J Am Osteopath Assoc.* 1990;90:810-823.

68. Roos DB. Thoracic outlet syndrome is underdiagnosed. *Muscle Nerve.* 1999;22:126-129.

69. Wilbourn AJ. The thoracic outlet syndrome is overdiagnosed. *Muscle Nerve.* 1999;22:130-136.

70. Wilbourn AJ, Ferrante MA. Plexopathies. In: Pourmand R, ed. *Neuromuscular Disease: Expert Clinicians' Views.* Boston MA: Butterworth Heinemann; 2001:493-527.

71. Cuetter AC, Bartoszek DM. The thoracic outlet syndrome: controversies, overdiagnosis, overtreatment, and recommendations for management. *Muscle Nerve.* 1989;12:410-419.

72. Washington State Department of Labor and Industries. Medical Treatment Guidelines: Shoulder Surgery and Thoracic Outlet Surgery. Olympia, WA: Washington State Dept of Labor and Industries; 2002.

73. Ambrad-Chalela E, Thomas GI, Johansen KH. Recurrent neurogenic thoracic outlet syndrome. *Am J Surg.* 2004;187:505-510.

74. Tolson TD. "EMG" for thoracic outlet syndrome. *Hand Clin.* 2004;20:37-42,vi.

75. Svendsen SW, Bonde JP, Mathiassen SE, et al. Work related shoulder disorders: quantitative exposure-response relations with reference to arm posture. *Occup Environ Med.* 2004;61:844-853.

76. Wickizer TM, Franklin G, Gluck JV, et al. Improving quality through identifying inappropriate care: the use of guideline-based utilization review protocol in the Washington State Compensation system. *J Occup Environ Med.* 2004;4693:198-204.

77. Cohen SA, Stabile MJ, Warfield CA. pain in the extremities. In: Warfield CA, Bajwa ZH, eds. *Principles and Practice of Pain Medicine.* 2nd ed. New York, NY: McGraw-Hill Companies Inc; 2004:330-331.

78. Jovanović J, Jovanović M. Neurotoxic effects of organic solvents among workers in paint and lacquer manufacturing industry [in Serbian]. *Med Pregl.* 2004;57:22-25.

79. Jovanović JM, Jovanović MM, Spasic MJ, Lukic SR, et al. Peripheral nerve conduction study in workers exposed to a mixture of organic solvents in paint and lacquer industry. *Croat Med J.* 2004;45:769-774.

80. Centers for Disease Control and Prevention. n-Hexane-related peripheral neuropathy among automotive technicians: California, 1999-2000. *MMWR Morb Mortal Wkly Rep.* 2001;50:1011-1013.

81. Page EH, Pajeau AK, Arnold TC, et al. Peripheral neuropathy in workers exposed to nitromethane. *Am J Ind Med.* 2001;40:107-113.

82. Kuang S, Huang H, Liu H, Chen J, Kong L, Chen B. A clinical analysis of 102 cases of chronic n-hexane intoxication [in Chinese]. *Zhonghua Nei Ke Za Zhi.* 2001;40:329-331.

83. Lotti M. Low-level exposures to organophosphorus esters and peripheral nerve function. *Muscle Nerve.* 2002;25:492-504.

84. Ray D, Richards P. The potential for toxic effects of chronic, low dose exposure to organophosphates. *Toxicol Lett.* 2001;120:343-351.

85. Glynn P. A mechanism for organophosphate-induced delayed neuropathy. *Toxicol Lett.* 2006;162:94-97.

86. Lotti M, Moretto A. Organophosphate-induced delayed polyneuropathy. *Toxicol Rev.* 2005;24:37-49.

87. Gochfeld M. Chemical agents. In: Brooks S, Gochfeld M, Herzstein J, et al, eds. *Environmental Medicine.* St Louis, MO: Mosby; 1995:592-614.

88. Hall A. Chronic arsenic poisoning. *Toxicol Lett.* 2002;128:69-72.

89. Hathaway G, Proctor N, Hughes J. Arsenic and arsine. In: *Proctor and Hughes' Chemical Hazards of the Workplace.* 3rd ed. New York, NY: Van Nostrand Reinhold Co; 1991:92-96.

90. Lagerkvist B, Zetterlund B. Assessment of exposure to arsenic among smelter workers: a 5 year follow-up. *Am J Ind Med.* 1994;25:477-488.

91. Tseng H, Wang Y, Wu M, et al. Association between chronic exposure to arsenic and slow nerve conduction velocity among adolescents in Taiwan. *J Health Popul Nutr.* 2006;24:182-189.

92. Letz R, Gerr F, Cragle D. Residual neurologic deficits 30 years after occupational exposure to elemental mercury. *Neurotoxicology.* 2000;21:459-474.

93. Hsu L, Lee H, Chia S. Acute mercury vapor poisoning in a shipyard worker: case report. *Ann Acad Med Singapore.* 1999;28:294-298.

94. Rubens O, Logina I, Kravale I. Peripheral neuropathy in chronic occupational inorganic lead exposure: a clinical and electrophysiological study. *J Neurol Neurosurg Psychiatry.* 2001;71:200-204.

95. Eghte M, Veide A, Bake MA, et al. Health consequence of occupational exposure to lead in Latvia. Proceedings of the Latvian Academy of Science, Section B 1998;52:205-207.
96. London Z, Albers J. Toxic neuropathies associated with pharmaceutic and industrial agents. *Neurol Clin.* 2007;25:257-276.
97. Moore D, House I, Dixon A. Thallium poisoning: diagnosis may be elusive but alopecia is the clue. *BMJ.* 1993;306:1527-1529.
98. Herrero F, Fernandez E, Gomez J, et al. Thallium poisoning presenting with abdominal colic, paresthesia, and irritability. *J Toxicol Clin Toxicol.* 1995;33:261-264.
99. Stanton-Hicks M, Janig W, Hassenbusch S, Haddox JD, Boas R, Wilson P. Reflex sympathetic dystrophy: changing concepts and taxonomy. *Pain.* 1995;63:127-133.
100. Ribbers GM, Geurts AC, Stam HJ, Mulder T. Pharmacologic treatment of complex regional pain syndrome, I: a conceptual framework. *Arch Phys Med Rehabil.* 2003;84:141-146.
101. Grabow TS, Guarino AH, Raja SN. Complex regional pain syndromes: diagnosis and treatment. In: Benzon HT, Raja SN, Molloy RE, Liu SS, Fishman SM, eds. *Essentials of Pain Medicine and Regional Anesthesia.* 2nd ed. New York, NY: Elsevier; 2005.
102. Huygen FJ, De Bruijn AG, De Bruin MT, et al. Evidence for local inflammation in complex regional pain syndrome type 1. *Mediators Inflamm.* 2002;11:47-51.
103. Fishbain DA. Approaches to treatment decisions for psychiatric comorbidity in the management of the chronic pain patient. *Med Clin North Am.* 1999;83:737-760, vii.
104. Washington State Department of Labor and Industries. Complex Regional Pain Syndrome (CRPS). Olympia, WA: Washington State Dept of Labor and Industries; 2002.
105. Quisel A, Gill JM, Witherell P. Complex regional pain syndrome underdiagnosed. *J Fam Pract.* 2005;54:524-532.
106. Perez RS, Keijzer C, Bezemer PD, Zuurmond WW, de Lange JJ. Predictive value of symptom level measurements for complex regional pain syndrome type I. *Eur J Pain.* 2005;9:49-56.
107. Yung Chung O, Bruehl SP. Complex regional pain syndrome. *Curr Treat Options Neurol.* 2003;5:499-511.
108. Hicks MD. Complex regional pain syndrome: a new name for reflex sympathetic dystrophy. In: Aronoff GM, ed. *Evaluation and Treatment of Chronic Pain.* 3rd ed. Baltimore, MD: Williams & Wilkins; 1998.
109. Bruehl S, Harden RN, Galer BS, et al. External validation of IASP diagnostic criteria for complex regional pain syndrome and proposed research diagnostic criteria. International Association for the Study of Pain. *Pain.* 1999;81:147-154.
110. State of Colorado Department of Labor and Employment, Division of Workers' Compensation. Colorado Rule XVII, Exhibit 7, Complex Regional Pain Syndrome Medical Treatment Guideline. Denver, CO: State of Colorado Dept of Labor and Employment; January 1, 2006.
111. Rowbotham MC. Pharmacologic management of complex regional pain syndrome. *Clin J Pain.* 2006;22:425-429.
112. Ramamurthy S, Hoffman J, Guanethidine Study Group. Intravenous regional guanethidine in the treatment of reflex sympathetic dystrophy/causalgia: a randomized, double-blind study. *Anesth Analg.* 1995;81:718-723.

113. Cepeda M, Carr D, Lau J. Local anesthetic sympathetic blockade for complex regional pain syndrome. *Cochrane Database Syst Rev.* 2005 ;(Oct.19;4): CD004598. Accessed month/date/year.

114. Mailis A, Furlan A. Sympathectomy for neuropathic pain. *Cochrane Database Syst Rev.* 2003;(2):CD002918. Accessed month/date/year.

115. Kemler MA, Barendse GA, van Kleef M, et al. Spinal cord stimulation in patients with chronic reflex sympathetic dystrophy. *N Engl J Med.* 2000 31;343:618-624.

116. Mailis-Gagnon A, Furlan A, Sandoval J, Taylor R. Spinal cord stimulation for chronic pain. *Cochrane Database Syst Rev.* 2004;(3):CD003783.

117. Harke H, Gretenkort P, Ladleif HU, Rahman S. Spinal cord stimulation in sympathetically maintained complex regional pain syndrome type I with severe disability: a prospective clinical study. *Eur J Pain.* 2005;9:363-373.

118. Taylor RS, Buyten JP, Buchser E. Spinal cord stimulation for complex regional pain syndrome: a systematic review of the clinical and cost-effectiveness literature and assessment or prognostic factors. *Eur J Pain.* 2006;10:91-101.

119. Stanton-Hicks M. Complex regional pain syndrome: manifestations and the role of neurostimulation in its management. *J Pain Symptom Manage.* 2006;31(4 suppl): S20-S24.

120. Sahin F, Yilmaz F, Kotevoglu N, Kuran B. Efficacy of salmon calcitonin in complex regional pain syndrome (type 1) in addition to physical therapy. *Clin Rheumatol.* June 25, 2005;25:143-148.

121. Oerlemans HM, Oostendorp RA, de Boo T, et al. Pain and reduced mobility in complex regional pain syndrome, I: outcome of a prospective randomized controlled clinical trial of adjuvant physical therapy versus occupational therapy. *Pain.* 1999;83:77-83.

122. van Lankveld W, Naring G, van't Pad Bosch P, et al. The negative effect of decreasing the level of activity in coping with pain in rheumatoid arthritis: an increase in psychological distress and disease impact. *J Behav Med.* 2000;23:377-391.

123. Stewart WF, Ricci JA, Chee E, Morganstein D, Lipton R. Lost productive time and cost due to common pain conditions in the US workforce. *JAMA.* 2003;290:2443-2454.

124. Boseman J. Disability management: application of a nurse based model in a large corporation, *AAOHN J.* 2001;49:176-186.

CHAPTER 14

CHAPTER 15

Rheumatologic Diseases

Mark H. Hyman, MD, and David Silver, MD

Rheumatologic diseases are among the most complex and difficult to diagnose. Because rheumatic diseases are predominantly due to symptomatic joint or organ system abnormalities, prospective double-blinded trials of causation are essentially impossible to perform. Thus, physicians must depend on retrospective or observational data, in combination with the available research into physiologic mechanisms, to determine the role of a particular event in disease causation. Nevertheless, studies show that fatigue, a common problem in patients with rheumatologic disease, is associated with lost productivity.[1] This chapter examines some of the more common rheumatologic diseases that manifest in the workplace and the evidence of a possible work relationship.

Osteoarthritis

Osteoarthritis (OA) is the most common of all arthritic conditions, affecting approximately 70 million Americans.[2] Classification of OA is based on the American College of Rheumatology criteria (Tables 15-1, 15-2, and 15-3).

TABLE 15-1   Criteria for Classification of Idiopathic Osteoarthritis (OA) of the Knee[3]

Clinical and laboratory	Clinical and radiographic	Clinical†
Knee pain	Knee pain	Knee pain
+ at least 5 of these 9:	+ at least 1 of these 3:	+ at least 3 of these 6:
• Age >50 y	• Age >50 y	• Age >50 y
• Stiffness <30 min	• Stiffness <30 min	• Stiffness <30 min
• Crepitus	• Crepitus	• Crepitus
• Bony tenderness	+ Osteophytes	• Bony tenderness
• Bony enlargement		• Bony enlargement
• No palpable warmth		• No palpable warmth
• ESR <40 mm/h		
• RF titer, <1:40		
• SF OA		

Abbreviations: ESR, erythrocyte sedimentation rate; RF, rheumatoid factor; and SF, synovial fluid

---

TABLE 15-2   Clinical (History, Physical Examination, and Laboratory) Classification Criteria for Osteoarthritis of the Hip, Classification Tree Format[4]

---

1. Hip pain and

2a. Hip internal rotation <15° and

2b. ESR 45 mm/h
   (If ESR not available, substitute hip flexion ≤115°)

or

3a. Hip internal rotation ≥15° and

3b. Pain on hip internal rotation and

3c. Morning stiffness of the hip ≤60 min and

3d. Age >50 y

Abbreviation: ESR, erythrocyte sedimentation rate.

TABLE 15-3   Classification Criteria for Osteoarthritis of the Hand[5]

Hand pain, aching, or stiffness and three or four of the following features:

• Hard tissue enlargement of ≥2 of 10 selected joints

• Hard tissue enlargement of ≥2 DIP joints*

• <3 swollen MCP joints

• Deformity of at least 1 of 10 selected joints

Abbreviations: DIP, distal interphalangeal; MCP, metacarpal phalangeal joint.
*The 10 selected joints are the second and third DIP, the second and third proximal interphalangeal, and the first carpometacarpal joints of both hands.

CHAPTER 15

The development of OA starts with trauma to the cartilage. The body attempts to repair the cartilage, but with age, continued trauma, or local susceptibility, increased activity of metalloproteinases and collagenases leads to degradation of cartilage, the beginning hallmark of OA. Inflammation has a significant role in the development of OA. Up-regulation of inflammatory cytokines, the *COX*-2 (cyclooxygenase-2) gene, and nitric oxide synthase, all seems to have a role in cartilage destruction.[6]

Predisposition to OA may be genetically mediated.[7,8] Osteoarthritis predominantly affects people older than 50 years, and the incidence increases with age. Women seem to be more likely to develop OA than men, and about 70% of people with OA are women, which is possibly related to women's increased life expectancy compared with that of men. Obesity is an independent risk factor, as is the presence of a sensory neuropathy.[9] Muscular deconditioning and hypermobility can have an important role in cartilage damage.[10,11] People report greater symptoms based on changes in barometric pressure or ambient temperature.[12]

Joint trauma can be seen with a specific injury or repetitive low-grade trauma to the joints. An occupation that requires increased joint loading or repetitive body movements that damage a joint can increase the risk of OA.[13] Although clearly a laborer involved in heavy lifting and frequent bending throughout the day is at high risk of cartilage damage, there is no certain safe level below which repetitive low-grade trauma avoids microdamage to the cartilage and the eventual development of arthritic joints.[14-16]

The greatest difficulty is determining the role of work in the development of a disease that is common in the general population and increases in incidence with age. Clearly, if a specific industrial injury to a joint occurred, future development of OA, especially if premature, would allow for a reasonable industrial contribution. Low-level work activities, such as minimal typing, filing, and light carrying can be more difficult to ascribe as causative in the development of OA, especially if the person is in his or her 60s or 70s.

Rheumatoid Arthritis

Rheumatoid arthritis (RA) is an autoimmune disease that predominantly affects the joints, including the synovium, cartilage, and subchondral bone. The following criteria were established in 1988 by the American Rheumatism Association to standardize the diagnosis of RA[78]:
1. Morning stiffness in and around the joints lasting more than 1 hour
2. Arthritis of three or more joint areas

3. Arthritis of the hand joints (wrist, MCP, or proximal interphalangeal (PIP) joints)
4. Symmetric arthritis
5. Rheumatoid nodules
6. Serum rheumatoid factor level (titer)
7. Radiographic changes (erosion or juxta-articular osteopenia)

To qualify, criteria 1 through 4 need to be present for at least 6 weeks, and a patient must meet four of the seven criteria. Newer laboratory tests, such as the anticitrullinated peptide antibody test, seem to be more specific than the standard rheumatoid factor measurement and may help to predict disease severity.[17,18] Other laboratory findings that support the diagnosis of RA include microcytic anemia, thrombocytosis, increased sedimentation rate, increased C-reactive protein (CRP) level, and a positive antinuclear antibody (ANA) test result.[19]

Genetic factors, specifically presence of the HLADR4 allele, seem to confer susceptibility to developing RA, but only in some ethnic groups and they only explain a small portion of the risk for RA.[20,21] Like most of the rheumatoid diseases, RA is seen predominantly in women (2 to 4:1),[22] with initial onset of disease most commonly occurring between the ages of 20 and 40 years. Surprisingly, the incidence of RA has been diminishing during the past 40 years and has decreased by almost 50%.[23]

Although in most cases RA predominantly affects the joints and can lead to profound disability on that basis alone, other organ systems may become involved. Patients with RA are at increased risk of infections, cancer (specifically, lymphomas), hematologic abnormalities, cutaneous vasculitis, pleural and interstitial lung disease, pericarditis, and coronary artery disease. Patients with RA die an average of 8 to 10 years earlier than age- and sex-matched control subjects.

The causes of RA are largely unknown, although many risk factors have been described. Smoking has been established as a risk factor for the development of seropositive RA.[24] There is insufficient evidence that environmental tobacco smoke increases the risk of developing RA. Numerous infections over the years have been linked to RA, and many patients claim infections as a trigger event, but there is no evidence to establish RA with any single infectious agent or event. Parvovirus B19 in adults can lead to clinical manifestation of RA, but the symptoms usually dissipate within 6 months. Occasionally, the symptoms may last longer and be virtually indistinguishable from those of RA.[25]

Trauma is often reported as a prelude to RA, and it has been suggested that up to 50% of patients with RA describe a physical trauma preceding their first episode of RA,[26] but there is no high-quality evidence in the literature to substantiate a relationship between trauma and RA. More medically probable is that physical trauma unmasks previously quiescent RA. However, studies have demonstrated that patients with RA who perform jobs that require extensive hand use have greater hand pain than patients whose jobs require moderate hand use. There is a concern that patients who stress an already inflamed or damaged joint are more likely to exacerbate the joint condition.[27] Although appropriate, moderate physical activity can help with symptoms of RA, heavy lifting, excessive typing, and improper ergonomics can worsen existing disease.

The weight of evidence from a number of studies strongly suggests that emotional stress has a role in the induction and exacerbation of RA and may significantly affect the disease severity and progression in RA. Stress alters immune responsiveness, but the role of this alteration in the progression of RA is unclear. Quantifying the magnitude of emotional stress needed to affect RA is not well defined, and emotional stress cannot be found in the literature as a factor that aggravates the RA disease state.

Finally, occupational exposures to silica dust have been strongly associated with the development of autoimmune diseases, including RA.[28] Solvent and pesticide exposure have shown weak associations, and farmers may be at higher risk. Enhanced proinflammatory responses and increased apoptosis of lymphocytes may explain the association with these exposures and the development of RA.

Systemic Lupus Erythematosus

Systemic lupus erythematosus (SLE) is a disease that can manifest in almost any organ of the body. Simply put, the immune system attacks the rest of the body. The target organ or tissue is damaged by pathogenic autoantibodies and immune complexes.[29] Although it seems that genetic factors have a role in the development of disease, no clear single gene candidate can explain the presence of SLE.[30]

The criteria for the diagnosis of SLE are as follows[31]:
- Malar rash
- Discoid rash
- Photosensitivity
- Ulcers in the mouth or nose
- Arthritis
- Pericarditis, confirmed by physical examination or electrocardiogram, or pleuritis, confirmed by physical findings or chest X-ray

- Kidney disorder, confirmed by high levels of protein in the urine or other specific urine abnormalities, especially red blood cells, suggesting inflammation in the kidney
- Neurologic disorder, including seizures or psychosis
- Blood disorder, including anemia, leukopenia, or thrombocytopenia
- Immune disorder established by the finding of certain antibodies in the blood, which may include positive results of an anti–double-stranded DNA test, an anti-Smith antibody test, a test for syphilis even though the person does not have syphilis, or an antiphospholipid antibody test (an antibody associated with miscarriage and blood clots).
- A positive ANA test result

Of the 11 criteria, 4 must be present for a definite diagnosis of SLE, and the presence of 3 of 11 is considered an indication of probable SLE in the correct clinical setting. Women make up the vast majority of people with SLE (9:1 compared with men), although after menopause, the ratio drops to 3:1, implying a role for sex hormones. The ANA test result is positive in more than 98% of patients with SLE, but the presence of the ANA is common (in 5%-10% of healthy women) and does not signify SLE without the presence of other diagnostic criteria.

Numerous environmental agents have been linked with the development of SLE. The strongest association is with UV-B light.[32] Not only has UV-B light been demonstrated in induced flare-ups of SLE, but research has shown that UV-B light can alter the DNA in the skin and lead to the development of autoantibodies. Patients who work in occupations where there is significant sun exposure are at increased risk for the development of SLE and discoid lupus, a cutaneous form of the disease.

Chemicals have been described that cause SLE. Aromatic amines and hydrazines are used in the synthesis of numerous products, including plastics, anticorrosives, rubber, herbicides, pesticides, preservatives, textiles, dyes, and pharmaceuticals. These same chemicals are also found in tobacco.[33,34] Patients who are "slow acetylators," i.e., they metabolize aromatic amines and hydrazines at a lower kinetic rate, are at increased risk for the development of SLE.[35]

Exposures to the heavy metals mercury,[36] gold,[37] and cadmium[38] have been shown to lead to an immune-mediated glomerulonephropathy that mimics SLE. In particular, miners and battery workers have significant cadmium exposure. Questions have been raised with regard to paraffin and silicone exposure as possible risk factors for SLE.[79]

Numerous medications have been linked to the development of so-called drug-induced SLE. More than 400 medications have been demonstrated to lead to ANA positivity.[39-41] The presence of the antihistone antibodies are indicative of drug-induced SLE. Hydralazine, procainamide, and quinidine are the most commonly described drugs in association with drug-induced SLE, and discontinuation of the medication usually leads to resolution of symptoms.

Infectious agents have been described as possible triggers for SLE, but no single agent has been definitively identified.[42,43] Dietary factors, specifically ingestion of alfalfa sprouts, have been linked to development or worsening of SLE.[44]

The role of physical trauma and emotional stress is commonly debated in the cause of SLE.[45-47] Both can affect immune system function, specifically T-cell immune function and probably B-cell hyperreactivity. Physical trauma has been shown to exacerbate the symptoms of SLE, and studies have shown worsening of disease following motor vehicle accidents. In addition, lesions of discoid lupus are often seen following superficial trauma and lacerations. Studies have indicated that when compared with healthy control subjects, patients with SLE experienced significantly higher levels of stress before the onset of their disease than seriously ill hospitalized patients.[46,48] Other studies have supported the concept of stress precipitating the initial onset or flare-up of SLE.[49] These data support the assertion that SLE and its variants may be triggered or aggravated by physical trauma or emotional stress.

Fibromyalgia Syndrome

Fibromyalgia is defined by the American College of Rheumatology[50] as diffuse body pain, above and below the waist, on both sides of the body, and, specifically, in the back. The pain must not be a direct result of some other condition. The patient should have 11 or more of 18 positive predefined tender points, with concomitant fatigue and sleep disturbance. Some patients with fibromyalgia may have as few as 7 positive tender points, and not all patients with 11 or more tender points will necessarily have fibromyalgia. Numerous other symptoms are seen in conjunction with fibromyalgia and are listed in Table 15-4.

TABLE 15-4	Conditions and Symptoms That Accompany Fibromyalgia[51]

- Nonrestorative sleep (alpha wave intrusion into delta wave sleep, with decreased stage IV and rapid eye movement sleep)
- Daytime fatigue
- Cognitive impairment
- Irritable bowel syndrome
- Irritable bladder
- Temporal mandibular joint disease
- Headaches
- Posturally mediated hypotension
- Anxiety/panic disorder

Risk factors that exist for the development of fibromyalgia include the following[52,53]:

- Female sex
- Increasing Age (with a possible middle age peak)
- Genetics
- History of physical or sexual abuse
- Physical or psychological trauma
- Infectious exposure
- Autoimmune disease
- Diabetes

Fibromyalgia was originally thought to be a musculoskeletal disorder, but it may best be thought of as a disorder of the central nervous system.[54-56] Abnormalities have been described in the hypothalamic-pituitary-adrenal axis, primarily with abnormal responses to adrenocorticotropic hormone, as have decreases in growth hormone, insulin-like growth factor (IGF-1), androgen levels, serotonin, and substance P levels.[57] Many of these abnormalities are similar to those seen in chronic stress and can be different from the patterns seen in depression. In addition, decreases in certain brain neurotransmitters have been described. Up-regulation of certain inflammatory cytokines, including interleukins 1 and 8 have been described,[58,59] and although fibromyalgia is not thought to be an inflammatory condition, these cytokines may have a role in pain sensitivity and transmission.

Abnormalities in autonomic nervous function have been described, with relative hyperactivity of the sympathetic nervous system and failure to activate the parasympathetic nervous system at night.[60] These autonomic abnormalities may help to explain some of the symptoms of sleep disturbance, irritable bowel symptoms, urinary bladder complaints, and anxiety that are seen in fibromyalgia. These autonomic changes seem distinct from the changes seen in patients with depression. Future studies using time-frequency domain on 24-hour Holter monitoring may clarify the autonomic effects.

The greatest source of controversy with regard to fibromyalgia in the workplace is its relationship with physical or psychological trauma. Prospective trials in this area are lacking. The best study to date looking at this issue found that head or neck trauma was 13 times more likely to lead to fibromyalgia than lower extremity trauma.[61] However, this study considered tender points primarily around the neck. Additional evidence suggests that motor vehicle accidents can lead to fibromyalgia.[62] Authors have suggested that emotional trauma can lead, in a susceptible person, to central pain sensitization and the development of widespread pain as seen in fibromyalgia.[63] The proposed central mechanism described seems to form a reasonable construct to support the concept that trauma can lead to the development of fibromyalgia in susceptible people, although more research is needed. Furthermore, determinations in this area are complicated by secondary gains in a legal environment and can make determination of a relationship between physical or psychological trauma and the fibromyalgia syndrome difficult to identify.[64]

There is very strong evidence that women are significantly more likely to have fibromyalgia than men, and epidemiologic studies place the ratio at about 9:1.[80] There additionally is strong evidence that patients with autoimmune diseases are at significantly higher risk and that fibromyalgia can often confound diagnosis of exacerbations of these diseases.[81] Clearly, if the work environment contributes to the development or exacerbation of an autoimmune disease, the subsequent fibromyalgia needs to be considered potentially exacerbated as well.

Numerous infections have been implicated in the development of fibromyalgialike symptoms, including influenza, parvovirus, hepatitis C,[65] and Lyme disease. Infections may represent a physical stress that triggers the same physiologic mechanisms that trauma does. People with diabetes also seem to be at increased risk for fibromyalgia. Vitamin D deficiency also manifests with diffuse musculoskeletal pain[66] and should be considered in the causation of fibromyalgia syndrome.

Osteoporosis

In the United States, an estimated 8 million women and 2 million men have osteoporosis, with 34 million having low bone mass.[67] In patients older than 50 years, one fourth of men and half of the women will sustain an osteoporosis-related fracture within their lifetime.[68,69]

White and Asian postmenopausal women are at increased risk for osteoporosis.[70] In addition, risk factors for osteoporosis include the following[70]: personal history of fracture in adulthood; first-degree relative with osteoporotic fracture; small, thin body frame; cigarette smoking; advancing age; poor general medical condition; impaired vision; dementia; early-onset estrogen deficiency; frequent falls; lifetime low intake of calcium; low level of physical activity; excessive alcohol consumption; elevated thyroid hormone level; bariatric surgery; inadequate nutrition; vitamin D deficiency; stroke; spinal cord injuries; anorexia nervosa; type 1 diabetes mellitus; organ transplantation; and parathyroid, inflammatory bowel, celiac, liver, advanced renal, or advanced chronic obstructive pulmonary disease. Medications used to treat other conditions that are known to contribute to osteoporosis include prolonged use of corticosteroids and the use of thiazolidinedione, valproic acid, aromatase inhibitors, gonadotropin-releasing hormone agonists, lithium, medroxyprogesterone, and immunosuppressive and chemotherapy agents. Although increased weight is usually viewed as protective of osteoporosis,[71] increased marrow fat deposition is not.[72] Osteopenia has similar but less well-studied risk factors.[73]

Assessing the risk for osteoporosis requires consideration of screening procedures, using standardized dual X-ray absorptiometry. Other methods, although not as generally available, may be useful for noninvasive examination of bone quality.[74] Pertinent to occupational considerations is that imposed immobilization for a prolonged period, usually more than 3 months, can contribute to the development of osteoporosis. Medication used to treat other occupational conditions, such as corticosteroids, can contribute to the development of osteoporosis as well.

Less Common Rheumatic Diseases

Specific occupational exposures have been linked to other rheumatic diseases. The strongest evidence relates to silica dust and scleroderma.[75] Some studies have demonstrated that more than 50% of patients with prolonged exposure to silica dust show evidence of sclerodermalikepulmonary fibrosis on chest X-ray. Workers exposed to polyvinyl chloride and vinyl chloride can develop

CHAPTER 15

sclerodermalike skin changes and Raynaud phenomenon.[76] These chemicals are commonly used in the plastics industry.

In workers with extended exposure to hydrocarbon solvents, used in paint, jet propulsion fuels, degreasing solvents, and hair sprays, Goodpasture syndrome, a rare, life-threatening condition causing renal failure and pulmonary hemorrhage, has developed.[77] Eosin, a chemical used in laboratories for tissue staining, can lead to a photosensitive rash.

References

1. Ricci JA, Chee E, Lorandeau Al, et al. Fatigue in the US workforce: prevalence and implications for lost productive work time. *J Occup Environ Med.* 2007;49:1-10.
2. Centers for Disease Control and Prevention. Oct. 25, 2002. *MMWR Morb Mortal Wkly Rep.* 2002;51(42);948-950.
3. Altman R, Asch E, Bloch D, et al. The American College of Rheumatology criteria for the classification and reporting of osteoarthritis of the knee. *Arthritis Rheum.* 1986;29:1039-1049.
4. Altman R, Alarcon G, Appelrouth D, et al. The American College of Rheumatology criteria for the classification and reporting of osteoarthritis of the hip. *Arthritis Rheum.* 1991;34:505-514.
5. Altman R, Alarcón G, Appelrouth D, et al. The American College of Rheumatology criteria for the classification and reporting of osteoarthritis of the hand. *Arthritis Rheum.* 1990;33:1601-1610.
6. Crofford LJ. COX-2 in synovial tissues. *Osteoarthritis Cartilage.* 1999;7:406-408.
7. Spector TD, Cicuttini F, Baker J, et al. Genetic influences on osteoarthritis in women: a twin study. *BMJ.* 1996;312:940-943.
8. Felson DT, Anderson JJ, Lange ML, et al. Should improvement in rheumatoid arthritis clinical trials be defined as fifty percent or seventy percent improvement in core set measures, rather than twenty percent? *Arthritis Rheum.* 1998;41: 1564-1570.
9. Kraus VB. Pathogenesis and treatment of osteoarthritis. *Med Clin North Am.* 1997;81:85-112.
10. Karpouzas GA, Terkeltaub RA. New developments in the pathogenesis of articular cartilage calcification. *Curr Rheumatol Rep.* 1999;1:121-127.
11. Jordan JM, Kingston RS, Lane NE, et al. Systemic risk factors for osteoarthritis. *Ann Intern Med.* 2000;133:637-639.
12. McAlindon T, Formica M, Schmid CH, et al. Changes in barometric pressure and ambient temperature influence osteoarthritis pain. *Am J Med.* 2007;120:429-434.
13. Felson DT. Preventing knee and hip OA. *Bull Rheum Dis.* 1998;47:1-4.
14. Cooper C. Occupational activity and the risk of osteoarthritis. *J Rheum.* 1995;43(suppl):10-12.

15. Maetzel A, Makela M, Hawker G, et al. Osteoarthritis of the hip and knee and mechanical occupational exposure: a systematic overview of the evidence. *J Rheumatol.* 1997;24:1599-1607.

16. Brandt KD. *Diagnosis and Management of Osteoarthritis.* 2nd ed.: Caddo, OK: Profession Communications; 2000.

17. Vincent C, Nogueira L, Sebbag M, et al. Detection of antibodies to deiminated recombinant rat filaggrin by enzyme-linked immunosorbent assay: a highly effective test for the diagnosis of rheumatoid arthritis. *Arthritis Rheum.* 2002;46:2051-2068.

18. Nishimura K, Sugiyama D, Kogata Y, et al. Meta-analysis: diagnostic accuracy of anti-cyclic citrullinated peptide antibody and rheumatoid factor for rheumatoid arthritis. *Ann Intern Med.* 2007;146:797-808.

19. Ballou SP, Kushner I. Laboratory evaluation of inflammation. In: Harris ED, Budd RC, Genovese MC, et al, eds. *Kelley's Textbook of Rheumatology.* 7th ed. New York, NY: WB Saunders and Co.; 2005:xx-xx.

20. Fries, JF, Wolfe F, Apple R, et al. HLA-DRB1 genotype associations in 793 white patients from a rheumatoid arthritis inception cohort: frequency, severity, and treatment bias. *Arthritis Rheum.* 2002;46:2320-2329.

21. Plenge RM, Padyukov L, Remmers EF, et al. Replication of putative candidate-gene associations with rheumatoid arthritis in >4,000 samples from North America and Sweden: association of susceptibility with PTPN22, CTLA4, and PADI4. *Am J Hum Genet.* 2005;77:1044-1060.

22. Weyand CM, Schmidt D, Wagner U, et al. The influence of sex on the phenotype of rheumatoid arthritis. *Arthritis Rheum.* 1998;41:817-822.

23. Linos A, Worthington JW, O'Fallon WM, et al. The epidemiology of rheumatoid arthritis in Rochester, Minnesota: a study of incidence, prevalence, and mortality *Am J Epidemiol.* 1980;111:87-98.

24. Karlson EW, Lee IM, Cook NR, et al. A retrospective cohort study of cigarette smoking and risk of rheumatoid arthritis in female health professionals. *Arthritis Rheum.* 1999;42:910-917.

25. Naides SJ. Rheumatic manifestations of parvovirus B19 infection. *Rheum Dis Clin North Am.* 1998;24:375-401.

26. Wallace DJ. The role of stress and trauma in rheumatoid arthritis and systemic lupus erythematosus. *Semin Arthritis Rheum.* 1987;16:153-157.

27. Allaire S, Wolfe F, Niu J, et al. Extent of occupational hand use among persons with rheumatoid arthritis. *Arthritis Rheum.* 2006;55:294-299.

28. Cooper GS, Miller FW, Germolec DR. Occupational exposures and autoimmune diseases. *Int Immunopharmacol.* 2002;2:303-313.

29. Wallace DJ, Hahn BH, eds. *Dubois' Lupus Erythematosus.* 6th ed. Philadelphia, PA: Lippincott Williams & Wilkins; 2002.

30. Tsao BP, Cantor RM, Kalunian KC, et al. The genetic basis of systemic lupus erythematosus. *Proc Assoc Am Physicians.* 1998;110:113-117.

31. Tan EM, Cohen AS, Fries JF, et al. The 1982 revised criteria for the classification of systemic lupus erythematosus. *Arthritis Rheum.* 1982;25:1271-1277.

32. Wysenbeek AJ, Block DA, Fries JF. Prevalence and expression of photosensitivity in systemic lupus erythematosus. *Ann Rheum Dis.* 1989;48:461-463.

33. Reidenberg MM. Aromatic amines and the pathogenesis of lupus erythematosus. *Am J Med.* 1983;75:1037-1042.

34. Reidenberg MM. The chemical induction of systemic lupus erythematosus and lupus-like illnesses. *Arthritis Rheum.*1981;24:1004-1009.
35. Perry HM, Tan EM, Carmody S, et al. Relationship of acetyl transferase activity to antinuclear antibodies and toxic symptoms in hypertensive patients treated with hydralazine. *J Lab Clin Med.* 1970;76:114-125.
36. Lindqvist KJ, Makene WJ, Shaba JD, et al. Immunofluorescence and electron microscopic studies of kidney biopsies from patients with nephrotic syndrome, possibly induced by skin lightening creams containing mercury. *E Afr Med J.* 1974;51:168-169.
37. Silverberg DS, Kidd EG, Shnitka TK, et al. Gold nephropathy: a clinical and pathologic study. *Arthritis Rheum.* 1970;13:812-825.
38. Joshi BC, Dwivedi C, Powell A, et al. Immune complex nephritis in rats induced by long-term oral exposure to cadmium. *J Comp Pathol.* 1981;91:11-15.
39. Rubin RL. Drug-induced lupus. *Toxicology.* 2005;209:135-147.
40. Rubin RL. Etiology and mechanisms of drug-induced lupus. *Curr Opin Rheumatol.* 1999;11:357-363.
41. Rich MW. Drug-induced lupus: the list of culprits grows. *Postgrad Med.* 1996;100:299-302.
42. Seve P, Ferry T, Koenig M, et al. Lupus-like presentation of parvovirus B19 infection. *Semin Arthritis Rheum.* 2005;34:642-648.
43. Tabechian D, Pattanaik D, Suresh U, et al. Lupus-like nephritis in an HIV-positive patient: report of a case and review of the literature. *Clin Nephrol.* 2003; 60:187-194.
44. Bardana EJ, Malinow MR, Houghton DC, et al. Diet-induced systemic lupus erythematosus (SLE) in primates. *Am J Kidney Dis.* 1982;1:345-352.
45. McClary AR, Meyer E, Weitzman EL. Observations on the role of the mechanism of depression in some patients with disseminated lupus erythematosus. *Psychosom Med.* 1955;17:311-321.
46. Ropes MW. *Systemic Lupus Erythematosis.* Cambridge, MA: Harvard University Press; 1976.
47. Blumemfield M. Psychological aspects of systemic lupus erythematosus. *Primary Care.* 1978;5:159-171.
48. Otto R, Mackey IR. Psycho-social and emotional disturbance in systemic lupus erythematosus. *Med J Aust.* 1967;2:488-493.
49. Wallace DJ. The role of stress and trauma in rheumatoid arthritis and systemic lupus erythematosus. *Semin Arthritis Rheum.* 1987:16:153-157.
50. Wolfe F, smythe HA, Yunus MB, et al. The American College of Rheumatology 1990 criteria for the classification of fibromyalgia: report of the Multicenter Criteria Committee. *Arthritis Rheum.* 1990;33:160-172.
51. Silver DS, Wallace DJ. The management of fibromyalgia-associated syndromes. *Rheum Dis Clin North Am.* 2002;28:405-417.
52. Wolfe F, Ross K, Anderson J, et al. The prevalence and characteristics of fibromyalgia in the general population. *Arthritis Rheum.* 1995;38:19-28.
53. Yunus M, Masi AT, Calabro JJ, et al. Primary fibromyalgia (fibrositis): clinical study of 50 patients with matched normal controls. *Semin Arthritis Rhuem.* 1981;11:151-171.
54. Bradley LA, McKendree-Smith NL, Alarcon GS, et al. Is fibromyalgia a neurologic disease? *Curr Pain Headache Rep* .2002;6:106-114.

CHAPTER 15

55. Cohen H, Neumann L, Kotler M, et al. Autonomic nervous system derangement in fibromyalgia syndrome and related disorders. *Isr Med Assoc J.* 2001;3:755-760.
56. Graven-Nielson T, Arendt-Nielsen L. Peripheral and central sensitization in musculoskeletal pain disorders: an experimental approach. *Curr Rheumatol Rep.* 2002;4:313-321.
57. Bennett RM. Disordered growth hormone secretion in fibromyalgia: a review of recent findings and a hypothesized etiology. *Z Rheumatol.* 1998;57(suppl 2):72-76.
58. Lucas HJ, Brauch CM, Settas L, theoharides TC. Fibromyalgia: new concepts of pathogenesis and treatment. *Int J Immunopathol Pharmacol.* 2006;19:5-10.
59. Wallace D, Linker-Israeli M, Hallegua D, et al. Cytokines play an aetiopathogenetic role in fibromyalgia: a hypothesis and pilot study. *Rheumatology (Oxford).* 2001;40:743-749.
60. Silverman SL, Silver DS, Charuvastra E, et al. Absence of circadian increase of parasympathetic function using spectral analysis of heart rate variability in fibromyalgia [Abstract 117]. *Arthritis Rheum.* 2005;48(suppl):S78.
61. Buskila D, Neumann L, Vaisberg G, et al. Increased rates of fibromyalgia following cervical spine injury: a controlled study of 161 cases of traumatic injury. *Arthritis Rheum.* 1997;40:446-452.
62. McLean SA, Williams DA, Clauw DJ. Fibromyalgia after motor vehicle collision: evidence and implications. *Traffic Inj Prev.* 2005;6:97-104.
63. Gupta A, Silman AJ. Psychological stress and fibromyalgia: a review of the evidence suggesting a neuroendocrine link. *Arthritis Res Ther.* 2004;6:98-106.
64. Abeles AM, Pillinger MH, Solitar BM, et al. Narrative review: the pathophysiology of fibromyalgia. *Ann Intern Med.* 2007;146:726-734.
65. Park JH, Niermann KJ, Olsen N. Evidence for metabolic abnormalities in the muscles of patients with fibromyalgia. *Curr Rheumatol Rep.* 2000;2:131-140.
66. Plotnikoff GA, Quigley JM. Prevalence of severe hypovitaminosis D in patients with persistent, nonspecific musculoskeletal pain. *Mayo Clin Proc.* 2003;78: 1463-1470.
67. National Osteoporosis Foundation. America's Bone Health: The State of Osteoporosis and Low Bone Mass in Our Nation.Washington, D.C.:National Osteoporosis Foundation; 2002.
68. Chrischilles EA, Butler CD, Davis CS, Wallace RB. A model of lifetime osteoporosis impact. *Arch Intern Med.* 1991;151:2026-2032.
69. Burge R, Dawson-Hughes B, Solomon DH, et al. Incidence and economic burden of osteoporosis-related fractures in the United States, 2005-2025. *J Bone Miner Res.* 2007;22:465-475.
70. Siris ES, Brenneman SK, Miller PD, et al. Predictive value of low BMD for 1-year fracture outcomes is similar for postmenopausal women ages 50-64 and 65 and older: results from the National Osteoporosis Risk Assessment (NORA). *J Bone Miner Res.* 2004;19:1215-1220.
71. Ettinger B, Black DM, Mitlak BH, et al. Reduction of vertebral fracture risk in postmenopausal women with osteoporosis treated with raloxifene: results from a 3-year randomized clinical trial. Multiple Outcomes of Raloxifene Evaluation (MORE) Investigators. *JAMA.*1999;282:637-645.
72. Griffith JF, Yeung DKW, Antonio GE, et al. Vertebral marrow fat content and diffusion and perfusion indexes in women with varying bone density: MR evaluation. *Radiology.* 2006;241:831-838.

CHAPTER 15

73. Khosla S, Melton LJ. Osteopenia. *N Engl J Med.* 2007;356:2293-2300.

74. Boutry S, Bouxsein ML, Munoz F, Delmas PD. In vivo assessment of trabecular bone microarchitecture by high-resolution quantitative computed tomography. *J Clin Endocrinol Metab.* 2005;90:6508-6515.

75. Steen VD. Occupational scleroderma. *Curr Opin Rheumatol.* 1999;11:490-494.

76. Nietert PJ, Silver RM. Systemic sclerosis: environmental and occupational risk factors. *Curr Opin Rheumatol.* 2000;12:520-526.

77. Beirne GJ, Brennan JT. Glomerulonephritis associated with hydrocarbon solvents: mediated by antiglomerular basement membrane antibody. *Arch Environ Health.* 1972;25:365-369.

78. Arnett FC, et al.: 1988 Revised American Rheumatism Association Criteria for Classificatrion of Rheumatoid Arthritis. Arthritis Rheum 1988; 31:315.

79. Kaiser W, et al. Human Adjuvent Disease: Remission of silicone induced autoimmune disease after explanation of breast augmentation. Ann Rheum Disease 1990; 49:937-8.

80. Wolff F, et al. The prevalence and characteristics of fibromyalgia in the general population. Arthritis Rheum 1995:38:19-25.

81. Koopman WJ, Dennis WB, Gustavo H. *Clinical Primer of Rheumatology.* Philadelphia, PA: Lippincott Williams & Wilkins; 2003: 35-39.

CHAPTER 16

Mental Illness

Robert J. Barth, PhD

The Special Difficulty of Establishing Legal Causation for Mental Illness

Chapter 2 offered the observation that medical-scientific causation is a radically different concept from legal causation and that the two concepts may actually cancel one another out. That problem is intensified to an extreme degree by the novel nature of mental illness. There are numerous fundamental obstacles to establishing a cause-and-effect relationship between some adult life experience (as a cause) and a claimed mental illness (as an effect).

For example, unlike all other health specialty areas, the diagnostic system for mental illness is not based on the cause of the disorders.[1] This "abnormal" approach to diagnosis has been made necessary by the simple fact that most mental illnesses do not have an identifiable cause.[2]

Chapter 2 also specified that to establish causation, two elements must be shown—medical-scientific cause and proximate cause. Given the lack of definitive causation information for most mental illnesses, it is doubtful that either of these elements could be credibly claimed for any individual case.

The National Institute for Occupational Safety and Health (NIOSH) criteria that were delineated in Chapter 4 create what seems to be an insurmountable obstacle to claiming work-relatedness for mental illness. For example, criterion 3 asks: "What evidence, particularly objective, is there that the level of exposure is of the frequency, intensity, and duration to rise to the level that would support a work-relatedness determination?" For mental illness, there simply is no objective method for establishing such level of exposure considerations for the types of causes that are typically claimed in workers' compensation (or in tort claims).

Findings from scientific studies have actually made it even more difficult to credibly claim that adult life experience is a cause of mental illness, by indicating a lack of relationship or an inverse relationship (e.g., work seems to be a protective factor against psychological dysfunction rather than a cause of it; psychopathology can be a cause of adult life events rather than vice versa). Examples of such findings are provided later in this chapter in the discussions of several specific mental illnesses.

The information from Chapters 2 and 4 is consistent with the legal requirements from most judicial and administrative systems, which place the burden of proof on the claimant's or plaintiff's side of the argument. Given this burden of proof issue and given the aforementioned causation considerations, it is clear that it will be an uphill battle, in any individual case, to establish work-relatedness, injury-relatedness, or any relationship that involves adult life events as a cause of mental illness. This chapter illuminates the steep nature of that hill and offers examples of the obstacles that must be overcome if a claim of causation is to be credibly attempted.

Justification for this Chapter

From a scientific perspective, a credible argument could be made that there is no place for claims of mental illness in the occupational injury and tort systems and, subsequently, no need for this chapter. That argument would be based on the lack of definitive causation science for mental illness (as discussed earlier). That argument would also be based on the fact that a great deal of scientific research has been conducted on the subject of the causes of mental illness, and the findings have often failed to indicate any role for occupational exposures or any other type of adult life experience. That history of scientific findings is actually reflected in the foreword of this book, which specifies depression as a nonoccupational causative agent rather than as an occupational health consequence.

So why does this chapter exist? Because claims of mental illness have somehow become common in some occupational injury and tort systems, despite the lack of scientific support. That phenomenon has made this chapter necessary. Scientific investigation has reliably indicated that involvement in workers' compensation and tort systems leads to worse clinical outcomes (worse than the outcomes obtained when the same health problems do not become involved in workers' compensation or litigation). [3-5] It might not be possible to save a claimant from the detrimental health effects of those systems when occupational exposure or some tort-relevant circumstance has truly had a causative role. But whenever a lack of relevant causation can be demonstrated (as will usually be the case for a claim of mental illness), an opportunity is created to prevent involvement in those systems and to thereby produce a better health outcome for the afflicted person. That opportunity is the justification for this chapter.

The Necessity for Independent Evaluation

The starting point of causation analysis for any individual claim of occupational or tort-relevant mental illness is an independent evaluation. Professional standards prevent mental health clinicians who are treating the affected persons from credibly offering causation conclusions, thereby necessitating independent evaluation whenever causation needs to be addressed.

Discussions of the relevant standards have been published by the American Psychological Association,[6] the American Psychiatric Association,[7] and the American Medical Association.[8] Detailed discussions of this issue have been provided in the listed references. For the purposes of this chapter, the following summary is provided: Mental health clinicians who are treating people for mental illness should refrain from forensic conclusions (including causation) about the people they are treating, because engaging in the generation of such conclusions results in the following: creates a financial conflict of interest that is unique to the treating clinicians; compromises the quality of the treatment that the clinician is attempting to provide; and deprives administrative and legal systems of the objectivity they need to work properly. Additional literature has explained that it would be a violation of the ethics guidelines of the American Psychological Association and the American Psychiatric Association for a treating clinician to offer conclusions about causation (or any other forensic issues).[9]

The Importance of Not Relying on an Examinee's Self-reported History

Evaluators might be tempted to conclude that a manifestation of mental illness is work- or tort-related because an examinee reports that the mental illness was not manifested until some adult life experience occurred. Scientific findings have indicated that such reports are not a scientifically credible basis for causation conclusions.

Research findings have indicated that reliance on an examinee's self-reported history is always a less-than-credible practice because of a tendency for examinees to underreport preexisting symptoms, and because of a tendency for reported histories to be influenced by an examinee's beliefs about the causes of his or her current problem.[10] Research findings have indicated that these natural human tendencies are compounded by an additional tendency among claimants to endorse an artificially low level of general difficulties for the period of their life that preceded a medical-legal claim (abnormally low compared with nonclaimants).[11] This tendency is consistent with an effort to disproportionately attribute currently claimed difficulties to the circumstances that make the claimant eligible for benefits (circumstances such as an occupational injury). Given such scientific findings, a claimant's self-reported history of preclaim vs postclaim differences in his or her health cannot credibly be used for attempting to establish occupational or tort-relevant causation.

The Fundamental Importance of a Credible Diagnosis

A scientifically credible causation analysis requires a review of the scientific literature about the cause of the mental illness in question. There is a wealth of such literature available. For the most part, it is organized by diagnosis. Once a diagnosis is credibly established, the literature can be reviewed to determine if anything of relevance to the claim has been established as a risk factor for that mental illness.

For a diagnosis to be even minimally credible, it must be based on the protocols that have been specified in the American Psychiatric Association's *Diagnostic and Statistical Manual of Mental Disorders (DSM)*.[12] This manual provides a comprehensive listing of all recognized mental illnesses and diagnostic protocols for each disorder. These protocols are the "gold standard" for the diagnosis of mental illness.

Psychological testing can be used as an adjunct to the diagnostic process to add an element of objectivity. The diagnostic protocols do not actually incorporate consideration of psychological testing, instead, it is a combination of the subjective reports of the examinee and subjective observations of the examiner. In contrast to the complete subjectivity of the diagnostic protocols, psychological testing provides an objective element by providing standardized data that can be compared directly with scientific literature. Testing can be used to determine whether an examinee's manifestations are objectively consistent with the claimed diagnostic manifestations in terms of differentiating between normal and psychopathological states, contrasting with other diagnostic possibilities, and differentiation of honest vs fraudulent presentations of mental illness.

In addition, the American Psychiatric Association's diagnostic system incorporates guidelines for the assessment of malingering,[12] and the guidelines are largely dependent on the use of psychological testing. For example, the guidelines call for consideration of the examinee's level of cooperation with the examination, and psychological testing is the only objective, standardized, and reliable means of assessing cooperation. In addition, the malingering guidelines call for examiners to consider any discrepancies between subjective complaints and objective findings, and psychological testing would be the primary source of any objective findings.

Diagnostic accuracy can be further enhanced through consideration of collateral information, such as reports from people familiar with the examinee (such reports should be collected separate from any meetings with the examinee), and a comprehensive review of health care records (especially preclaim records).

The Importance of Considering the Entire Clinical Picture, Rather Than an Isolated Diagnosis

Although a credible diagnosis is essential, discussion of any isolated diagnosis is often an artificial exercise. To develop an informed conceptualization of causation for any one diagnostic claim, the entire clinical history and presentation must be considered.

A relatively simple example of this issue involves the comorbidity between major depressive disorder (MDD) and generalized anxiety disorder. If an injured person becomes depressed, meets diagnostic criteria for MDD, and blames the depression on the injury, an uninformed evaluator might conclude that the MDD is caused by the injury. But if that person also has a history of generalized anxiety disorder, this uninformed conclusion would lack scientific credibility. One element of the lack of credibility stems from scientific findings that 70% of people with generalized anxiety disorder eventually demonstrate MDD.[13] Given such findings, the scientific probability is that MDD would have manifested for this examinee, regardless of whether he or she had experienced an injury. The manifestation of MDD would be a normal and expected development for this claimant, rather than representing some abnormal development that might require an explanation (an explanation such as claiming it to be a consequence of an injury).

The central role of personality disorders is another relatively simple example of the importance of considering the entire picture. Evaluating for a personality disorder is a standard part of the American Psychiatric Association's diagnostic system.[12] The manual defines personality disorders as "an enduring pattern of inner experience and behavior that deviates markedly from the expectations of the individual's culture, is pervasive and inflexible, has an onset in adolescence or early adulthood, is stable over time, and leads to distress or impairment." In other words, personality disorders are a pervasive form of mental illness that reliably leads to distress or impairment regardless of whether an occupational or tort-relevant exposure has occurred. Furthermore, personality disorders will usually be, by definition, a preexisting condition when considered within the context of most claims (because of the onset in adolescence or early adulthood). Given these considerations, the identification of a personality disorder creates an obstacle to credibly claiming occupational or tort-relevant causation for any manifestation of distress or impairment. The critical importance of this standard part of the diagnostic process is illustrated by scientific findings that 70% of workers' compensation claimants with claims of low back pain were found to have a personality disorder (when the possibility was actually assessed).[14] This finding is consistent with a long history of research findings that have revealed a high percentage of personality disorders among patients with chronic pain.[15]

A more complex example of the need to consider a claimant's entire history and all manifestations is the often-claimed scenario of chronic pain purportedly leading to a mood disorder. The rationale behind such claims involves a belief that an injury caused the chronic pain and the chronic pain subsequently caused a mood disorder, thereby establishing occupational or tort-relevant causation for the mood disorder. One major shortcoming of such claims is the scientific finding that mood disorders are predictive of a lack of general medical findings for the pain complaints.[16] Therefore, the development of a mood disorder is an indication *against* an injury (or any general medical condition) being the cause of the pain complaints. A simultaneous manifestation of chronic pain and a mood disorder moves the entire clinical picture away from injury-relatedness, rather than justifying a claim of occupational or tort-relevant mental illness.

The Pervasive Lack Of Credible Diagnostic Claims Within Workers' Compensation

Chapter 4 of this book specified the following issue as a primary part of the assessment in the process of determining work-relatedness: "What certainty is there that the diagnosis is correct?" Empirical investigations, conducted specifically for this book, indicated a pervasive lack of diagnostic accuracy for mental illness claims within workers' compensation.

For example, several agencies that obtain workers' compensation data nationally were asked to tabulate and report the most frequent occupational mental illness claims. The reports from each of these agencies included "diagnoses" that are not actually mental illnesses, such as *depression, neurotic depression, situational depression, postconcussional disorder, chronic pain, mood disorder due to chronic pain, chronic pain syndrome*, and *mood disorder due to work-related injury.*

Readers who are not mental health specialists might be surprised to find that these diagnostic labels are not actually mental illnesses. The gold standard for diagnosis of mental illness is found in the American Psychiatric Association's *DSM.*[12] This manual contains a comprehensive listing of all recognized mental illnesses. That list does *not* include depression, postconcussional disorder, chronic pain syndrome, or any of the other diagnoses mentioned in the preceding paragraph.

To illustrate the importance of this issue, several examples are discussed in greater detail. For example, depression can be a perfectly normal part of human existence and, as such, it would not represent a mental illness. Depression can also be a symptom of many different mental illnesses, but it is not a mental illness on its own. When it is a manifestation of mental illness, a diagnostic claim of "depression" does not provide a focus that would be sufficient to conduct a causation analysis. That lack of focus is demonstrated by a textbook's account that depression is a symptom of at least 41 mental illnesses.[17] Because the scientific research regarding causation of mental illness is stratified by diagnosis, a nondiagnosis such as depression actually creates an obstacle to conducting a causation analysis and to claiming work-relatedness.

Postconcussional disorder is documented in the *DSM*[12] as having been considered as a diagnostic entity by the American Psychiatric Association, but it was rejected. The protocol that was rejected is specified in an appendix of the *DSM*. Given the data reported herein, it would seem that many clinicians who had relied on the appendix may not have fully read it and may not have realized that this diagnostic concept was rejected.

Similarly, chronic pain syndrome is not on the list of recognized mental illnesses. The AMA's *Guides to the Evaluation of Permanent Impairment*[18] actually specifies that this diagnosis is not official nomenclature. The *Guides* further specify that chronic pain syndrome is a non–injury-related and non–general medical syndrome that can be best conceptualized as an excessive adoption of a behavioral sick role. These definitional considerations clearly place any such manifestations into the realm of mental illness, but a diagnosis of chronic pain syndrome still leaves a mystery about which mental illness is responsible.

Data from two insurance companies and two state workers' compensation funds suggest that physician's may be asked to create diagnoses that suggest mental illness when no accurate diagnosis can be made. Because the data are reliant on the International Classification of Diseases codes provided, the data would make it appear that the diagnosis was accurate when in fact there was no mental illness diagnosis.

To understand the actual nature of diagnostic claims within workers' compensation, I reviewed a sample of files from workers' compensation claims that were in my possession. The samples that were analyzed included 632 claims of occupational mental illness, which involved a diagnostic evaluation conducted by a mental health specialist.

Analysis of the clinical documentation from those files revealed that approximately 43% involved a diagnosed mental illness that does not actually exist. Frequent examples included diagnostic claims that were similar to the nondiagnosis labels that were discussed earlier, as well as *anxiety, occupational stress, anxiety disorder due to work-related injury, depression due to work-related injury, personality change due to occupational trauma, alcohol abuse due to occupational stress, work-related drug abuse, chronic pain due to work-related injury,* and *substance abuse due to work-related pain.* Subsequently, based on this sampling and the aggregate reports from the various agencies, it is clear that occupational mental illness claims are afflicted by a trend toward nondiagnosis diagnoses. Such nondiagnoses obstruct attempts at causation analysis and thereby prevent credibility for claims of occupational causation.

This sampling of files also provided systematic verification of another trend that had been informally noted: a pervasive lack of use of diagnostic protocols, even when a recognized diagnosis was claimed. The American Psychiatric Association's *DSM* provides a diagnostic protocol for every known mental illness. These protocols are the gold standards for determining whether a person has a mental illness and which mental illness is involved. To justify a diagnosis of mental illness, the diagnostician must (at a minimum) document use of the relevant protocol and a description of how the examinee's manifestations satisfy the requirements of that protocol. In the sample that was reviewed for this book, it was found that when an actual mental illness was being claimed, documentation of the protocol that would be necessary to justify that diagnosis was absent 91% of the time. Even when a recognized mental illness is being claimed, the claim is almost never justified at even a minimal level.

Despite the critical importance of assessing for personality disorders (as illustrated in the previous section), the file sampling that was conducted for this book revealed that this standard part of the diagnostic process was omitted or was not performed. In almost every file that was reviewed (>99%), this portion of the diagnostic process was either "deferred" without explanation and without documented follow-up, but was concluded with a claim that there was no personality disorder and without documentation to prove the use of the diagnostic protocols that would have been necessary to justify this conclusion, or it's simply not mentioned.

Many of the sampled files have been part of the utilization-review processes, which gave me the opportunity to contact the clinicians who created the documentation and asked why this critical portion of the evaluation process had been left uncompleted or missing. Most responses fell into one of the following four categories: (1) The clinician apparently did not understand the question and therefore offered nonresponsive opinions. (2) The clinician realized that any personality disorder would, by definition, not be a work-related condition, and he or she subsequently omitted, skipped, or overlooked that portion of the diagnostic process in order to avoid mixing work-related services with non–work-related services. The obvious problem with this response is that such an approach could lead to misdirected conclusions of occupational causation (owing to a personality disorder being overlooked) and, subsequently, to unnecessary exposure of the claimant to the reliably detrimental health effects of involvement in the workers' compensation system. (3) This standard portion of the evaluation process had been omitted, skipped, or overlooked because of the limitations placed on the evaluator by the workers' compensation payers. These clinicians typically acknowledged that their work is less than complete based on this limitation. (4) The clinician specified that he or she omitted, skipped or overlooked investigating the possibility of a personality disorder because finding a personality disorder would have caused the claim to be identified as non–work-related. Consistent with the pervasive lack of diagnostic adequacy discussed earlier, these findings reveal a severe obstacle to credible causation analysis and to credibly claim occupational causation.

The issues that have been discussed in this section warrant the establishment of the following warning: Any claims of occupational mental illness are probably going to be based on an inadequate diagnostic evaluation and should subsequently be intensely scrutinized.

Specific Diagnostic Examples

Posttraumatic Stress Disorder

Posttraumatic stress disorder (PTSD) appeared on the recruited tabulations of mental illnesses that most commonly show up in workers' compensation. This is not a surprising result because the definition and diagnostic protocol for PTSD are of a nature that readily lends itself to an assumption that traumatic experiences, such as severe occupational injuries or workplace catastrophes, are the cause for this disorder. However, such assumptions have failed scientific tests.

The attempts to claim that PTSD is caused by traumatic events stem from the text of the American Psychiatric Association's *DSM*,[12] such as the following passage: "The essential feature of Posttraumatic Stress Disorders the development of characteristic symptoms *following* exposure to an extreme traumatic stressor involving direct personal experience of an event that involves actual or threatened death or serious injury, or other threat to one's physical integrity; or witnessing an event that involves death, injury, or threat to the physical integrity of another person; or learning about unexpected or violent death, serious harm, or threat of death or injury experienced by a family member or other close associate."

Apparently, the word *following* in the preceding quotation is regularly misinterpreted as meaning *caused by.* The vulnerability of this concept to such misinterpretation has resulted in exploitation that the American Psychiatric Association's literature has characterized as a "growth industry" of "burgeoning litigation."[19] Scientific findings that clarify that *following* should not be interpreted as meaning *caused by* are discussed subsequently.

For example, an incredible amount of research has been conducted on the cause of PTSD, the first line of the resulting evidence table would reveal that a search of PTSD and causation in PubMed produced 1,233 articles (accessed May 15, 2007). However, most of that research is flawed by a technicality that makes the findings less useful for the purpose of this book. Specifically, the diagnostic protocol for PTSD requires the person to have experienced a trauma that fits the quoted *DSM* description. In other words, this technicality means that a person cannot be given this diagnosis unless he or she has experienced such trauma, even if he or she has every symptom of PTSD and the manifestations satisfy all of the other diagnostic criteria. This is a very unfortunate set of circumstances for causation analysis because it creates a definitional confounding of trauma with the symptoms. Therefore, if a research design does not somehow overcome this definitional confounding, the only possible research outcome is a misleading finding that PTSD is always associated with trauma. This is analogous to concluding that all cars are blue after a research project that excluded, from the beginning, any cars that were not blue.

It is only recently that research designs have emerged that allow for consideration of the symptomatic nature of PTSD apart from this definitional confounding with trauma. That research has reliably produced results that indicate that there is no actual correlation between a protocol-type trauma and the symptoms of PTSD.

For example, if a traumatic experience is actually the cause of PTSD, the symptoms of PTSD should be more common among people who report that they have experienced such trauma. Research findings have indicated that this is not the case. Such findings have actually included a lower rate of PTSD symptoms among people who reported that they had experienced a protocol-type trauma (and, correspondingly, a higher incidence among people who had not experienced such a trauma).[20,21] In addition, significantly fewer people who had experienced a protocol-type trauma satisfied symptom requirements for a PTSD diagnosis (and, correspondingly, people who did not experience a protocol-type trauma were actually more likely to satisfy symptom requirements for PTSD).[20] In other words, scientific investigation has repeatedly produced findings that are the exact opposite of what would be expected if trauma were the cause of PTSD symptoms.

CHAPTER 16

Reports from the research participants in these studies indicated that normal life stress is more strongly associated with PTSD symptoms than is the experience of trauma. Such findings are consistent with previously published reports from different designs.[22-25]

The PTSD investigations reported herein are population-based studies rather than being based on mental health patients. But clinical research has produced similar results. Research that was limited to people who sought mental health care revealed that rates of PTSD symptoms were the same for people who had not experienced a protocol-type trauma as for people who had.[26] In other words, the results indicated that the complex of symptoms that have been included in the diagnostic protocol for PTSD is not actually correlated with trauma. The symptoms of PTSD seem to be a generic manifestation of mental illness, which does not manifest any more often among people who have experienced trauma than among people who have not.

Consistent with the recent findings that trauma is not a necessary cause of PTSD symptoms, attempts to comprehensively review the relevant literature had previously indicated that a traumatic experience is also not a sufficient cause of PTSD. For example, research has consistently revealed that PTSD is not likely to follow trauma.[7,19,27,28] Scientific analysis has also indicated that exposure to any specifically claimed trauma is not even the most important risk factor for PTSD.[27] Therefore, when considered in its entirety, the history of relevant scientific efforts indicates that trauma is neither a necessary nor a sufficient cause of PTSD symptoms.

Consistent with all of the preceding information, scientific investigation has demonstrated that there is not a reliable dose-response gradient for any supposed relationship between severity of an occupational trauma (e.g., as experienced by firefighters) and the development of PTSD.[29] The absence of such a reliable dose-response gradient provides additional evidence against a causative role for trauma.

Scientific research has further indicated the lack of work-relatedness in regard to PTSD when an issue of great significance to workers' compensation is considered—permanent impairment. Specifically, scientific investigations have indicated that trauma does not have any predictive role in the manifestation of long-term symptoms of PTSD (This finding emerged even without a research design that could overcome the definitional confounding of trauma with symptoms.).[30] The findings indicated that the only predictor of such long-term PTSD symptoms is preexisting psychopathology. Such findings create yet another obstacle to credibly claiming that adult life events can have a causative role in the development of permanent impairment from PTSD.

Scientific studies of PTSD also provide an illustration of the fundamental role of genetics in the causation of mental illness. Relevant research findings include genetic factors accounting for up to 34% of the variance for the development of PTSD symptoms and specifically accounting for more symptoms than did trauma exposure (even without controlling for the definitional confounding of trauma and symptoms).[31]

The scientific findings regarding PTSD provide another valuable opportunity for illustrating the demands of causation analysis in that a credible analysis requires thorough consideration of alternative explanations for the clinical manifestations. In this discussion, this means consideration of potential causes other than occupational or tort-relevant causation. One example of an alternative cause is eligibility for compensation. Research has revealed that eligibility for compensation has a much more profound role than trauma does in determining whether a diagnosis of PTSD will be made. Although PTSD is diagnosed in only 7% to 12% of people in the general population who are exposed to accidents,[32] rates of 85% have been documented when the accident created an opportunity to seek compensation.[33] In other words, the indication from such science is that 73% of the claims of PTSD would be more likely attributable to benefit eligibility than to trauma. Subsequently, in an artificial exercise that considers only exposure to trauma and eligibility for benefits as potential causes of PTSD, eligibility for benefits would overwhelmingly be the more probable cause.

Major Depressive Disorder

Major depressive disorder was prominent on the recruited lists of mental illnesses that frequently appear in workers' compensation claims. From a scientific perspective, the appearance of MDD on these lists is surprising. For MDD to appear on those lists, there must be some assumption within workers' compensation that work is a cause of MDD. Current research has repeatedly indicated that such an assumption is false.

Research findings have reliably indicated that work is a protective agent in regard to MDD.[17] It is not a risk factor and, therefore, not a cause. This is not even a matter of there being a lack of relationship between work and MDD. Instead, work has repeatedly been demonstrated to have an inverse relationship with MDD—MDD is approximately three times less common among people who are working as opposed to people who are not working.

Research has also clarified actual risk factors for MDD, thereby inadvertently providing an understanding of what it is that work is protecting vulnerable people (who are vulnerable to certain mental illness) from. For example, as is the case with most forms of mental illness, genetics have a dominant role in the cause of MDD.[7] Childhood experience also seems to have a "compelling" role.[17] Work apparently buffers the effects of such factors, so that the symptoms of the mental illness are manifested less often or less severely.

Research also provides some clues about *how* work protects vulnerable people from MDD. Important factors seem to include the manner in which work improves a person's financial state, self-esteem, social connectedness, motivation, and sense of purpose. In addition, work provides a mental respite from internal and external correlates of mood disturbance.[34]

Another obstacle to establishing occupational or tort-relevant causation for MDD is the chronic nature of this disorder. Any person who has had one major depressive episode at any point in his or her life is probably going to experience, or has already had, other major depressive episodes.[12] In most cases, MDD is going to be a chronic, recurring illness rather than a focused response to some specific experience. Subsequently, it becomes extremely difficult to justify a claim of recent causation for a major depressive episode. If a history of a previous episode is acknowledged, any new episode would be a normal and expected manifestation of the preexisting disorder rather than an unexpected event that might require an explanation (an explanation such as occupational or tort-relevant causation). It would actually be unusual and more worthy of explanation if the new episode had not occurred. The situation does not benefit from the examinee denying previous episodes, given the repeated scientific findings that indicate that such denials are not a credible basis for clinical decision making.[10,11]

The data that were collected and reviewed specifically for this chapter indicated a trend for work-relatedness to be claimed for MDD because MDD is being attributed to chronic pain complaints, and work-relatedness is also being claimed for the chronic pain complaints. Attempts to credibly establish occupational causation for such claims face numerous obstacles, including scientific findings that indicate that any combination of chronic pain and a mood disorder raises the probability that there will be no objective general medical explanation for the pain complaints, thereby moving the entire claim farther away from occupational causation [16]; and denials of preexisting mood disturbance from a claimant cannot be credibly used in clinical decision making.[10,11] Another obstacle to justifying such arguments is the fact that the many attempts to comprehensively review the scientific literature on the cause of MDD reliably fail to mention pain as a cause of MDD.[7,17,35] In addition, research findings have indicated that mood disorders tend to precede chronic pain complaints rather than follow them,[36] and even a family history of mood disorder tends to predispose people to the development of complaints of chronic pain.[37] Subsequently, scientific findings more easily support a conclusion that mood disorders are a cause of complaints of chronic pain rather than an argument that the complaints of chronic pain caused the mood disorder and, subsequently, established occupational or tort-related causation for the mood disorder.

Dysthymic Disorder

Another mental illness that was prominent in the tabulations recruited for this book was dysthymic disorder. Much of what has been previously discussed in this chapter applies to any effort to establish occupational or tort-relevant causation for dysthymic disorder. Attempts to credibly establish such causation for dysthymic disorder also face additional obstacles.

For any individual case of dysthymic disorder, the probability is that the illness is preexisting rather than a work- or tort-relevant illness. This probability is because of the scientific findings that the illness is usually apparent in childhood or adolescence rather than manifesting as a consequence of adult life experience.[38]

Similarly, scientific discussions of the causes of dysthymic disorder emphasize risk factors that do not involve occupational or tort-relevant issues. Examples of established risk factors include certain types of sleep disorders, thyroid abnormalities, faulty personality development, social disappointment early in life, and dysfunctional fantasies.[17]

Similarly, scientific study of adult life trauma revealed that such trauma was not associated with increased rates of dysthymic disorder.[39]

Pain Disorder

Pain disorder appeared on the list of mental illnesses that are common in workers' compensation claims.

Pain disorder is a somatoform disorder, which means that it is a mental illness characterized by physical complaints. As such, it is definitionally impossible to attribute pain disorder to an occupational injury. The definition of all somatoform disorders specifies that they cannot be accounted for by any general medical condition (such as an occupational or tort-relevant injury).[12]

Direct interviewing of some clinicians who claimed work-relatedness for pain disorder revealed some clues about how this definitionally non–injury-related mental illness has found its way into the workers' compensation system. Specifically, there seems to be prominent confusion among mental health specialists about the nature of pain disorder and the definitional ramifications that can accompany variations in the use of this phrase. For example, the American Psychiatric Association's *DSM*[12] discusses a concept of "pain disorder associated with a general medical condition." This concept is defined by pain that is primarily attributable to a general medical condition. Clinicians who were claiming occupational causation for pain disorder actually reported that they were referring to that passage from the *DSM*. Unfortunately, these clinicians did not realize that the concept of "pain disorder associated with a general medical condition" is specified in the manual as not being a mental illness or a diagnosis (e.g., there is no diagnostic code associated with this concept, and if this concept is to be used, the underlying general medical diagnosis and its associated diagnostic code are to be used).

In addition to the definitional lack of relationship between physical injury and pain disorder, attempts to establish occupational or tort-relevant causation also face the obstacle of the nonoccupational and non–tort-relevant nature of the risk factors that have been identified for pain disorder. Potential causative factors that have been listed in attempts to comprehensively review the relevant literature include the following[17]:

- The pain is an expression of some internal conflict.
- The examinee is unable to use words to describe his or her feelings.
- The examinee is creating the pain complaints
  - so that he or she will have a legitimate claim to the fulfillment of his or her dependency needs,
  - to atone for perceived sins,
  - as an expression of guilt,
  - as an expression of aggression,
  - because he or she believes that he or she deserves to suffer,
  - as a means of obtaining love,
  - as a way of identifying with a loved one who also has pain complaints,
  - because the pain complaints are being rewarded in some way (such as the solicitous and attentive behavior of others, monetary gain, or avoidance of distasteful activities), and/or
  - as a means of manipulation and gaining advantage in personal relationships.
- The pain disorder is caused by preexisting anatomic or biochemical abnormalities that produce, otherwise unexplainable experiences of pain.

Substance Abuse

Various forms of substance-related disorders appeared in the tabulations of the most common mental illnesses in workers' compensation. A review of several files indicated a trend for work-relatedness to be claimed because narcotic medication was being abused and the medication had been prescribed within the context of a workers' compensation claim.

However, this simplistic approach to claiming occupational causation is contradicted by scientific findings. Research has repeatedly indicated that neither complaints of chronic pain nor the prescription of narcotic medications is associated with an elevated risk of substance abuse. Instead, the findings indicate that when substance abuse occurs within the context of chronic pain and/or prescription narcotics, the substance abuse is more likely to have preceded that context rather than to be a consequence of it.[40-44] In other words, if there is a causative relationship, it is more likely that substance abuse tendencies are the cause of the complaints of chronic pain (and subsequent prescription of narcotic medications) rather than vice versa.

Considerations About Application of the NIOSH Process to Claims of Mental Illness

Chapter 4 provided a review of NIOSH's six step process for the determination of work-relatedness. This section provides some direction for applying that process to claims of occupational mental illness.

1. *Evidence of disease. What is the disease? Is the diagnosis correct? Does the evidence (history, physical examination, and supporting studies) support or fail to support the diagnosis?*

   The previous sections of this chapter have illustrated the elevated jeopardy of a false diagnosis when occupational mental illness is being claimed. Given such jeopardy, any attempt to claim occupational-relatedness (or tort-relatedness) should involve strict adherence to the diagnostic protocols from the American Psychiatric Association's *DSM*[12] a comprehensive review of all records that can be obtained from the examinee's entire life (especially preclaim records), collateral input, and thorough, objective use of psychological testing.

2. *Epidemiologic data: What is the epidemiologic evidence for that disease or condition? Do the data support a relationship with work?*

   This part means that any credible attempt to claim work-relatedness (or tort-relatedness) for a mental illness must involve a presentation of credible and reliable scientific findings that indicate that the claimed exposure is a cause of that specific mental illness. Any such attempt must also demonstrate why any scientific findings that indicate against such a causative relationship are not relevant to the case being evaluated. For claims of work-related mental illness, this part of the process means that an evaluator who is claiming work-relatedness must credibly explain why the scientific indications that work actually protects against psychological disturbance do not apply to the case being evaluated.

3. *Evidence of exposure: What evidence, predominantly objective, is there that the level of occupational environmental exposure (frequency, intensity, and duration) could cause the disease?*

As discussed previously in this chapter, this part of the process often brings attempts to claim work-relatedness (or tort-relatedness) to a halt for any claim of mental illness. There are multiple obstacles to completing this step when the examined disease is a mental illness. For example, before attempts are undertaken to objectify the level of exposure to the suspected causative issue, the examiner should first establish a credible scientific basis for identifying any occupational (or tort-relevant) issue as being causative (part 2 of the NIOSH process). Establishing such a basis will usually not be possible, given the lack of definitive causative information for most mental illnesses,[2] scientific findings that have indicated that adult life experience does not have a role in the genesis of mental illness (examples discussed earlier), and the scientific findings that work has a protective role against manifestations of psychological disturbance.[17]

Therefore, a credible evaluator will usually be unable to move past step 2 in the process. But the review of files that was conducted for this chapter revealed that clinicians regularly ignore step 2 and claim causative agents that do not have epidemiologic support. However, that noncredible practice pattern would then be thwarted by step 3 because there is no objective method for establishing level of exposure considerations for the types of causes that are typically claimed for mental illness within workers' compensation claims (or in tort claims).

4. *Other relevant factors. What other relevant factors are present in this case? Are there individual risk factors other than the occupational environmental exposure that could contribute to the development of the disease?*

When step 1 confirms a diagnosis, step 2 can be used to identify the scientifically credible risk factors for the disorder. Such scientific findings can be applied to the individual case to determine whether any of the nonoccupational (and non–tort-relevant) risk factors for the disorder are evident for this examinee. For a conclusion of work- or tort-relatedness to be credible, the examiner must provide a comprehensive review of how such non-related risk factors do not apply or how they apply to a less significant extent than claim-related factors.

Step 4 also reflects the discussion that was provided in the section of this chapter entitled "The Importance of Considering the Entire Clinical Picture, Rather Than an Isolated Diagnosis." Subsequently, any credible attempt to claim work-relatedness (or tort-relatedness) for a mental illness must involve a thorough diagnostic evaluation of all potentially relevant mental illnesses (rather than a focus on a single mental illness for which relatedness is being claimed). Any evaluator who is claiming work-relatedness (or tort-relatedness) must be able to demonstrate that the claimed mental illness is truly an unexpected development caused by the claimed life experience, rather than a normal and expected manifestation of the examinee's general psychological nature.

In addition, if stress is being claimed as the cause of a mental illness, any credible attempt to claim work- or tort-relatedness must involve the following: a comprehensive analysis of other sources of stress in the examinee's life, an objective analysis of the relative levels of supposedly related stress vs unrelated stress, and a credible explanation for why the work- or tort-related stress is emphasized as opposed to unrelated stress.

5. *Validity of the evidence. Is there confounding or conflicting evidence to suggest information obtained in the assessment is inaccurate?*

This part of the process is most effectively addressed as a component of each of the preceding four steps. In other words, for mental illness, any attempt to claim work- or tort-relatedness will probably be confronted by confounding or conflicting evidence during each step in this process. By addressing this issue within each step, rather than waiting to address it as a separate fifth step, the efficiency of the process can be elevated. For example, steps 2 through 6 will often be unnecessary, given the tendency discussed previously in this chapter for noncredible diagnoses to emerge from workers' compensation claims. Similarly, steps 3 through 6 will often be unnecessary based on epidemiologic evidence that contradicts claims of work- or tort-relatedness.

6. *Evaluation and conclusions.*

This part of the assessment process calls for a previous section of this chapter, "The Necessity for Independent Evaluation," to be emphasized. For mental health specialists, professional standards universally indicate that treating clinicians should not engage in causation analysis. Therefore, for conclusions of work- or tort-relatedness to be credible, they must come through independent review (rather than from treating clinicians). Any clinician who offers a conclusion of work- or tort-relatedness must ensure that that he or she has never had a direct relationship with the examinee, and must permanently avoid entering into any such relationship with the examinee.

Application of the NIOSH Process to an Individual Claim of Mental Illness

The following hypothetical case is based on features from several files that involved claims of occupational mental illness: A man's hand was traumatically amputated in an occupational accident. For 12 years after that accident, workers' compensation benefits were provided for mental health care focused on complaints of depression that the claimant states are due to the amputation.

1. Evidence of disease

For the entire 12 years of this workers' compensation claim, there had never been any diagnosis for the complaint of depression or the associated treatment. Medical records, without exception, had listed the diagnosis as "depression" (which, as was explained above, is not a mental illness or a diagnosis). Records also indicated that there had never been any attempt to provide this claimant with a diagnostic workup for the complaint of depression. Subsequently, a causation analysis could stop at this first part in the process because there was no evidence of disease and no diagnosis.

But the referral process authorized a comprehensive independent evaluation to determine whether there was a mental illness, what any diagnosis might be, and whether there was any work-relatedness. Use of the American Psychiatric Association's diagnostic system revealed consistency with a diagnosis of dysthymic disorder (the examinees' manifestations did not satisfy criteria for any other mental illness or for malingering). This diagnostic impression was objectively supported by the results of psychological testing. Psychological testing did not produce clear indications of malingering. The diagnostic impression was also supported by reports that were obtained from the claimant's mother. Records were roughly consistent with this diagnosis and did not provide clearly contradictory information.

2. Epidemiologic data

As was discussed above, epidemiologic evidence for dysthymic disorder does not support a causative role for work or for physical injury. Therefore, the causation analysis could stop here owing to the claim's lack of epidemiologic support.

3. Evidence of exposure

For this case, there is no opportunity to use this part of the process to establish work-relatedness because parts 1 and 2 failed to provide any reason to suspect a relationship between the clinical manifestations and exposure to any potential occupational cause. If the evaluation process had ignored part 2 and accepted the examinee's claim that the amputation had been the cause of his mental illness, then any credible claim of work-relatedness would have to involve some objective measurement of exposure. Such measurement would have to provide an objective answer to the following question: Was this examinee's exposure to injury and amputation of a level that could account for the difference between him and other people who experience traumatic amputations but do not fit the criteria for dysthymic disorder? It is doubtful that such measurement or such objective explanation could be given. Subsequently, if the effort to establish work-relatedness proceeds this far, it could reasonably stop here owing to the lack of ability to satisfy the demands of this step.

4. Other relevant factors

A variety of nonoccupational risk factors for dysthymic disorder were discussed earlier in this chapter. The scientific findings can be compared with an individual case such as this to determine whether the nonoccupational risk factors are relevant to the examinee. For this case, the claimant's reported childhood experiences were found to have involved the type of social disappointments that have been scientifically linked to dysthymic disorder.

5. Validity of the evidence

In this case, examples of conflicting evidence included the inconsistency between the typical nature of dysthymic disorder and this examinee's claim that his mental illness began after his injury. A diagnosis of dysthymic disorder means that his mental illness was probably preexisting. (Readers are reminded that the examinee's denial of preexisting mental illness does not provide a credible basis for clinical decision making.) Medical records from the examinee's entire life were requested. The records obtained documented preinjury visits to physicians with complaints of depression and subsequent treatment for depression. There was no diagnosis in the records, but the reports were generally consistent with dysthymic disorder. In addition, the examinee's mother was interviewed as a source of collateral information. She reported that the examinee had been depressed throughout his life (the depression was evident during childhood, decades before the occupational injury). Her description of his preinjury depression satisfied diagnostic criteria for dysthymic disorder. She also reported that his current depression seemed less severe than his preinjury depression.

When asked about this discrepancy between his reports and the other sources of information, the claimant readily admitted that his reports had been incorrect, explained that he had denied the preexisting nature of his depression because he simply did not want to think about that depressed portion of his life, and insightfully admitted that it was easier to blame his depression on his injury than to acknowledge that he has a mental illness. He also endorsed his mother's report that his preinjury depression had actually been more severe than his current experience of depression.

6. Evaluation and conclusions

The findings that have been presented provide a sound basis for concluding that work-relatedness cannot be credibly claimed for this case and for subsequently recommending a removal of the man's mental health care from the workers' compensation system (to spare him from further exposure to the reliably detrimental health effects of involvement in that system).

Acknowledgements

Gratitude is extended to the following agencies and people who provided reports in regard to the claims of mental illness that most frequently appear within workers' compensation:

Sue Twigg, CWC, ACA, Oasis Outsourcing

Christopher R. Brigham, MD, Brigham and Associates, Inc.

Four additional agencies that asked to remain anonymous (they represent two insurance claims data and two state workers' compensation claims data).

References

1. Hyman SE. Foreword, In: Phillips KA, First MB, Pincus HA, eds. *Advancing DSM: Dilemmas in Psychiatric Diagnosis.* Washington, DC: American Psychiatric Association; 2003.
2. Caine ED. Determining causation in psychiatry. In: Phillips KA, First MB, Pincus HA, eds. *Advancing DSM: Dilemmas in Psychiatric Diagnosis.* Washington, DC: American Psychiatric Association; 2003.
3. Rohling ML, Binder LM, Langhinrichsen-Rohling J. Money matters: a meta-analytic review of the association between financial compensation and the experience and treatment of chronic pain. *Health Psychol.* 1995;14:537-547.
4. Binder LM, Rohling ML. Money matters: a meta-analytic review of the effects of financial incentives on recovery after closed head injury. *Am J Psychiatry.* 1996;153:7-10.
5. Harris I, Multford J, Solomon M, van Gelder JM, Young J. Association between compensation status and outcome after surgery. *JAMA.* 2005;293:1644-1652.
6. Greenberg SA, Shuman DW. Irreconcilable conflict between therapeutic and forensic rules. *Prof Psychol Res Pr.* 1997;28:50-57.
7. Hales RE, Yudofsky SC. *The American Psychiatric Publishing Textbook of Clinical Psychiatry, Fourth Edition.* Washington, DC: American Psychiatric Publishing; 2002.
8. Barth RJ, Brigham CR. Who is in the better position to evaluate, the treating physician or an independent evaluator. *The Guides Newsletter.* September/October 2005:8-11.
9. Reid WH. Treating clinicians and expert testimony. *J Pract Psychiatry Behav Health.* 1998;4:121-123.
10. Barsky AJ. Forgetting, fabricating, and telescoping: the instability of the medical history. *Arch Intern Med.* 2002;162:981-984.
11. Lees-Haley PR, Williams CW, English LT. Response bias in self-reported history of plaintiffs compared with non-litigating patients. *Psychol Rep.* 1996;79:811-818.
12. American Psychiatric Association. *Diagnostic and Statistical Manual of Mental Disorders, Fourth Edition, Text Revision.* Washington, DC: American Psychiatric Association; 2000.
13. Breslau N, Davis GC. DSM-III generalized anxiety disorder: an empirical investigation of more stringent criteria. *Psychiatry Res.* 1985;15:231-238.
14. Dersh J, Gatchel RJ, Polatin P, Temple OR. Prevalence of psychiatric disorders in patients with chronic disabling occupational spinal disorders. *Spine.* 2006;31:1156-1162.
15. Gatchel RJ, Weisberg JN. *Personality Characteristics of Patients With Pain.* Washington, DC: American Psychological Association; 2000.
16. Magni G. On the relationship between chronic pain and depression when there is no organic lesion. *Pain.* 1987;31:1-21.
17. Sadock BJ, Sadock VA. *Kaplan and Sadock's Synopsis of Psychiatry.* 9th ed. Philadelphia, PA: Lippincott Williams & Wilkins; 2003.
18. Cocchiarella L, Anderson G, eds. *Guides to the Evaluation of Permanent Impairment.* 5th ed. Chicago, IL: American Medical Association; 2001:567-569.

CHAPTER 16

19. Simon RI, ed. *Posttraumatic Stress Disorder in Litigation: Guidelines for Forensic Assessment.* 2nd ed. Washington, DC: American Psychiatric Publishing; 2003.

20. Gold SD, Marx BP, Soler-Baillo JM, Sloan DM. Is life stress more traumatic than traumatic stress? *J Anxiety Disord.* 2005;19:687-698.

21. Mol SS, Arntz A, Metsemakers JF, Dinant GJ, Vilters-van Montfort PA, Knottnerus JA. Symptoms of post-traumatic stress disorder after non-traumatic events: evidence from an open population study. *Br J Psychiatry.* 2005;186:494-499.

22. Helzer JE, Robins L, McEvoy L. Post-traumatic stress disorder in the general population: findings of the epidemiological catchment area survey. *N Engl J Med.* 1987;317:1630-1634.

23. Burstein A. Post-traumatic stress disorder. *J Clin Psychiatry.* 1985;46:554-556.

24. Scott MJ, Stradling SG. Post-traumatic stress disorder without the trauma. *Br J Clin Psychol.* 1994;33:71-74.

25. Olff M, Koeter MWJ, Van Haaften EH, Kersten PH, Gersons BPR. Impact of a foot and mouth disease crisis on post-traumatic stress symptoms in farmers. *Br J Psychiatry.* 2005;186:165-166.

26. Bodkin JA, Pope HG, Detke MJ, Hudson JI. Is PTSD caused by traumatic stress? *J Anxiety Disord,* 2007;21:176-182.

27. Yehuda R, ed. *Risk Factors for Posttraumatic Stress Disorder.* Washington, DC: American Psychiatric Press; 1999.

28. Yehuda R, ed. *Psychological Trauma.* Washington, DC: American Psychiatric Press; 1998.

29. McFarlane AC. The aetiology of post-traumatic stress disorders following natural disasters. *Br J Psychiatry.* 1988;152:116-121.

30. McFarlane AC. The aetiology of post-traumatic morbidity: predisposing, precipitating and perpetuating factors. *Br J Psychiatry.* 1989;154:221-228.

31. True WR, Rice J, Eisen SA, et al. A twin study of genetic and environmental contributions to liability for posttraumatic stress symptoms. *Arch Gen Psychiatry.* 1993;50:257-264.

32. Breslau N. The epidemiology of posttraumatic stress disorder: what is the extent of the problem? *J Clin Psychiatry.* 2001;62(suppl 17):16-22.

33. Rosen GM. The *Aleutian Enterprise* sinking and posttraumatic stress disorder: misdiagnosis in clinical and forensic settings. *Prof Psychol Res P.* 1995;26:82-87.

34. Rothman EF, Hathaway J, Stidsen A, de Vries HF. How employment helps female victims of intimate partner violence: a qualitative study. *J Occup Health Psychol.* 2007;12:136-143.

35. Sadock BJ, Sadock VA. *Kaplan and Sadock's Comprehensive Textbook of Psychiatry.* 8th ed. Philadelphia, PA: Lippincott Williams & Wilkins; 2004.

36. Polatin PB, Kinney RK, Gatchel RJ, Lillo E. Psychiatric illness and chronic low back pain: the mind and the spine: which goes first? *Spine.* 1993;18:66-71.

37. Raphael KG, Janal MN, Nayak S, Schwartz JE, Gallagher RM. Familial aggregation of depression in fibromyalgia: a community-based test of alternate hypotheses. *Pain.* 2004;110:449-460.

38. US Department of Health and Human Services. *Mental Health: A Report of the Surgeon General: Executive Summary.* Rockville, MD: Dept of Health and Human Services, Substance Abuse and Mental Health Services Administration, Center for Mental Health Services, National Institutes of Health, National Institute of Mental Health; 1999.

39. Winfield I, George LK, Swartz M, et al. Sexual assault and psychiatric disorders among women in a community population. *Am J Psychiatry.* 1990;147:335-341.
40. Brown RL, Patterson JJ, Rounds LA, Papasouliotis O. Substance abuse among patients with chronic back pain. *J Fam Pract.* 1996;43:152-160.
41. Martell BA, O'Connor PG, Kerns RD, et al. Systematic review: opioid treatment for chronic back pain: prevalence, efficacy, and association with addiction. *Ann Intern Med.* 2007;146:116-127.
42. Breckenridge J, Clark JD. Patient characteristics associated with opioid versus nonsteroidal anti-inflammatory drug management of chronic low back pain. *J Pain.* 2003;4:344-350.
43. Von Korff M, Crane P, Lane M, et al. Chronic spinal pain and physical-mental comorbidity in the United States: results from the National Comorbidity Survey Replication. *Pain.* 2005;113:331-339.
44. Dersh J, Gatchel RJ, Polatin P. Prevalence of psychiatric disorders in patients with chronic work-related musculoskeletal pain disability. *J Occup Environ Med.* 2002;44:459-468.

CHAPTER 17

Genitourinary Problems

Fred Kuyt, MD, William Ackerman, MD and Mark H. Hyman, MD

Vesicoureteral Reflux

It has always been a urologic principle that protecting the kidneys and, therefore, preserving renal function, is uppermost in priority. A delicate balance exists in the pressure differential between the upper urinary tract (kidneys and ureters) and the lower urinary tract (bladder and urethra). This gradient is a prerequisite to normal renal function and, thus, must be maintained and protected. In other words, for the nephrons to carry out fluid balance functions within the body, a low-pressure system within the upper urinary tract must exist so that the rate of urine production and its antegrade flow through the upper tracts is facilitated. Any condition that increases pressure within the urinary bladder may potentiate reflux or retrograde flow of urine. If unidentified and unchecked, vesicoureteral reflux can cause an increase in intrarenal pressure, reflux nephropathy, and renal failure. These latter conditions can lead not only to electrolyte imbalances with all their incumbent physiologic effects, but also to hypertension.

Among the most common conditions that cause urinary reflux encountered by industrial medical examiners are those categorized as anatomic or physiologic obstruction of the urinary bladder. Anatomic injuries to the urethra via blunt trauma incurred with straddle injury, pelvic fracture, or the presence of an indwelling urinary catheter can result in a urethral stricture.[1-4] This stricture decreases the urinary flow rate and increases the resistance to that flow, eventually causing bladder impairment, bladder muscle fatigue, and subsequent inability of the bladder to empty itself. As the residual urinary volume increases, the pressure inside the bladder increases and eventually causes a breach in function of the physiologic valve between the bladder and ureters. Reflux ensues, and kidney damage often follows. Analogously, an enlarged prostate can propagate a similar course.

The physiologic causes of bladder outflow obstruction are neurologic injuries that have occurred at various levels of the spinal cord through disc herniation, spinal cord trauma, or complications of spinal surgery.[5,6] Neurologic bladder control comes from above the sacral (S2-S4) micturition center up to the micturition center in the brain stem, referred to as the pontine micturition center. These areas have a role in allowing the sphincter muscles within the lower urinary tract to relax. The result of any injury to these neurologic areas is varying degrees of inability of the urinary sphincter valves to relax. With uncoordinated sphincter activity, there is an increase in the resistance to urinary flow, followed by bladder fatigue and decompensation, which increase urinary residual volumes and bladder pressure. Again, the end results are vesicoureteral reflux and renal impairment. Another problem that can result from injury to the area above the sacral micturition center is unopposed bladder wall contraction, often associated with a lack of coordination in voluntary relaxation of the external sphincter or involuntary relaxation of the internal sphincter.[6-8] This condition in its entirety is known as *detrusor* (the bladder wall muscle) *sphincter dyssynergia.*

Micturition

The activating and inhibiting components of coordinated voiding require the detrusor muscle to contract, while both urinary sphincters relax in sequence. The relaxation of the sphincter muscles is facilitated via signals carried through inhibitory pathways that descend down the spinal cord originating from the brain stem. Any injury above the sacral micturition center, within the "upper motor neuron segment," impairs sphincter relaxation to varying degrees and causes dyssynergia between the detrusor muscle and the sphincter muscles. These same types of injuries could leave bladder contraction relatively unopposed, resulting in detrusor hyperactivity. The classic symptoms of these conditions are urinary urgency, urge urinary incontinence, frequency, and nocturia.

Injury to the sacral micturition center, which, under normal conditions, causes not only the bladder to contract, but also the external sphincter to contract in response to the Valsalva maneuver (e.g., when coughing, sneezing, and laughing), can result in stress urinary incontinence. The ability of the external urinary sphincter to coapt in response to the Valsalva maneuver and heavy lifting is dependent not only on an intact nerve supply, but also on proper anatomic configuration. When there is vaginal herniation that promotes bladder descensus and ineffective external sphincter closure, stress urinary incontinence occurs.[9] Stress urinary incontinence is related to multiple pregnancies and obesity.[10-14] Repeated heavy lifting, multiple pregnancies, and obesity can cause vaginal herniation.[15] In a nulliparous woman who is not obese, heavy lifting for a long period can cause stress urinary incontinence.

Sexual Function

Erectile dysfunction can be caused by hypertension, diabetes, vascular disease, and the medications used to treat these conditions. There are possible circumstances in which industrial injury can contribute to the process.[16-20] Straddle injury to the nerve supply of the erectile mechanism, spinal cord injury, and industrially related vascular injury, such as found with pelvic fracture, are examples.[21-24]

Retrograde ejaculation with possible infertility can occur with the anterior spinal cord approach to surgery via disturbances to the sympathetic pathways.[25,26] Blunt testicular trauma can also cause infertility.[27,28] Pain can cause erectile dysfunction, such as pain related to a back injury or prostatitis or the pain of postoperative nerve entrapment found with inguinal hernia repairs.[29,30]

Exposure to Chemicals and Solvents

Upper Tract Disease

Chemicals used in industry are usually metabolized by the liver and excreted by the kidneys. However, exposure to chemicals can have an adverse effect on the kidneys. Environmental pollutants such as arsenic, lead, and cadmium are known to induce chronic renal disease.[31] The nephrotoxic effects of these metals occur because urinary elimination is the main route of excretion, and the proximal tubules are especially sensitive owing to their high reabsorptive activity. The renal pathologic effects of these metals vary with the chemical form of the metal, the dose, and whether the exposure is short- or long-term.[31]

Occupational exposure to vapors, gases, and aerosols promotes an increase in the incidence of renal disease.[32] In a survey of patients with idiopathic membranous glomerulonephritis, the predominance of the condition among men could be at least partly explained by an increased risk of exposure to organic solvents and heavy metals in the course of their work.[33] For example, renal disease can occur in battery workers exposed to cadmium and lead.[34,35] Environmental and industrial exposures to lead continue to pose major public health problems in children and adults. Short-term exposure to high concentrations of lead can result in proximal tubular damage with characteristic histologic features.[36] Cadmium is widely dispersed in the environment owing to occupational and cigarette emissions.[37,38] Chronic lead nephropathy occurs as a result of years of exposure to lead.[39,40]

Occupational exposure to organic solvents has been found to be associated with the development and progression of tubulointerstitial fibrosis and chronic renal failure.[41-43] Substantially more cases of tubular damage were found among patients with renal cell carcinoma who had been exposed to high levels of trichloroethylene for many years than among patients with renal cell carcinoma who had not been exposed to trichloroethylene.[44,45]

An occupational survey was done in patients with end-stage renal failure to determine their exposure to hydrocarbon-based compounds.[46] Approximately 59% of patients with renal failure due to glomerulonephritis had significant contact with hydrocarbons compared with 25% of patients with renal failure due to other causes. Occupational exposure to hydrocarbons may account for the male predominance in glomerulonephritis. Goodpasture syndrome may be caused by benzene exposure.[47] Membranous nephropathy from exposure to mercury in the fluorescent-tube-recycling industry may occur in workers exposed to this metal.[48-50] Glomerulonephritis has also been reported to be associated with hydrocarbon solvents.[51,52] Technical dinitrotoluene (DNT) is a mixture of 2,4- and 2,6-DNT. In humans, industrial or environmental exposure can occur orally, by inhalation, or by skin contact. Recent data point to the carcinogenicity of DNT on the urinary tract of exposed humans.[53]

Kidney autoimmunity can occur with environmental and occupational exposure to metal.[54] Metals, present in the environment or administered for therapeutic reasons, are prototypical xenobiotics that cause decreases or enhancements of immune responses. In particular, exposure to gold and mercury may result in autoimmune responses to various self-antigens and autoimmune disease of the kidney and other tissues.

Rapidly progressive renal failure can develop in patients exposed to silica.[55] Progressive renal failure with a syndrome of rapidly progressive glomerulonephritis has been reported to develop in coal miners with silicosis.[56] Renal biopsies reveal crescentic glomerulonephritides associated with angiitis.

Some workers may be exposed to fluoride. The prognosis for fluoride inhalation is poor owing to the extreme toxicity of the substance and lack of satisfactory treatment.[57] A transient restriction in renal function or acute renal failure will occur following fluoride exposure.

Exposure to depleted uranium can result from external irradiation and internal contamination. The associated risks are of a chemical-toxicologic cause, and the target organ is the kidney.[58] Mysterious deaths of archeologists related to kidney disease have occurred after the archeologists opened Egyptian tombs; these deaths have been suspected to be secondary to inhalation of mycotoxins.[59]

Lower Tract Disease

There can be a risk of testicular cancer associated with occupation. For example, occupational exposures to fertilizers, phenols, and fumes or smoke and trauma to the testis can increase the risk for testicular cancer.[60] For bladder tumors, personal habits and exogenous carcinogens have a causative role.[61] Bladder cancer is increased in workers exposed to polycyclic aromatic hydrocarbons, diesel smoke, and aromatic amines.[62] Exposure to silica and to electromagnetic fields may have an increased risk of bladder cancer.[63]

Lifestyles have an important role in the causality of bladder cancer, and occupational exposure probably has less impact in the occurrence of the disease in the general population.[64] This study reported an increased cancer risk in smokers.[64] An association exists between occupational exposure to polycyclic aromatic hydrocarbons and bladder cancer.[65] Cigarette smoking is associated with a twofold excess risk of bladder cancer, whereas alcohol consumption has no association with bladder cancer risk.[66]

When occupations are examined individually, motor vehicle operators, truck drivers, vehicle mechanics, other mechanics, and janitors are among those employees most likely to be diagnosed with high-grade or late-stage bladder tumors.[67] Excesses of bladder cancer are reported in female workers compared with male workers in the rubber industry.[68] With regard to a priori high-risk industries, ever-employment in the rubber, plastics, synthetics, dyestuff, paints, mining, and printing industries and secondary processing was associated with significantly higher relative risks, and a statistically significant trend in risk with increasing duration of employment was found for the first three industries mentioned.[69] For job-related exposures to specified substances, the relative risks observed for increasing duration of exposure suggest that exposures to petroleum, oils, chromium or chromate, spray paints, and zinc, which correspond to exposures involved in the occupations showing a higher relative risk in this study, are associated with a higher risk for cancer of the lower urinary tract. Excess mortality was found for workers on ships and railways, in electrical and electronics occupations, shoemakers, and tobacco workers.[70] An excess of cases also occurred among food workers, particularly workers in the bread and flour or confectionary industry or involved in the extraction of animal and vegetable oils and fats.

An increased risk of bladder cancer was observed after an adjustment for smoking, for physicians, administrators, managers, clerical workers, sales agents among men, and nursing assistants among women.[71] For physicians, the reason may be early diagnosis; for the other groups, a sedentary type of work may have a role in the cause of bladder cancer. Another study reported that higher risks were observed for specific categories of painters; metal, textile, and electrical workers; miners; transport operators; excavating-machine operators; and nonindustrial workers such as concierges and janitors.[72] Industries entailing a high risk included salt mining and manufacture of carpets, paints, plastics, and industrial chemicals.

Sexual Dysfunction

Injuries can cause sexual dysfunction.[74] Evidence suggestive of harmful effects of occupational exposure on the reproductive system and related outcomes has gradually accumulated in recent decades, and is further strengthened by persistent endocrine-disruptive chemicals in the environment.[73] Chemicals such as dioxin, 4'-diaminostilbene-2,2'-disulfonic acid, and toluene have been found to interfere with the function of the endocrine system, which is responsible for growth, sexual development, and many other essential physiologic functions.[74-76] Occupations involving exposure to chemicals that are not easily degradable or to bioaccumulative chemicals, heat, radiation, toxic solvents, and fumes are reported to be associated with reproductive dysfunction.[77] Some of the chemical factors implicated in the study include metals, mineral oils, pesticides, herbicides, neurotoxins, vinyl chloride and its analogs, and carbon disulfide.[77]

References

1. Izumi K, Konaka H, Seto C, et al. A case of bilateral testicular calcifications in a bicycle motocross rider accompanied by bulbar urethral injury. *Hinyokika Kiyo.* 2006;52:383-385.

2. Culty T, Boccon-Gibod L. Anastomotic urethroplasty for posttraumatic urethral stricture: previous urethral manipulation has a negative impact on the final outcome. *J Urol.* 2007;177:1374-1377.

3. Culty T, Ravery V, Boccon-Gibod L. Post-traumatic rupture of the urethra: a series of 105 cases. *Prog Urol.* 2007;17:83-91.

4. Basta AM, Blackmore CC, Wessells H. Predicting urethral injury from pelvic fracture patterns in male patients with blunt trauma. *J Urol.* 2007;177:571-575.

5. Grigoleit U, Pannek J. Urological rehabilitation of spinal cord injury patients [in German]. *Urologe A.* 2006;45:W1549-W1558.

6. Langmayr JJ, Ortler M, Obwegeser A, Felber S. Quadriplegia after lumbar disc surgery: a case report. *Spine.* 1996;21:1932-1935.

7. Dong D, Xu Z, Shi B, et al. Urodynamic study in the neurogenic bladder dysfunction caused by intervertebral disk hernia. *Neurourol Urodyn.* 2006; 25:446-450.

8. Nishio Y, Takane K, Hasegawa T, et al. Dissociated micturitional disturbance in a patient with cervical spondylotic myelopathy [in Japanese]. *Rinsho Shinkeigaku.* 2005;45:226-229.

9. Paraiso MF, Walters MD. Laparoscopic surgery for stress urinary incontinence and pelvic organ prolapse. *Clin Obstet Gynecol.* 2005;48:724-736.

10. Perucchini D, Fink D. Urinary stress incontinence in the female: comparison of incontinence theories and new tension-free surgical procedures [in German]. *Gynakol Geburtshilfliche Rundsch.* 2002;42:133-140.

11. Browning A. Risk factors for developing residual urinary incontinence after obstetric fistula repair. *BJOG.* 2006;113:482-485.

12. Rogers RG, Lebkuchner U, Kammerer-Doak DN, et al. Obesity and retropubic surgery for stress incontinence: is there really an increased risk of intraoperative complications? *Am J Obstet Gynecol.* 2006;195:1794-1798.

13. Rubenstein AH. Obesity: a modern epidemic. *Trans Am Clin Climatol Assoc.* 2005;116:103-113.

14. Goldberg RP, Kwon C, Gandhi S, et al. Urinary incontinence after multiple gestation and delivery: impact on quality of life. *Int Urogynecol J Pelvic Floor Dysfunct.* 2005;16:334-336.

15. Gedymin K, Starczewski A, Torbe A. The influence of individual and total lifted objects on the equilibrium of the uterus. *Med Pr.* 1986;37:333-336.

16. Miner MM, Kuritzky L. Erectile dysfunction: a sentinel marker for cardiovascular disease in primary care. *Cleve Clin J Med.* 2007;74(suppl 3):S30-S37.

17. Falkensammer J, Hakaim AG, Falkensammer CE, et al. Prevalence of erectile dysfunction in vascular surgery patients. *Vasc Med.* 2007;12:17-22.

18. Blanker MH. Re: Erectile dysfunction: an observable marker of diabetes mellitus? A large national epidemiological study: P. Sun, A. Cameron, A. Seftel, R. Shabsigh, C. Niederberger and A. Guay. *J Urol.* 2006;176:1081-1085 [letter]. *J Urol.* 2007;177:1588.

19. Reffelmann T, Kloner RA. Sexual function in hypertensive patients receiving treatment. *Vasc Health Risk Manag.* 2006;2:447-455.
20. Paick JS, Yang JH, Kim SW, Ku JH. Severity of erectile dysfunction in married impotent patients: interrelationship with anthropometry, hormones, metabolic profiles and lifestyle. *Int J Urol.* 2007;14:48-53.
21. Sramkova T, Filipinsky J, Sutory M, et al. Erectile dysfunction after traumatic pelvic injury [in Spanish]. *Rozhl Chir.* 2005;84:299-302.
22. Tang YX, Jiang XZ, Tan J, et al. Erectile dysfunction induced by pelvic fracture urethral injury [in Chinese]. *Zhong Nan Da Xue Xue Bao Yi Xue Ban.* 2004;29: 478-479, 493.
23. Harwood PJ, Grotz M, Eardley I, Giannoudis PV. Erectile dysfunction after fracture of the pelvis. *J Bone Joint Surg Br.* 2005;87:281-290.
24. Leibovitch I, Mor Y. The vicious cycling: bicycling related urogenital disorders. *Eur Urol.* 2005;47:277-287.
25. Inamasu J, Guiot BH. Laparoscopic anterior lumbar interbody fusion: a review of outcome studies. *Minim Invasive Neurosurg.* 2005;48:340-347.
26. Sasso RC, Kenneth Burkus J, LeHuec JC. Retrograde ejaculation after anterior lumbar interbody fusion: transperitoneal versus retroperitoneal exposure. *Spine.* 2003;28:1023-1026.
27. Culty T, Ravery V. Scrotal trauma: management strategy [in French]. *Ann Urol (Paris).* 2006;40:117-125.
28. Kukadia AN, Ercole CJ, Gleich P, et al. Testicular trauma: potential impact on reproductive function. *J Urol.* 1996;156:1643-1646.
29. Muller A, Mulhall JP. Sexual dysfunction in the patient with prostatitis. *Curr Urol Rep.* 2006;7:307-12.
30. Beutel ME, Weidner W, Brahler E. Chronic pelvic pain and its comorbidity [in German]. *Urologe A.* 2004;43:261-267.
31. Madden EF, Fowler BA. Mechanisms of nephrotoxicity from metal combinations: a review. *Drug Chem Toxicol.* 2000;23:1-12.
32. Khamitova RIa, Sigitova ON, Zabbarova AT. Early signs of renal pathology in small intensity chemical exposure [in Russian]. *Gig Sanit.* November 1993:27-29.
33. Harrison DJ, Thomson D, MacDonald MK. Membranous glomerulonephritis. *J Clin Pathol.* 1986;39:167-171.
34. Adams RG, Harrison JF, Scott P. The development of cadmium-induced proteinuria, impaired renal function, and osteomalacia in alkaline battery workers. *Q J Med.* 1969;38:425-443.
35. Albahary C, Richet G, Guillaume J, Morel-Maroger L. The kidney in occupational lead poisoning [in French]. *Arch Mal Prof.* 1965;26:5-19.
36. Loghman-Adham M. Renal effects of environmental and occupational lead exposure. *Environ Health Perspect.* 1997;105:928-939.
37. Cao XJ, Chen R, Li AP, Zhou JW. JWA gene is involved in cadmium-induced growth inhibition and apoptosis in HEK-293T cells. *J Toxicol Environ Health A.* 2007;70:931-937.
38. Grisler R, Gobbi A. Cadmium-induced nephropathy [in Italian]. *Med Lav.* 1978;69:576-593.
39. Benjelloun M, Tarrass F, Hachim K, Medkouri G, Benghanem MG, Ramdani B. Chronic lead poisoning: a "forgotten" cause of renal disease. *Saudi J Kidney Dis Transpl.* 2007;18:83-6.

40. Bennett WM. Lead nephropathy. *Kidney Int.* 1985;28:212-220.

41. Al-Ghamdi SS, Raftery MJ, Yaqoob MM. Toluene and p-xylene induced LLC-PK1 apoptosis. *Drug Chem Toxicol.* 2004;27:425-432.

42. Bertelli G, Farina G, Alessio L. Glomerular disease caused by solvents: an emerging problem [in Italian]. *Med Lav.* 1982;73:175-186.

43. Ehrenreich T, Yunis SL, Churg J. Membranous nephropathy following exposure to volatile hydrocarbons. *Environ Res.* 1977;14:35-45.

44. Bruning T, Golka K, Makropoulos V, Bolt HM. Preexistence of chronic tubular damage in cases of renal cell cancer after long and high exposure to trichloroethylene. *Arch Toxicol.* 1996;70:259-260.

45. David NJ, Wolman R, Milne FJ, van Niekerk I. Acute renal failure due to trichloroethylene poisoning. *Br J Ind Med.* 1989;46:347-349.

46. Finn R, Fennerty AG, Ahmad R. Hydrocarbon exposure and glomerulonephritis. *Clin Nephrol.* 1980;14:173-175.

47. Klavis G, Drommer W. Goodpasture syndrome and the effects of benzene [in German]. *Arch Toxikol.* 1970;26:40-55.

48. Aymaz S, Gross O, Krakamp B, et al. Membranous nephropathy from exposure to mercury in the fluorescent-tube-recycling industry. *Nephrol Dial Transplant.* 2001;16:2253-2255.

49. Barregard L, Svalander C, Schutz A, et al. Cadmium, mercury, and lead in kidney cortex of the general Swedish population: a study of biopsies from living kidney donors. *Environ Health Perspect.* 1999;107:867-871.

50. Barregard L, Sallsten G, Conradi N. Tissue levels of mercury determined in a deceased worker after occupational exposure. *Int Arch Occup Environ Health.* 1999;72:169-173.

51. Beirne GJ, Brennan JT. Glomerulonephritis associated with hydrocarbon solvents: mediated by antiglomerular basement membrane antibody. *Arch Environ Health.* 1972;25:365-369.

52. Bell GM, Gordon AC, Lee P, et al. Proliferative glomerulonephritis and exposure to organic solvents. *Nephron.* 1985;40:161-165.

53. Bruning T, Thier R, Bolt HM. Nephrotoxicity and nephrocarcinogenicity of dinitrotoluene: new aspects to be considered. *Rev Environ Health.* 2002; 17:163-172.

54. Bigazzi PE. Metals and kidney autoimmunity. *Environ Health Perspect.* 1999;107(suppl 5):753-765.

55. Bolton WK, Suratt PM, Strugill BC. Rapidly progressive silicon nephropathy. *Am J Med.* 1981;71:823-828.

56. Dracon M, Noel C, Wallaert B, et al. Rapidly progressive glomerulonephritis in pneumoconiotic coal miners [in French]. *Nephrologie.* 1990;11:61-65.

57. Braun J, Stoss H, Zober A. Intoxication following the inhalation of hydrogen fluoride. *Arch Toxicol.* 1984;56:50-54.

58. Cantaluppi C, Degetto S. Civilian and military uses of depleted uranium: environmental and health problems. *Ann Chim.* 2000;90:665-676.

59. Di Paolo N, Guarnieri A, Loi F, et al. Acute renal failure from inhalation of mycotoxins. *Nephron.* 1993;64:621-625.

60. Haughey BP, Graham S, Brasure J, et al. The epidemiology of testicular cancer in upstate New York. *Am J Epidemiol.* 1989;130:25-36.

61. Akdas A, Kirkali Z, Bilir N. Epidemiological case-control study on the etiology of bladder cancer in Turkey. *Eur Urol.* 1990;17:23-26.

62. Audureau E, Karmaly M, Daigurande C, et al. Bladder cancer and occupation: a descriptive analysis in Haute Normandie in 2003 [in French]. *Prog Urol.* 2007;17:213-218.

63. Band PR, Le ND, MacArthur AC, et al. Identification of occupational cancer risks in British Columbia: a population-based case-control study of 1129 cases of bladder cancer. *J Occup Environ Med.* 2005;47:854-858.

64. Bento MJ, Barros H. Life style and occupational risk factors in bladder carcinoma [in Portuguese]. *Acta Med Port.* 1997;10:39-45.

65. Bonassi S, Merlo F, Pearce N, Puntoni R. Bladder cancer and occupational exposure to polycyclic aromatic hydrocarbons. *Int J Cancer.* 1989;44:648-651.

66. Brownson RC, Chang JC, Davis JR. Occupation, smoking, and alcohol in the epidemiology of bladder cancer. *Am J Public Health.* 1987;77:1298-1300.

67. Brooks DR, Geller AC, Chang J, Miller DR. Occupation, smoking, and the risk of high-grade invasive bladder cancer in Missouri. *Am J Ind Med.* 1992;21:699-713.

68. Carpenter L, Roman E. Cancer and occupation in women: identifying associations using routinely collected national data. *Environ Health Perspect.* 1999; 107(suppl 2):299-303.

69. Claude JC, Frentzel-Beyme RR, Kunze E. Occupation and risk of cancer of the lower urinary tract among men: a case-control study. *Int J Cancer.* 1988; 41:371-379.

70. Dolin PJ, Cook-Mozaffari P. Occupation and bladder cancer: a death-certificate study. *Br J Cancer.* 1992;66:568-578.

71. Ji J, Granstrom C, Hemminki K. Occupation and bladder cancer: a cohort study in Sweden. *Br J Cancer.* 2005;92:1276-1278.

72. Kogevinas M, 't Mannetje A, Cordier S, et al. Occupation and bladder cancer among men in Western Europe. *Cancer Causes Control.* 2003;14:907-914.

73. Kumar S. Occupational exposure associated with reproductive dysfunction. *J Occup Health.* 2004;46:1-19.

74. Wissing M. Dioxins: current knowledge about health effects [in French]. *Rev Med Brux.* 1998;19:A367-A371.

75. Quinn MM, Wegman DH, Greaves IA, et al. Investigation of reports of sexual dysfunction among male chemical workers manufacturing stilbene derivatives. *Am J Ind Med.* 1990;18:55-68.

76. Singer R, Scott NE. Progression of neuropsychological deficits following toluene diisocyanate exposure. *Arch Clin Neuropsychol.* 1987;2:135-144.

77. Steeno OP, Pangkahila A. Occupational influences on male fertility and sexuality, I. *Andrologia.* 1984;16:5-22.

18

CHAPTER

Causation in Common Gastrointestinal Problems

Elizabeth Genovese, MD, and Mark H. Hyman, MD

Claims are often made about the exacerbation or aggravation of gastrointestinal syndromes directly by work stressors or indirectly, owing to the effects of medication or other treatments required for management of a work-related injury. Dyspepsia, gastritis, ulcers, and gastroesophageal reflux disease (GERD) are the upper gastrointestinal problems most commonly described as caused or exacerbated by work-related factors. Irritable bowel syndrome (IBS) and inflammatory bowel disease (IBD) are the corresponding lower gastrointestinal problems. Hernias are also discussed.

Dyspepsia, Ulcers, and Gastritis

Dyspepsia or "upset stomach," also termed *functional* or *non-ulcer dyspepsia,* is pain or discomfort in the epigastrium without a clear anatomic cause.[1] Gastritis and ulcer disease also can manifest with epigastric pain or discomfort, but the latter conditions differ in that there is, in both, objective radiologic, endoscopic, and/or serologic (*Helicobacter pylori*) evidence of disease.

There is no clear evidence-based method to use history alone as the basis for distinguishing symptoms of functional or nonulcer dyspepsia from those of ulcer disease, GERD, or gastritis,[2] although careful questioning about symptoms may be of value. Diagnostic criteria for functional dyspepsia are based on the Rome III consensus document[3] and characterized by the presence of one or more symptoms originating from the gastroduodenal region in the absence of organic, systemic, and metabolic disease. Newer terminology also separates dyspepsia into two subgroups of symptoms: epigastric pain syndrome and postprandial distress syndrome.

Causes of the functional dyspeptic conditions are usually multifactorial, but a direct positive correlation with body mass index[4] is commonly found and may be mediated through hyperglycemia.[5,6] Psychological causes are also well described as associated with functional dyspepsia syndromes,[7] but the strength of the causal relationship between stress and functional dyspepsia requires further study. Data on the benefit of psychological treatment are insufficient to use as the basis for asserting the existence of a causal relationship.[8]

There is extensive literature about the causal relationship between ulcer disease and gastritis and factors that include advancing age, genetics, alcohol use, smoking cigarettes, using nonsteroidal anti-inflammatory drugs (NSAIDs),[9,10] and *H pylori* infection.[11-16] As a corollary, cessation of the use of alcohol, cigarettes, and NSAIDs and treatment of *H pylori* infection improves outcomes,[17] with literature suggesting that *H pylori* infection should be identified and eradicated before initiating therapy with NSAIDs.[18,19] The strength of the causal relationship between use of NSAIDs and gastritis or ulcer disease is particularly relevant to workers' compensation because these agents are often prescribed to treat compensable musculoskeletal injuries. As was the case for functional dyspepsia, psychological stress has been advanced as another cause of ulcer disease and gastritis,[20] with severe environmental societal stressors precipitating an increased incidence of community diagnosis of these conditions.[21] The association between stress and ulcer disease requires further study.[22] No occupation seems to be at increased risk for dyspepsia, ulcer disease, or gastritis. *Helicobacter pylori* infection also has no clear industrial causation because the infection is most commonly acquired in childhood, through municipal water sources or possibly fecal-oral contamination.[46] The use of NSAIDs is the main work-related factor documented as causally related to ulcer disease, although the contribution of concomitant risk factors must be considered, especially when other factors are of greater prominence or duration.

Gastroesophageal Reflux Disease

Although many classic symptoms such as dysphagia, odynophagia, globus sensation, hiccups, and heartburn suggest the presence of GERD, the cardinal symptom is heartburn.[23] In addition, GERD is the most common cause of non-cardiac chest pain[24] and can be suggested by the presence of cough or worsening asthma,[25] especially if nocturnal. Hiatal hernia is one anatomic cause of symptoms, with a poor correlation between symptoms and anatomic evidence of esophageal erosion.[26-28] Numerous additional causes of esophageal symptoms range from primary smooth muscle disease, neuromuscular diseases and cancers, to infections. The NSAIDs have been demonstrated as etiologic in some cases of esophagitis and stricture formation.[29] The definitive presence of GERD is determined by pH monitoring,[30] with capsule or invasive endoscopy being reliable indicators.[31,32] Grading systems for severity have been offered.[33] Empiric treatment of GERD does not ensure the diagnosis,[34] and nonacidic reflux can continue despite therapy.[35] Surgical therapy for GERD also has equivocal anatomic and symptom-relief results.[36-38]

Lifestyle factors are often cited as the most common cause of GERD. These factors include alcohol use; smoking cigarettes; sleeping position; and ingestion of caffeine, chocolate, citrus, spicy food, late-evening meals, and peppermint or spearmint. Yet there is inadequate evidence for the benefit of addressing these conditions.[39,40] Obesity is the one lifestyle factor that has a direct positive correlation with GERD and with improvement in symptoms once treated.[41-43] Interestingly, the presence of concurrent *H pylori* infection lowers the risk of GERD.[44]

A final area of intense interest regarding the causes of GERD revolves around the relationship between psychological factors and symptoms. Most studies show a poor correlation between patient-reported impact of stress or psychological problems on symptoms and objective evidence of changes GERD as measured by changes in pH, esophageal motility, or prediction of response to treatment.[45-49] A fair interpretation of the literature would identify psychological factors as having, at best, only a weak correlation with symptoms or underlying pathologic changes.[50,51] There have been reports suggesting that psychological interventions may be helpful for patients having antireflux surgery.[52]

No clear occupation is associated with increased risk for the development of GERD. Heavy isometric weight lifting or more than 100 sit-ups per day have been cited as associated with this condition,[53] but no causal relationship has been demonstrated.

Irritable Bowel Syndrome

Irritable bowel syndrome has been defined by the Rome III criteria[54,55] as at least 3 months, with the onset at least 6 months previously, of recurrent abdominal pain or discomfort associated with two or more of the following:

- Improvement with defecation
- Onset associated with a change in frequency of stool
- Onset associated with a change in form (appearance) of stool

Differentiating IBS from more clearly established "organic disease" requires careful evaluation of the symptomatic person,[56,57] with IBS the paradigmatic gastrointestinal condition for the spectrum of functional somatic syndromes.[58,59] The impact of IBS on health-related quality of life and health care services utilization can be considerable and is driven predominantly by the extraintestinal manifestations of disease such as fatigue, headache, and other constitutional symptoms.[60,61]

The causes of IBS are multifactorial, with genetic predisposition being important. Postinfectious gastroenteritis is a well-documented cause of IBS.[62] Bacterial overgrowth contributes to IBS, and treatment of the overgrowth leads to a decrease in symptoms.[63-65] There are studies associating body mass index with IBS, which parallel those linking it with dyspepsia.[35,66] Some have advocated analgesics and food additives as etiologic in IBS, although the data are not clear.[67] It is, however, most useful to consider three interrelated factors as the underlying mechanism for IBS(1) altered gut reactivity (motility, secretion) in response to luminal (e.g., meals, gut distention, inflammation, bacterial factors) or provocative environmental (psychosocial stress) stimuli; (2) a hypersensitive gut with enhanced visceral perception and pain; and (3) dysregulation of the brain-gut axis, possibly associated with greater stress reactivity and altered perception and/or modulation of visceral afferent signals.[68]

Early life stress, inadequate childhood rearing, affluent childhood, inadequate social support, maladaptive coping styles, and physical or sexual abuse[69-73] have also been shown to be associated with the development of symptoms in at-risk people. Thus, even though the pathogenesis of IBS has not been fully elucidated, ie, a direct and consistent relationship to altered motility has not been shown, relief of symptoms from the use of smooth muscle relaxants and antidepressant medication suggests that intrinsic muscular and psychological factors contribute to the pathogenesis of this condition.[74-76] The use of an integrative biopsychosocial model in evaluating patients with IBS to understand the multiple factors that contribute to the genesis and continuation of symptoms is warranted.[50,77]

There is no occupation associated with an increased risk for IBS despite its well-documented impact on employer costs.[78] Although stress may be described by workers as increasing symptoms of IBS, it has not been demonstrated as causative per se. Shift work has also been claimed to affect the severity of symptoms in people with this disorder.[79] Although physiologic changes to correlate with the increase in symptoms have not been found, given the biopsychosocial model described previously, it is reasonable, when developing a treatment strategy, to consider the possibility that psychological stressors, at work and at home, may be contributing to symptoms.

Inflammatory Bowel Disease

Inflammatory bowel disease consists of two entities, Crohn disease (CD) and ulcerative colitis (UC). Although definitive diagnosis requires pathologic confirmation, diagnosis and monitoring are being aided by capsule endoscopy.[80,81] Causation is principally genetic,[82-84] although it can by moderated by environmental factors. Active smoking decreases risk for UC and increases the risk for CD. Appendectomy decreases risk for UC, breast-feeding decreases risk for CD, and perinatal infection increases risk for IBD. Inflammatory bowel disease is more prevalent in people with higher economic status and in Western countries and northern latitudes, although this trend may be changing.[85] Bacteria are also important factors in the development of IBD.[86] Analgesic ingestion and oral contraception may contribute to relapse of IBD, but the data are weak.[87,88]

Occupational risk has been suggested from evidence that IBD is more common in white-collar workers from higher social class. One study showed a low male prevalence of IBD among bricklayers, road construction workers, unskilled workers in brick and stone, unskilled laborers, and security personnel. Low rates were found among women employed in cleaning and maintenance and in women without an occupation. In contrast, a high male prevalence was found among instrument makers, electricians, bakers, and technical assistants. Among female employees, IBD was significantly associated with sales representatives, office workers, health care workers, and hairdressers.[89] Another study showed that IBD mortality by occupation was significantly reduced among farmers, mining machine operators, and laborers. A nonsignificant increase was found among salespeople and secretaries. Mortality associated with IBD by industry was significantly reduced in agricultural production of livestock, mining, grocery store occupations, and work in private households. A nonsignificant increase was found in food production, investment and insurance businesses, and administration.[90] Both studies suggest that the incidence and mortality of IBD are low in occupations associated with manual work and outdoor work and relatively high in sedentary occupations associated with indoor work. Similar findings demonstrating an association between IBD and sedentary work have been identified.[91] Because people with IBD would be expected to choose sedentary indoor jobs as opposed to jobs requiring a higher level of physical conditioning or environmental tolerance, the significance of these associations is unclear.

There is conflicting evidence in the literature about the contribution of psychological stress to symptoms of IBD, precluding a determination whether this factor has a true evidence-based impact on IBD.[28,92-96] A recent set of recommendations for safety personnel indicated that IBD was not considered stress-related,[97] which seems reasonable when one considers that true evidence of IBD disease exacerbation requires pathologic confirmation.

Hernias

The discussion in this chapter applies to ventral, umbilical, inguinal, and femoral hernias. Hernia diagnosis is usually not a diagnostic dilemma.[98] Genetic and developmental factors are the primary etiologic factors, although conditions that lead to chronically increased abdominal pressure such as obesity, ascites, and pregnancy are associated with causing hernia formation.[99] The abdominal musculature has protective mechanisms recruited during lifting to help prevent hernia formation. This is why there are no good studies showing an increased risk of hernia formation in laborers.[100] Nevertheless, traumatic events involving severe abdominal blows necessitating hospitalization and exploratory surgery have been associated with hernia formation.[101] Likewise, it is reasonable to assume that sudden increases in intra-abdominal pressure may cause herniations in people who already have a baseline weakness in the supportive tissues and are predisposed to this disease. Smoking is a risk factor for hernia formation and incisional hernias.[102,103]

Assessing the Contribution of Occupational Risk Factors for Gastrointestinal Disease

We can state with some degree of confidence that the use of NSAIDs for management of work-related injuries is causally associated with the development of peptic ulcer disease in some people and that episodic heavy lifting is most likely associated with the development of abdominal and inguinal herniations.

Although psychological and physiologic stress may increase symptoms of dyspepsia, IBS, and IBD, stressors are not generally limited to the workplace, and people who experience work-related stress do not necessarily have symptoms. Thus, one should be cautious in imputing a causal relationship between work-related factors and the severity of symptoms in these disorders. Modification of presumptive contributory factors should be attempted if possible; a subsequent, clear-cut improvement in surrogate markers for disease severity (such as medication use) and function should serve as the impetus for further clarification of how best to optimize the work environment. However, as is the case for most disease processes perceived as more symptomatic in the presence of "stress," there are individual variations in the response to stress and the degree to which a given situation is perceived as stressful. Therefore, it would seem unreasonable to conclude that work-related stress is the only cause of nonspecific upper or lower gastrointestinal tract symptoms and, perhaps, more reasonable to conclude that the presence of disease processes worsened by stress may represent a relative contraindication for choosing certain jobs.

References

1. Talley NJ, Stranghellini V, Heading C, et al. Functional gastrointestinal disorders. *Gut.* 1999;45:1137-1142.
2. Moayyedi P, Talley NJ, Fennerty MB, et al. Can the clinical history distinguish between organic and functional dyspepsia? *JAMA.* 2006;295:1566-1576.
3. Tack J, Talley NJ, Camilleri M, et al. Functional gastroduodenal disorders. *Gastroenterology.* 2006;130:1466-1479.
4. Crowell MD, Cheskin LJ, Musial F. Prevalence of gastrointestinal symptoms in obese and normal weight binge eaters. *Am J Gastroenterol.* 1994;89:387-391.
5. Bytzer P, Talley NJ, Hammer J, et al. GI symptoms in diabetes mellitus are associated with both poor glycemic control and diabetic complications. *Am J Gastroenterol.* 2002;97:604-611.
6. Bulpitt CJ, Palmer AJ, Battersby C, et al. Association of symptoms of type 2 diabetic patients with severity of disease, obesity, and blood pressure. *Diabetes Care.* 1998;21:111-115.
7. Talley SJ, Bytzer P, Hammer J, et al. Psychological distress is linked to gastrointestinal symptoms in diabetes mellitus. *Am J Gastroenterol.* 2001; 96:1033-1038.
8. Soo S, Moayyedi P, Deeks J, et al. Psychological interventions for non-ulcer dyspepsia. *Cochrane Database Syst Rev.* 2005;2:CD002301.
9. Lee EL, Feldman M. Gastritis and gastropathies. In: Feldman M, Friedman LS, Brandt LJ, eds. *Feldman:Sleisenger and Fordtran's Gastrointestinal and Liver Disease.* 8th ed. New York, NY: Saunders/Elsevier; 2006:1068 -1090.
10. Cryer B, Spechler SJ. Peptic ulcer disease. In: Feldman M, Friedman LS, Brandt LJ, eds. *Feldman:Sleisenger and Fordtran's Gastrointestinal and Liver Disease.* 8th ed. New York, NY: Saunders/Elsevier; 2006: 1091 - 1105.
11. Suerbaum S, Michetti P. *Helicobacter pylori* infection. *N Engl J Med.* 2002;347:1175-1186.
12. Delaney B, Ford AC, Forman D, et al. Initial management strategies for dyspepsia. *Cochrane Database Syst Rev.* 2005; 4:CD001961.
13. Jaakkimainen RL, Boyle E, Tudiver F. Is *Helicobacter pylori* associated with non-ulcer dyspepsia and will eradication improve symptoms? A meta-analysis. *BMJ.* 1999;319:1040-1044.
14. Mazzoleni LE, Sander GB, Ott EA, et al. Clinical outcomes of eradication of *Helicobacter pylori* in nonulcer dyspepsia in a population with a high prevalence of infection: results of a 12-month randomized, double blind, placebo-controlled study. *Dig Dis Sci.* 2006;51:89-98.
15. Graham DY, Sung JJY. *Helicobacter pylori.* In Feldman M, Friedman LS, Brandt LJ, eds. *Feldman:Sleisenger and Fordtran's Gastrointestinal and Liver Disease.* 8th ed. New York, NY: Saunders/Elsevier; 2006: 1049 -1063.
16. Bayyurt N, Abasiyanik MF, Sander E, Salih BA. Canonical correlation analysis of factors involved in the occurrence of peptic ulcers. *Dig Dis Sci.* 2007;52:140-146.
17. Meurer LN, Bower DJ. Management of *Helicobacter pylori* infection. *Am Fam Physician.* 2002;65:1327-1336.

18. Chang CC, Chen SH, Lien GS, et al. Eradication of *Helicobacter pylori* significantly reduced gastric damage in nonsteroidal anti-inflammatory drug–treated Mongolian gerbils. *World J Gastroenterol.* 2005;11:104-108.
19. McCarthy DM. *Helicobacter pylori* and NSAIDs: what interaction. *Eur J Surg suppl.* 2001;(586):56-65.
20. Levenstein S, Ackerman S, Kiecolt-Glaser JK, et al. Stress and peptic ulcer disease. [Editorial].*JAMA.* 1999;281:10-11.
21. Aoyama N, Kinoshita Y, Fujimoto S, et al. Peptic ulcers after the Hanshin-Awaji earthquake: increased incidence of bleeding gastric ulcers. *Am J Gastroenterol.* 1998;93:311-316.
22. Feldman M. Mental stress and peptic ulcers: an earthshaking association. [Editorial].*Am J Gastroenterol.* 1998;93:291-292.
23. DeVault KR. Symptoms of esophageal disease. In: Feldman M, Friedman LS, Brandt LJ, eds. *Feldman:Sleisenger and Fordtran's Gastrointestinal and Liver Disease.* 8th ed. New York, NY: Saunders/Elsevier; 2006: 109 – 117.
24. Richter JE, Bradley LA, Castell DO. Esophageal chest pain: current controversies in pathogenesis, diagnosis and therapy. *Ann Intern Med.* 1989;110:66-78.
25. Harding SM. Gastroesophageal reflux: a potential asthma trigger. *Immunol Allergy Clin North Am.* 2005;25:131-148.
26. Niemantsverdriet EC, Timmer R, Breumelhof R, et al. The roles of excessive gastro-oesophageal reflux, disordered oesophageal motility and decreased mucosal sensitivity in the pathogenesis of Barrett's oesophagus. *Eur J Gastroenterol Hepatol.* 1997;9:515-519.
27. Venables TL, Newland RD, Patel AC, et al. Omeprazole 10 mg once daily, omeprazole 20 mg once daily, or ranitidine 150 mg twice daily, evaluated as initial therapy for the relief of symptoms of gastro-oesophageal reflux disease in general practice. *Scand J Gastroenterol.* 1997;32:965-973.
28. Carlsson R, Galmiche JP, Dent J, et al. Prognostic factors influencing relapse of oesophagitis during maintenance therapy with antisecretory drugs: a meta-analysis of long-term omeprazole trials. *Aliment Pharmacol Ther.* 1997;11:473-482.
29. El-Serag HB, Sonnenberg A. Association of esophagitis and esophageal strictures with diseases treated with non-steroidal anti-inflammatory drugs. *Am J Gastroenterol.* 1997;92:52-56.
30. Cappell MS. Clinical presentation, diagnosis, and management of gastrointestinal reflux disease. *Med Clin North Am.* 2005;89:243-291.
31. Keuchel M. Video capsule endoscopy in the work-up of abdominal pain. *Gastrointest Endosc Clin N Am.* 2004;14:195-205.
32. Eisen GM. The economics of PillCam. *Gastrointest Endosc Clin N Am.* 2006;16:337-345.
33. Lundell LR, Dent J, Bennett JR, et al. Endoscopic assessment of oesophagitis: clinical and functional correlates and further validation of the Los Angeles classification. *Gut.* 1999;45:172-180.
34. Numans ME, Lau J, de Wit NJ, et al. Short-term treatment with proton-pump inhibitors as a test for gastroesophageal reflux disease. *Ann Intern Med.* 2004;140:518-527.
35. Vela MF, Camacho-Lobato L, Srinivasan R, et al. Reflux is nonacidic with omeprazole, but symptoms can persist. *Gastroenterology.* 2001;120:1599-1606.

CHAPTER 18

36. Fibbe C, Layer P, Keller J, et al. Esophageal motility in reflux disease before and after fundoplication: a prospective, randomized, clinical and manometric study. *Gastroenterology.* 2001;121:5-14.

37. Spechler SJ, Lee E, Ahnen D, et al. Long-term outcome of medical and surgical therapies for gastroesophageal reflux disease: follow-up of a randomized controlled trial. *JAMA.* 2001;285:2331-2338.

38. Richter JE. Surgery relieved symptoms but decreased survival more than medical treatment in gastroesophageal reflux disease. *ACP J Club.* 2002;136:17.

39. Kaltenbach T, Crockett S, Gerson LB. Are lifestyle measures effective in patients with gastroesophageal reflux disease? *Arch Intern Med.* 2006;166:965-971.

40. Wani S, Sharma P. Review: sparse evidence supports lifestyle modifications for reducing symptoms of gastroesophageal reflux disease. *ACP J Club.* 2006;145:44.

41. Shah A, Uribe J, Katz PO. Gastroesophageal reflux disease and obesity. *Gastroenterol Clin North Am.* 2005;34:35-43.

42. Hampel H, Abraham NS, El-Serag HB. Meta-analysis: obesity and the risk of gastroesophageal reflux disease and its complications. *Ann Intern Med.* 2005;143:199-211.

43. Jacobson BC, Somers SC, Fuchs CS, et al. Body-mass index and symptoms of gastroesophageal reflux in women. *N Engl J Med.* 2006;354:2340-2348.

44. Richter JE, Falk GW, Vaezi MF. *Helicobacter pylori* and gastroesophageal reflux disease: the bug may not be all bad. *Am J Gastroenterol.* 1998;93:1800-1802.

45. Baker LH, Lieberman D, Oehlke M. Psychological distress in patients with gastroesophageal reflux disease. *Am J Gastroenterol.* 1995;90:1797-1803.

46. Johnston BT, Lewis SA, Love AHG. Stress, personality and social support in gastro-oesophageal reflux disease. *J Psychosom Res.* 1995;39:221-226.

47. Wiklund I, Butler-Wheelhouse P. Psychosocial factors and their role in symptomatic gastroesophageal reflux disease and functional dyspepsia. *Scand J Gastroenterol.* 1996;31S:94-100.

48. Johnston BT, McFarland RJ, Collins JSA, et al. Effect of acute stress on oesophageal motility in patients with gastro-oesophageal reflux disease. *Gut.* 1996;38:492-497.

49. Lau GKK, Hui WM, Lam SK. Life events and daily hassles in patients with atypical chest pain. *Am J Gastroenterol.* 1996;91:2157-2162.

50. Drossman DA. Presidential address: gastrointestinal illness and the biopsychosocial model. *Psychosom Med.* 1998;60:258-267.

51. Stranghellini V. Relationship between upper gastrointestinal symptoms and lifestyle, psychological factors and comorbidity in the general population: results from the domestic/international gastroenterology surveillance study (DIGEST). *Scand J Gastroenterol.* 1999;34S:29-37.

52. Kamolz T, Granderath FA, Bammer T, et al. Psychological intervention influences the outcome of laparoscopic antireflux surgery in patients with stress-related symptoms of gastroesophageal reflux disease. *Scand J Gastroenterol.* 2001;36:800-805.

53. Richter JE. Let the patient beware: the evolving truth about laparoscopic antireflux surgery. *Am J Med.* 2003;114:71-73.

54. Drossman DA, ed. *Rome III: The Functional Gastrointestinal Disorders.* 3rd ed. McClean, VA: Degnon Associates; 2006.

55. Longstreth GF, Thompson WG, Chey WD, et al. Functional bowel disorders. *Gastroenterology.* 2006;130:1480-1491.
56. Talley NJ. Irritable bowel syndrome. In: Feldman M, Friedman LS, Brandt LJ, eds. *Feldman:Sleisenger and Fordtran's Gastrointestinal and Liver Disease.* 8th ed. New York, NY: Saunders/Elsevier; 2006: 2633 -2647.
57. Holten KB, Wetherington A, Bankston L. Diagnosing the patient with abdominal pain and altered bowel habits: is it irritable bowel syndrome? *Am Fam Physician.* 2003;67:2157-2162.
58. Barsky AJ, Borus JF. Functional somatic syndromes. *Ann Intern Med.* 1999;130:910-921.
59. Aaron LA, Buchwald D. A review of the evidence for overlap among unexplained clinical conditions. *Ann Intern Med.* 2001;134:868-881.
60. Spiegel BMR, Gralnek IM, Bolus R, et al. Clinical determinants of health-related quality of life in patients with irritable bowel syndrome. *Arch Intern Med.* 2004;164:1773-1780.
61. Jones R, Latinovic J, Charlton J, et al. Physical and psychological co-morbidity in irritable bowel syndrome: a matched cohort study using the general practice research database. *Aliment Pharmacol Ther.* 2006;24:879-886.
62. Ilnyckyj A, Balachandra B, Elliott L, et al. Post–traveler's diarrhea irritable bowel syndrome: a prospective study. *Am J Gastroenterol.* 2003;98:596-599.
63. Pimentel M, Chow EJ, Lin HC. Normalization of lactulose breath testing correlates with symptom improvement in irritable bowel syndrome: a double-blind, randomized, placebo-controlled study. *Am J Gastroenterol.* 2003; 98:412-419.
64. Pimentel M, Park S, Mirocha J, Kane SV, Kong Y. The effect of a nonabsorbed oral antibiotic (rifaximin) on the symptoms of the irritable bowel syndrome: a randomized trial. *Ann Intern Med.* 2006;145:557-563.
65. Lin HC. Small intestinal bacterial overgrowth. *JAMA.* 2004;292:852-858.
66. Saito YA, Locke GR, Talley NJ, et al. A comparison of the Rome and Manning criteria for case identification in epidemiological investigations of irritable bowel syndrome. *Am J Gastroenterol.* 2000;95:2816-2824.
67. Locke GR III, Zinsmeister AR, Talley NJ, et al. Risk factors for irritable bowel syndrome: role of analgesics and food sensitivities. *Am J Gastroenterol.* 2000;95:157-165.
68. American Gastroenterological Association medical position statement: irritable bowel syndrome. *Gastroenterology.* 2002;123:2105-2107.
69. Koloski NA, Talley NJ, Boyce PM. Predictors of health care seeking for irritable bowel syndrome and nonulcer dyspepsia: a critical review of the literature on symptom and psychosocial factors. *Am J Gastroenterol.* 2001;96:1340-1349.
70. Bennett EJ, Tennant CC, Piesse C, et al. Level of chronic life stress predicts clinical outcome in irritable bowel syndrome. *Gut.* 1998;43:256-261.
71. Welgan P, Meshkinpour H, Beeler M. Effect of anger on colon motor and myoelectric activity in irritable bowel syndrome. *Gastroenterology.* 1988; 94:1150-1156.
72. Gwee KA, Graham JC, McKendrick MW, et al. Psychometric scores and persistence of irritable bowel after infectious diarrhoea. *Lancet.* 1996;347: 150-153.

CHAPTER 18

73. Howell S, Talley NJ, Quine S, et al. The irritable bowel syndrome has origins in the childhood socioeconomic environment. *Am J Gastroenterol.* 2004;99:1572-1578.

74. Jailwala J, Imperiale TF, Kronke K. Pharmacologic treatment of the irritable bowel syndrome: a systematic review of randomized controlled trials. *Ann Intern Med.* 2000;133:136-147.

75. Poynard T, Regimbeau C, Benhamou Y. Meta-analysis of smooth muscle relaxants in the treatment of irritable bowel syndrome. *Aliment Pharmacol Ther.* 2001;15:355-361.

76. Jackson JL, O'Malley PG, Tomkins G, et al. Treatment of functional gastrointestinal disorders with antidepressant medications: a meta-analysis. *Am J Med.* 2000;108:65-72.

77. 77. McEwen BS. Stress, adaptation, and disease: allostasis and allostatic load. *Ann N Y Acad Sci.* 1998;840:33-44.

78. Leong SA, Barghout V, Birnbaum HG, et al. The economic consequences of irritable bowel syndrome. *Arch Intern Med.* 2003;163:929-935.

79. Zhen Lu W, Ann Gwee K, Yu Ho K. Functional bowel disorders in rotating shift nurses may be related to sleep disturbances. *Eur J Gastroenterol Hepatol.* 2006;18:623-627.

80. Lo SK. Capsule endoscopy in the diagnosis and management of inflammatory bowel disease. *Gastrointest Endosc Clin N Am.* 2004;14:179-193.

81. Elkaim R, Adler SN. Capsule video endoscopy in Crohn's disease: the European experience. *Gastrointest Endosc Clin N Am.* 2004;14:129-137.

82. Sands BE. Crohn's disease. In: Feldman M, Friedman LS, Brandt LJ, eds. *Feldman:Sleisenger and Fordtran's Gastrointestinal and Liver Disease.* 8th ed. New York, NY: Saunders/Elsevier; 2006:2459-2498.

83. Su C, Lichtenstein GR. Ulcerative colitis. In: Feldman M, Friedman LS, Brandt LJ, eds. *Feldman:Sleisenger and Fordtran's Gastrointestinal and Liver Disease.* 8th ed. New York, NY: Saunders/Elsevier; 2006: 2499-2539.

84. Annese V, Piepoli A, Latiano A, et al. HLA-DRB1 alleles may influence disease phenotype in patients with inflammatory bowel disease: a critical reappraisal with review of the literature. *Dis Colon Rectum.* 2005;48:57-64.

85. Zheng JJ, Zhu XS, Huanfu Z, et al. Crohn's disease in mainland China: a systematic analysis of 50 years of research. *Chin J Dig Dis.* 2005;6:175-181.

86. Bamias G, Nyce MR, De la Rue SA, et al. New concepts in the pathophysiology of inflammatory bowel disease. *Ann Intern Med.* 2005;143:895-904.

87. Forrest K, Symmons D, Foster P. Systematic review: is ingestion of paracetamol or non-steroidal anti-inflammatory drugs associated with exacerbations of inflammatory bowel disease? *Aliment Pharmacol Ther.* 2004;20:1035-1043.

88. Sandler RS, Loftus EV. Epidemiology of inflammatory bowel diseases. In: Sartor RB, Sandborn WJ, ed. *Kirsner's Inflammatory Bowel Diseases.* 6th ed. Philadelphia, PA: WB Saunders; 2004:245.

89. Sonnenberg A. Occupational distribution of inflammatory bowel disease among German employees. *Gut.* 1990;31:1037-1040.

90. Cucino C, Sonnenberg A. Occupational mortality from inflammatory bowel disease in the United States 1991-1996. *Am J Gastroenterol.* 2001;96:1101-1105.

91. Boggild H, Tuchsen F, Orhede E. Occupation, employment status and chronic inflammatory bowel disease in Denmark. *Int J Epidemiol.* 1996;25:630-637.

92. Li J, Norgard B, Precht DH, et al. Psychological stress and inflammatory bowel disease: a follow-up study in parents who lost a child in Denmark. *Am J Gastroenterol.* 2004;99:1129-1133.

93. Mawsley JE, Rampton DS. Psychological stress in IBD: new insights into pathogenic and therapeutic implications. *Gut.* 2005;54:1481-1491.

94. Maunder RG. Evidence that stress contributes to inflammatory bowel disease: evaluation, synthesis, and future directions. *Inflamm Bowel Dis.* 2005;11:600-608.

95. Sainsbury A, Heatley RV. Review article; psychosocial factors in the quality of life of patients with inflammatory bowel disease. *Aliment Pharmacol Ther.* 2005;21:499-508.

96. Bitton A, Sewitch MJ, Peppercorn MA, et al. Psychosocial determinants of relapse in ulcerative colitis: a longitudinal study. *Am J Gastroenterol.* 2003;98:2203-2208.

97. Goldberg, RL, Spillberg SW, Weyers SG. California Commission on Peace Officer Standards and Training (POST). Sacramento, CA: California Post:; 2004:113.

98. Jeyarajah R, Harford WV. Abdominal hernias and gastric volvulus. In: Feldman M, Friedman LS, Brandt LJ, eds. *Feldman:Sleisenger and Fordtran's Gastrointestinal and Liver Disease.* 8th ed. New York, NY: Saunders/Elsevier; 2006: 477 - 492.

99. Malangoni MA, Gagliardi RJ. Hernias. In: Townsend CM, Beauchamp RD, Evers BM, et al, eds. *Sabiston Textbook of Surgery.* 17th ed. Philadelphia, PA: WB Saunders; 2004: xx-xx.

100. Abrahamson J. Etiology and pathophysiology of primary and recurrent groin hernia formation. *Surg Clin North Am.* 1998;78:953-972.

101. Simpson J, Lobo DN, Shah AB, et al. Traumatic diaphragmatic rupture: associated injuries and outcome. *Ann R Coll Surg Engl.* 2000;82:97-100.

102. Sorensen LT, Friis E, Jorgensen T, et al. Smoking is a risk factor for recurrence of groin hernia. *World J Surg.* 2002;26:397-400.

103. Sorensen LT, Hemmingsen UB, Kirkeby LT, et al. Smoking is a risk factor for incisional hernia. *Arch Surg.* 2005;140:119-123.

CHAPTER 18

CHAPTER 19

Causation in Ear, Eye, Nose, and Throat Disorders and Sun Exposure

William Edward Ackerman, III, MD, Roger M. Belcourt, MD, and Marc T. Taylor, MD

This chapter addresses causation of work-related ear, eye, nose, and throat diseases and diseases related to sun exposure. Unlike an orthopedic fracture, causation of such diseases can be difficult to determine because of occupational and environmental risk factors. For example, hearing loss is a condition caused by environmental factors that damage structures involved in hearing, which may include ears, nerves, and the brain. Occupational hearing loss is a result of damage to the inner ear from noise or vibrations due to certain types of jobs and entertainment. However, hearing loss can also occur outside of one's work environment. Therefore, before attempting to determine causation, individual, occupational, and environmental risk factors must be addressed.

Hearing Loss

Hair cells in the cochlea in the inner ear detect sound waves and convert them into nerve signals. Exposure to loud sounds can occur in and out of the work place. The hair cells can be damaged by loud noises. These noises may be consistently loud or intermittent and brief. Acute noise injury can cause temporary and permanent damage. Long-term exposure to loud sounds causes permanent injury because hair cells are gradually lost. There are about 25,000 rows of hair cells in each ear, and each row responds to a particular pitch. As hair cells are lost, a person becomes unable to hear sounds at certain pitches. High-pitch rows are most easily injured. Guidelines have been established to assist in the diagnosis of noise-induced hearing loss (NIHL) in medicolegal settings.[1] Initially, a distinction needs to be made between possible and probable causes of NIHL. The amount of NIHL needed to qualify for that diagnosis is the amount that is reliably measurable and identifiable on the audiogram. The three main requirements for the diagnosis of NIHL are as follows: (1) high-frequency hearing impairment, (2) a potentially hazardous amount of noise exposure, and (3) an identifiable high-frequency audiometric notch or bulge. Four modifying factors also need consideration[1]: (1) the clinical picture; (2) compatibility with age and noise exposure; (3) the Robinson criteria for other causation; and (4) complications such as asymmetry, mixed disorder, and conductive hearing impairment.

Individual Risk Factors

Individual risk factors for hearing loss includes disease or infection,[2,3] ototoxic drugs,[4,5] exposure to noise, tumors,[6] trauma,[7] and the aging process.[8] **Meniere disease** affects the membranous inner ear and is characterized by deafness, vertigo, and tinnitus.[9] **Otosclerosis** is a disease involving the middle ear capsule, specifically affecting the movement of the stapes.[10] Some specific drugs known to be ototoxic are aminoglycoside antibiotics,[11] salicylates,[12] loop diuretics,[13] and chemotherapy agents.[14] An **acoustic neuroma** is an example of a tumor that causes unilateral hearing loss.[15] **Trauma** can also result in hearing loss. Examples include puncture of the eardrum by foreign objects and sudden changes in air pressure.[16] Loss of hearing as a result of the **aging process** involves degeneration of the cochlea.[17] Additional individual risk factors for hearing loss include loud music[18] and, possibly, exposure to carbon monoxide.[19] Furthermore, exposure to carbon monoxide combined with loud noise at monster truck and motocross shows may place people at risk for hearing loss.[20] Among the documented adverse effects of aspirin is the potential for ototoxicity.[21] Tinnitus and hearing loss, usually reversible, are associated with acute salicylate intoxication and long-term administration of salicylates.[22]

Occupational Risk Factors

Occupational risk factors for hearing loss include exposure to environmental agents and loud explosions (impulse noise >115 dB). Some jobs, such as construction, airline ground maintenance, farming, and jobs involving loud music or machinery, carry a high risk for hearing loss. Toxic solvents in car paints can act in synergism with moderate noise exposure, damaging the cochlear hair cells.[23] Farmers are exposed to noise that is potentially hazardous to hearing.[24] Toluene exposure can exacerbate hearing loss in a noisy environment, with the main impact on the lower hearing frequencies.[25]

The maximum occupational noise exposure is regulated by law. The Occupational Safety and Health Administration (OSHA) sets limits on occupational noise exposure.[26] A comparison of noise exposure measurements based on the recently revised noise exposure criteria recommended by the US National Institute for Occupational Safety and Health (NIOSH) and the current OSHA Hearing Conservation Amendment to the occupational noise standard was done.[27] The noise dose based on the NIOSH criteria was higher than the corresponding OSHA noise dose, with differences in noise exposures measured. The results of this study indicate that if the NIOSH criteria are to be adopted as an OSHA standard, there is likely to be a substantial increase in the number of workers in hearing-conservation programs. Currently, people exposed to 85 dB or more at work are required to wear some form of hearing protection. The length of exposure and the decibel level are considered for occupational exposure limits. If the sound is at or greater than the maximum levels recommended, protective measures are required. The NIOSH surveyed noise exposure for a professional stock car team at its race shop and during two races at one racetrack.[28] At the team's shop, area sound pressure levels (SPLs) were measured for various work tasks. Equivalent levels (Leqs) ranged from 58 to 104 dBA. Personal noise dosimetry was conducted for at least one employee for each job description in race car assembly (n = 9). The OSHA permissible exposure limit of 90 dBA for an 8-hour, 5-dB exchange rate time-weighted average was never exceeded, but in two cases, values exceeded the OSHA action level of 85 dBA for hearing-conservation implementation. The NIOSH recommended exposure limit (REL) of 85 dBA for a 3-dB exchange rate Leq was exceeded for five of the measured jobs. During the races, SPLs averaged more than 100 dBA in the pit area where cars undergo adjustments and refueling before and during the race. Peak levels reached 140 dB SPL. The NIOSH REL was exceeded for every personal noise dosimetry measurement.

Unilateral vs Bilateral Hearing Loss

Hearing loss can be unilateral or bilateral. In a study done to ascertain whether unilateral noise exposure causes unilateral hearing loss, shingle sawyers were exposed to noise predominantly from the left side.[29] This study examined the asymmetry in hearing loss among shingle sawyers and its possible relation to the difference in noise exposure to the two ears. The results suggest that the lateral difference in noise exposure in industry, even in the obvious case of a shingle sawyer, is small. Boilermakers, who may have high exposure to loud noise, can have high levels of hearing loss.[30]

Affected Populations

Hearing loss is more common in the aging population than in the young adult population. The hearing of older adults may, therefore, be at risk from causes not related to occupation.[31] Significant hearing difficulties and tinnitus, however, are quite common in men in the older working age range.[32] Both are strongly associated with years spent in a noisy occupation. Rail workers are also at a risk for occupational hearing loss.[33] Rail workers are at risk of NIHL from exposure to high-impact noise. Smoking may adversely affect hearing, and workers should be encouraged to refrain from smoking and exposure to unnecessary noise.[34]

It is not uncommon for aging firefighters to have significant hearing loss greater than that in the general national population.[35] This increased hearing loss with age for firefighters suggests occupational overexposure to noise. This effect is most noticeable in firefighters from the early 1980s and before, when wearing adequate hearing protection when riding on a truck was not common practice.

Musicians can develop occupational loss of hearing.[36] In this profession, a hearing loss can end a musician's career.

Other occupational risk factors include exposure to solvents in combination with exposure to noise.[37,38] Styrene is an aromatic solvent widely used as a precursor for polystyrene plastics in many factories that produce glass-reinforced plastic. This solvent has been shown to disrupt the auditory system in humans and animals.[37] Simultaneous exposure to carbon disulfide and noise has a combined effect on hearing impairment that was reported in a study from a rayon plant.[39] In addition, toluene exacerbates hearing loss in a noisy environment, with the main impact on the lower frequencies.[25] Solvents in car paints are a source of occupational ototoxicity. It has been shown that toxic solvents in car paints increase the risk associated with moderate noise exposure of less than 85 dB, with levels of NIHL similar to those in workers exposed only to loud noises between 92.5 and 107 dB.[23] Organic solvents may increase ototoxicity in a nonnoisy environment. For example, in an artist who painted large posters with different mixtures of organic solvents, including toluene, xylene, benzene, methyl ethyl ketone, toluene diisocyanate, acetone, and thinner, ototoxic hearing loss developed.[40]

Environmental Risk Factors

Environmental factors can contribute to hearing loss. Common environmental factors that contribute to hearing loss include harmful gases, such as carbon monoxide (CO).[19] Examples of sources of CO include air pollution, smoking and secondhand smoking, and occupational exposures. The main toxic mechanism of CO can lead to hypoxia due to the conversion of oxyhemoglobin to carboxyhemoglobin.[19] Patients with CO intoxication are at risk of hearing impairment; therefore, there is a need for audiometric follow-up.[41]

Loud noise can cause hearing deficits. Furthermore, an increased risk exists for promotion of NIHL by hydrogen cyanide.[42] Firefighters are at increased risk of NIHL as well, which may be related to CO exposure in addition to noise pollution.[43]

Heavy metals present in the environment as industrial pollutants or by-products can cause hearing loss.[44] A loud, intense burst of sound, such as a gunshot, can cause blast overpressure, or high-energy impulse noise. *Blast overpressure* is the sharp, instantaneous rise in ambient atmospheric pressure resulting from detonation of explosives or firing of weapons. Exposure to incident blast overpressure waves can cause auditory and nonauditory damage. The injury from blast overpressure has been attributed to its external physical impact on the body causing internal mechanical damage.[45]

When there is a sudden change in hearing ability owing to noise exposure, most people recover their hearing completely within 24 to 48 hours. When hearing returns, the hair cells are permanently damaged. Most cases of occupational hearing loss develop gradually.

Mercury is used in gold mining operations. Adults and children living near these operations are at risk of neurologic injury, including hearing loss from exposure to methylmercury owing to the consumption of contaminated food and, possibly, from inhalation of elemental mercury vapors formed during amalgam burning in the gold-extraction process.[46]

Exposure to lead in the environment from water sources, lead based paints, leaking old batteries etc., can also be a risk factor for hearing loss to those individuals who have contact with this element.[47] Arsenic exposure not only causes hearing loss, but also induces cardiovascular diseases, developmental abnormalities, neurologic and neurobehavioral disorders, diabetes, hematologic disorders, and various types of cancer. Although exposure may occur via the dermal and parenteral routes, the main pathways of exposure include ingestion and inhalation. The severity of adverse health effects is related to the chemical form of arsenic and is time- and dose-dependent. A recent report pointed out that arsenic poisoning seems to be one of the major pandemic public health problems in some countries.[48] Short- and long-term exposure to arsenic occurs in areas where a large proportion of drinking water (groundwater) is contaminated with high concentrations of arsenic. Manganese ingestion in the presence of anemia and loud noise may be associated with an increased risk of hearing loss.[49] These examples suggest that people exposed to noise along with one of the other environmental factors may experience more significant hearing loss.

Organic solvent exposure may also be a contributing factor to hearing loss in some people. It is suggested that there might be an ototraumatic interaction between solvents and noise.[50] In view of the neurotoxic effects of organic solvents, such an interaction is conceivable. Organic solvents can produce central vestibular organ impairments and extracochlear high-frequency hearing loss.[51] Although exposure to noise is the most significant contributor to occupational hearing loss, recent evidence points to solvents and their interactions as additional contributors to occupational deafness.[52] Furthermore, owing to the metabolic competitive inhibition between aromatic solvents and ethanol, the solvent toxicity is enhanced in certain circumstances. So, two dangerous interactions—noise and solvent interactions and solvent and ethanol interactions—deserve consideration when evaluating the causation of hearing loss.

Determining Work-Relatedness

Determining work-relatedness of hearing loss can be challenging. A clinician must first define the disease. Epidemiologic support for a relationship with work must be defined. There must also be evidence of exposure. Other relevant factors must be considered before occupational causation can be determined. Industrial hygiene surveys of ambient noise and the use of personal noise dosimeters can aid in this process.

Cataracts

Cataracts are the leading cause of blindness worldwide. Almost all elderly people develop lens opacities.[53] Age, a body mass index of more than 35 kg/m^2, and a low educational level were associated with the probability of having cataracts or undergoing surgery for cataracts.[54] Oxidative stress is the result of an imbalance of antioxidants and pro-oxidants. Opacity of the lens is a direct result of oxidative stress.[55]

Individual Risk Factors

Epidemiologic changes within the next decades will lead to an increase in the world population and life expectancy. These changes will, in turn, lead to an increase in age-correlated lens opacities and cataracts. In addition to the known risk factors (smoking, diabetes, and exposure to UV light) consistently identified for cataract development, increased attention is being given to oxidative processes that may provide means for cataract prevention.

There are only a few risk factors that satisfy the criteria for causal effect: smoking, which results in the increased risk of nuclear cataract; excessive UV-B exposure and diabetes, which increase the risk of cortical cataract; and steroid treatment, diabetes, and ionizing radiation, which lead to the formation of posterior subcapsular opacity.[56] Other risk factors for cataract formation include female sex, inadequate education, lower socioeconomic status, and heavy alcohol consumption.[57] Another possible factor in an increasing incidence of cataracts may be the increase in UV-B radiation due to ozone depletion.[58] Typically, changes in the old lens are caused by the failure of protective systems and an accumulation of metabolic end products and their influence on light transmission.[59] Evidence suggests that smoking increases the risk for incident nuclear cataract development threefold.[60] The association, according to the study's authors, fulfills the established criteria for cataract causality. Furthermore, smokeless tobacco use is more strongly associated with cataract formation.[61] Glucocorticoids have been widely used as a therapeutic drug for various diseases. However, there are many complications of glucocorticoid therapy, including cataracts.[62]

CHAPTER 19

Occupational Risk Factors

The occupational risk factors for cataract formation include working in sunlight.[63] In addition, in open hearth shop work, cataract development was proven to be directly dependent on length of employment: changes in the posterior capsule and opacifications of the posterior cortical segments of the lens were observed in workers whose labor record ranged from 10 to 15 years.[64] The association between the exposure to cosmic radiation in pilots and the risk of nuclear cataracts, adjusted for age, smoking status, and sunbathing habits, indicates that cosmic radiation may be a causative factor in nuclear cataracts among commercial airline pilots.[65]

Electrically induced injuries can have many ocular manifestations that may occur simultaneously or sequentially, occasionally occurring later than the inciting event. The most common ocular finding is cataract formation.[66] Lightning-caused cataracts may occur after industrial electrical accidents.[67]

Thermal cataract formation is an occupational disease in furnace workers.[68] In medical staff professionals, cataracts, when they occurred, were described as premature, and, therefore, ionizing radiation was considered a cofactor in premature cataract formation in this group of professionals.[69] In astronauts, low doses of space radiation may predispose crew members to [corrected] an increased incidence and early appearance of cataracts.[70] Exposure to intense optical radiation leads to the development of infrared cataracts in the workplace.[71] The risk of cataracts related to microwaves may be identified in radio linemen.[72]

Traumatic cataracts resulting from penetrating injuries occur most frequently from projectile metallic foreign bodies. The majority of intraocular foreign bodies cause sight-threatening damage, including traumatic cataract, in up to 25% of the cases.[73]

The prevalence of cataracts in workers exposed to trinitrotoluene was compared with that in a group of unexposed workers. Exposure to trinitrotoluene may cause a unique type of cataract in exposed workers, which a general ophthalmologist should be able to distinguish from other cataracts.[74]

Environmental Risk Factors

Environmental factors include sun exposure, in addition to some of the other risk factors previously mentioned. There is a link between sun exposure and nuclear cataract formation. The risk is highest, however, among people with high sun exposure at younger ages.[75] Areas with warmer ambient temperatures are reported to have a higher incidence of cataracts in aging people.[76] All relevant factors must be considered before determining causation.

Nose and Throat

Environmental and occupational risk factors can affect nose and throat diseases. As in the previous sections of this chapter, individual and occupational risk factors need to be addressed when attempting to determine causation.

Individual Risk Factors

Individual risk factors include psychosocial stress factors and personal factors such as sex, age, the presence of asthma, and indoor exposures.[77] A person's home environment must be considered. The number of complaints about the quality of indoor air has increased during the past two decades. The indoor exposures have been frequent enough that the terms *sick house syndrome* and *sick building syndrome* have been coined. Complaints are likely related to the increased use of synthetic organic materials in house, furnishing, and consumer products; building consumer products; and decreased ventilation for energy conservation in homes.[78] Approximately 1000 volatile chemicals have been identified in indoor air. The main sources of these chemicals are house materials, combustion fumes and cleaning compounds, and paints and stains. Exposure to high levels of these emissions and to others, coupled with the fact that most people spend more time indoors than outdoors, raises the possibility that there is a risk to human health from indoor air pollution. The complaints most frequently described are irritations of the eye, nose, and throat; cough and hoarseness of voice; headache; and mental fatigue.[77]

Microbes exist in indoor air in the home that cause nose and throat irritation.[77] As the air tightness of dwellings has increased, problems associated with indoor air pollution and dampness have become important environmental health issues.[79] The concentrations of formaldehyde, acetaldehyde, and 17 volatile organic compounds in new dwellings were measured. Toluene, butyl acetate, ethylbenzene, alpha-pinene, p-dichlorobenzene, nonanal, and xylene were significantly related to throat and respiratory symptoms.[79]

Occupational Risk Factors

Sinonasal malignancy is a rare disease in which a number of possible etiologic factors have been implicated, including occupational, social, and genetic factors.[80] This malignancy has a higher incidence in a number of occupations such as those involving wood, nickel, chrome, chemicals, shoes, and textiles. However, the exact causative agent has not been clarified.

A problem in determining causation with respect to occupational and environmental exposure in diseases of the upper and lower airways in many situations is related to similarities and common aspects of these pathologic entities that might be caused by chemical irritants or toxic or carcinogenic substances.[81] In other words, it can be difficult identifying where the exposure occurred in some situations.

Some occupations, however, are associated with an increased risk of developing nose and throat diseases. For example, chromium electroplating workers have an increased risk of perforation of the nasal septum and scar formation or ulceration of the nasal mucosa.[82] These workers were compared with workers from aluminum electroplating factories who had no abnormalities of the nasal septum. A consistent trend was noted between the degree of chromium exposure and the signs and symptoms related to the nose and throat. In addition, glassblowers are exposed to numerous noxious physical and chemical noxious at the workplace. Mucosal layers of the nose, oral cavity, pharynx, and larynx are vulnerable to the influence of hot gases, dust particles, and oral contact with glassblower's pipes. These are the most important causes of chronic inflammation of the upper respiratory tract.[83] There was a significantly higher prevalence of chronic laryngitis among glassblowers than among a control group of workers employed in the same plant. Sinonasal cancer has been found in employees in the leather industry as well. Chromium salts and natural tannins were indicated as possible etiologic agents.[84]

Industrial arts teachers may have complaints related to the eyes, nose, throat, and lower airways than a control group.[85] A higher occurrence of symptoms exists in shops with bad ventilation and dust-spreading machines and in shops where dust-spreading cleanup methods are used.[85]

There is strong evidence that exposure to mustard gas can cause cancers of the upper respiratory tract and some evidence that it can cause lung cancer and nonmalignant respiratory disease as well.[86] Workers exposed to copper and sulfuric acid are at risk for otorhinolaryngologic disease. In one study, 85.6% of the workers had diseases of the upper respiratory tract and the ears.[87] Olfactory disturbance were noted in 61.9% of the 118 workers who were examined.[87]

The sick building syndrome is a group of symptoms experienced by people working in modern office buildings. This syndrome defines illnesses related to nonindustrial and nonresidential buildings. Symptoms include irritation of skin and mucous membranes of the eyes, nose, and throat; headache; fatigue; and concentration difficulties.[88] This syndrome may be related to inadequate ventilation, humidity and temperature changes, and chemical and biological contaminants from indoor and outdoor sources.

Sun Exposure

Sun exposure can cause serious skin diseases. Nonmelanocytic skin cancer has long been regarded as one of the harmful effects of solar UV radiation on human health.[89] Skin cancer occurs mainly at sun-exposed body sites and in people who are sensitive to the sun. An occupational hazard can be sunburn for workers exposed to sunlight.

Sunburn occurs at a very high rate in the United States.[90] However, sunburn is a major preventable risk factor for skin cancer. A study determined when sunburn occurs and who experiences sunburn by using personal UV dosimetry that measured time-stamped doses continuously for a median of 119 days. People with skin type IV (burns minimally, always tans well to moderately brown) had fewer incidences of sunburn than people with types I through III (type I always burns, never tans; type II burns easily, tans minimally; and type III burns moderately, tans gradually to light brown). There were significant correlations between sunburn "size" and severity; sunburn and sunscreen use; and sunburn and sun-bed use.[91] Exposure to solar UV radiation is a major environmental factor implicated in the development of melanoma and other skin cancers and in eye damage and skin photoaging.[92] Individual risk factors include outdoor recreational activities.

As with the other sections in this chapter, determination of work-relatedness in skin lesions can be complex. However, Michailov et al[93] identified skin damage produced by sun exposure in workers as an occupational hazard.

References

1. Coles RR, Lutman ME, Buffin JT. Guidelines on the diagnosis of noise-induced hearing loss for medicolegal purposes. *Clin Otolaryngol Allied Sci.* 2000;25:264-273.
2. Lazarini PR, Camargo AC. Idiopathic sudden sensorineural hearing loss: etiopathogenic aspects. *Rev Bras Otorrinolaringol (Engl Ed).* 2006;72:554-561.
3. Sethi A, Sabherwal A, Gulati A, Sareen D. Primary tuberculous petrositis. *Acta Otolaryngol.* 2005;125:1236-1239.
4. Biro K, Noszek L, Prekopp P, et al. Detection of late ototoxic side effect of cisplatin by distortion otoacoustic emission (DPOAE). *Magy Onkol.* 2006; 50:329-335.
5. Shine NP, Coates H. Systemic ototoxicity: a review. *East Afr Med J.* 2005; 82:536-539.
6. Caye-Thomasen P, Dethloff T, Hansen S, et al. Hearing in patients with intracanalicular vestibular schwannomas. *Audiol Neurootol.* 2007;12:1-12.
7. Kojima H, Tanaka Y, Mori E, et al. Penetrating vestibular injury due to a twig entering via the external auditory meatus. *Am J Otolaryngol.* 2006;27:418-421.
8. Matas CG, Filha VA, Okada MM, Resque JR. Auditory evoked potentials in individuals over 50 years [in Portuguese]. *Pro Fono.* 2006;18:277-284.
9. Frykholm C, Larsen HC, Dahl N, et al. Familial Meniere's disease in five generations. *Otol Neurotol.* 2006;27:681-686.
10. Quaranta N, Bartoli R, Lopriore A, et al. Cochlear implantation in otosclerosis. *Otol Neurotol.* 2005;26:983-987.
11. Selimoglu E. Aminoglycoside-induced ototoxicity. *Curr Pharm Des.* 2007; 13:119-126.
12. Eddy LB, Morgan RJ, Carney HC. Hearing loss due to combined effects of noise and sodium salicylate. *ISA Trans.* 1976;15:103-108.
13. Wrzesniok D, Buszman E, Matusinski B. Drugs ototoxicity, part II: loop diuretics, nonsteroidal anti-inflammatory drugs, antineoplastic and antimalarial drugs [in Polish]. *Wiad Lek.* 2003;56:369-374.
14. Biro K, Noszek L, Prekopp P, et al. Characteristics and risk factors of cisplatin-induced ototoxicity in testicular cancer patients detected by distortion product otoacoustic emission. *Oncology.* 2006;70:177-814.
15. Meyer TA, Canty PA, Wilkinson EP, et al. Small acoustic neuromas: surgical outcomes versus observation or radiation. *Otol Neurotol.* 2006;27:380-392.
16. Densert B, Arlinger S, Densert O. Air-bone gap in Meniere's disease after exposure to overpressure. *Audiology.* 1987;26:339-347.
17. Wallhagen MI, Pettengill E, Whiteside M. Sensory impairment in older adults, part 1: hearing loss. *Am J Nurs.* 2006;106:40-69.
18. Hausler R. The effects of acoustic overstimulation [in German]. *Ther Umsch.* 2004;61:21-29.
19. Lacerda A, Leroux T, Morata T. Ototoxic effects of carbon monoxide exposure: a review [in Portuguese]. *Pro Fono.* 2005;17:403-412.
20. Morley JC, Seitz T, Tubbs R. Carbon monoxide and noise exposure at a monster truck and motocross show. *Appl Occup Environ Hyg.* 1999;14:645-655.

21. Brien JA. Ototoxicity associated with salicylates: a brief review. *Drug Saf.* 1993;9:143-148.
22. Cazals Y. Auditory sensori-neural alterations induced by salicylate. *Prog Neurobiol.* 2000;62:583-631.
23. El-Shazly A. Toxic solvents in car paints increase the risk of hearing loss associated with occupational exposure to moderate noise intensity. *B-ENT.* 2006;2:1-5.
24. Thelin JW, Joseph DJ, Davis WE, et al. High-frequency hearing loss in male farmers of Missouri. *Public Health Rep.* 1983;98:268-273.
25. Chang SJ, Chen CJ, Lien CH, Sung FC. Hearing loss in workers exposed to toluene and noise. *Environ Health Perspect.* 2006;114:1283-1286.
26. Middendorf PJ. Surveillance of occupational noise exposures using OSHA's Integrated Management Information System. *Am J Ind Med.* 2004;46:492-504.
27. Sriwattanatamma P, Breysse P. Comparison of NIOSH noise criteria and OSHA hearing conservation criteria. *Am J Ind Med.* 2000;37:334-338.
28. Van Campen LE, Morata T, Kardous CA, et al. Ototoxic occupational exposures for a stock car racing team, I: noise surveys. *J Occup Environ Hyg.* 2005;2:383-390.
29. Chung DY, Mason K, Willson GN, Gannon RP. Asymmetrical noise exposure and hearing loss among shingle sawyers. *J Occup Med.* 1983;25:541-543.
30. Hessel PA. Hearing loss among construction workers in Edmonton, Alberta, Canada. *J Occup Environ Med.* 2000;42:57-63.
31. Irwin J. What are the causes, prevention and treatment of hearing loss in the ageing worker? *Occup Med (Lond).* 2000;50:492-495.
32. Palmer KT, Griffin MJ, Syddall HE, et al. Occupational exposure to noise and the attributable burden of hearing difficulties in Great Britain. *Occup Environ Med.* 2002;59:634-639.
33. Landon P, Breysse P, Chen Y. Noise exposures of rail workers at a North American chemical facility. *Am J Ind Med.* 2005;47:364-369.
34. Palmer KT, Griffin MJ, Syddall HE, Coggon D. Cigarette smoking, occupational exposure to noise, and self reported hearing difficulties. *Occup Environ Med.* 2004;61:340-344.
35. Reischl U, Hanks TG, Reischl P. Occupation related fire fighter hearing loss. *Am Ind Hyg Assoc J.* 1981;42:656-662.
36. Zuskin E, Schachter EN, Kolcic I, et al. Health problems in musicians: a review. *Acta Dermatovenerol Croat.* 2005;13:247-251.
37. Campo P, Lataye R, Loquet G, Bonnet P. Styrene-induced hearing loss: a membrane insult. *Hear Res.* 2001;154:170-180.
38. Gagnaire F, Langlais C. Relative ototoxicity of 21 aromatic solvents. *Arch Toxicol.* 2005;79:346-354.
39. Chang SJ, Shih TS, Chou TC, et al. Hearing loss in workers exposed to carbon disulfide and noise. *Environ Health Perspect.* 2003;111:1620-1624.
40. Moshe S, Bitchatchi E, Goshen J, Attias J. Neuropathy in an artist exposed to organic solvents in paints: a case study. *Arch Environ Health.* 2002;57:127-129.
41. Michalska-Piechowiak T, Miarzynska M, Perlik-Gattner I. Sudden unilateral sensorineural hearing loss after carbon monoxide intoxication [in Polish]. *Przegl Lek.* 2004;61:374-376.
42. Fechter LD. Promotion of noise-induced hearing loss by chemical contaminants. *J Toxicol Environ Health A.* 2004;67:727-740.
43. Melius J. Occupational health for firefighters. *Occup Med.* 2001;16:101-108.

CHAPTER 19

44. Rybak LP. Hearing: the effects of chemicals. *Otolaryngol Head Neck Surg.* 1992;106:677-686.
45. Elsayed NM. Toxicology of blast overpressure. *Toxicology.* 1997;121:1-15.
46. Counter SA, Buchanan LH, Laurell G, Ortega F. Blood mercury and auditory neuro-sensory responses in children and adults in the Nambija gold mining area of Ecuador. *Neurotoxicology.* 1998;19:185-196.
47. Kamel NM, Ramadan AM, Kamel MI, et al. Impact of lead exposure on health status and scholastic achievement of school pupils in Alexandria. *J Egypt Public Health Assoc.* 2003;78:1-28.
48. Tchounwou PB, Centeno JA, Patlolla AK. Arsenic toxicity, mutagenesis, and carcinogenesis: a health risk assessment and management approach. *Mol Cell Biochem.* 2004;255:47-55.
49. Ray DE. Function in neurotoxicity: index of effect and also determinant of vulnerability. *Clin Exp Pharmacol Physiol.* 1997;24:857-860.
50. Barregard L, Axelsson A. Is there an ototraumatic interaction between noise and solvents? *Scand Audiol.* 1984;13:151-155.
51. Bazydlo-Golinska G. The effect of organic solvents on the inner ear. *Med Pr.* 1993;44:69-78.
52. Campo P, Lataye R. Noise and solvent, alcohol and solvent: two dangerous interactions on auditory function. *Noise Health.* 2000;3:49-57.
53. Shinohara T, White H, Mulhern ML, Maisel H. Cataract: window for systemic disorders. *Med Hypotheses.* 2007;69:669-677.
54. Navarro Esteban JJ, Gutierrez Leiva JA, Valero Caracena N, et al. Prevalence and risk factors of lens opacities in the elderly in Cuenca, Spain. *Eur J Ophthalmol.* 2007;17:29-37.
55. Vinson JA. Oxidative stress in cataracts. *Pathophysiology.* 2006;13:151-162.
56. Robman L, Taylor H. External factors in the development of cataract. *Eye.* 2005;19:1074-1082.
57. Virgolici B, Popescu L. Risk factors in cataract [in Italian]. *Oftalmologia.* 2006;50:3-9.
58. West SK, Longstreth JD, Munoz BE, et al. Model of risk of cortical cataract in the US population with exposure to increased ultraviolet radiation due to stratospheric ozone depletion. *Am J Epidemiol.* 2005;162:1080-1088.
59. Dawczynski J, Strobel J. The aging lens: new concepts for lens aging [in German]. *Ophthalmologe.* 2006;103:759-764.
60. Kelly SP, Thornton J, Edwards R, et al. Smoking and cataract: review of causal association. *J Cataract Refract Surg.* 2005;31:2395-2404.
61. Raju P, George R, Ve Ramesh S, et al. Influence of tobacco use on cataract development. *Br J Ophthalmol.* 2006;90:1374-1377.
62. Nishigori H. Steroid (glucocorticoid)-induced cataract [in Japanese]. *Yakugaku Zasshi.* 2006;126:869-884.
63. Mukesh BN, Le A, Dimitrov PN, et al. Development of cataract and associated risk factors: the Visual Impairment Project. *Arch Ophthalmol.* 2006;124:79-85.
64. Dorozhkin AV. "Cataract of metallurgists" in workers of the oxygen-converter production [in Spanish]. *Vestn Oftalmol.* 2003;119:31-34.
65. Rafnsson V, Olafsdottir E, Hrafnkelsson J, et al. Cosmic radiation increases the risk of nuclear cataract in airline pilots: a population-based case-control study. *Arch Ophthalmol.* 2005;123:1102-1105.

66. Miller BK, Goldstein MH, Monshizadeh R, et al. Ocular manifestations of electrical injury: a case report and review of the literature. *CLAO J.* 2002; 28:224-227.

67. Biro Z, Pamer Z. Electrical cataract and optic neuropathy. *Int Ophthalmol.* 1994;18:43-47.

68. Vos JJ, van Norren D. Thermal cataract, from furnaces to lasers. *Clin Exp Optom.* 2004;87:372-376.

69. Durovic B, Spasic-Jokic V.[Occupational exposure to ionizing radiation and the occurrence of cataract [in _____]. *Vojnosanit Pregl.* 2004;61:387-390.

70. Cucinotta FA, Manuel FK, Jones J, et al. Space radiation and cataracts in astronauts. *Radiat Res.* 2001;156:460-466.

71. Okuno T. Thermal effect of visible light and infra-red radiation (i.r.-A, i.r.-B and i.r.-C) on the eye: a study of infra-red cataract based on a model. *Ann Occup Hyg.* 1994;38:351-359.

72. Microwave cataract in radio-linemen [letter]. *Lancet.* 1984;2:760.

73. Kumar A, Kumar V, Dapling RB. Traumatic cataract and intralenticular foreign body. *Clin Experiment Ophthalmol.* 2005;33:660-661.

74. Kruse A, Hertel M, Hindsholm M, Viskum S. Trinitrotoluene (TNT)-induced cataract in Danish arms factory workers. *Acta Ophthalmol Scand.* 2005;83:26-30.

75. Neale RE, Purdie JL, Hirst LW, Green AC. Sun exposure as a risk factor for nuclear cataract. *Epidemiology.* 2003;14:707-712.

76. Miranda MN. Environmental temperature and senile cataract. *Trans Am Ophthalmol Soc.* 1980;78:255-264.

77. Yuan I, Xu J, Millar BC, et al. Molecular identification of environmental bacteria in indoor air in the domestic home: description of a new species of *Exiguobacterium. Int J Environ Health Res.* 2007;17:75-82.

78. Ando M. Indoor air and human health: sick house syndrome and multiple chemical sensitivity [in Japanese]. *Kokuritsu Iyakuhin Shokuhin Eisei Kenkyusho Hokoku.* 2002;(120):6-38.

79. Saijo Y, Kishi R, Sata F, et al. Symptoms in relation to chemicals and dampness in newly built dwellings. *Int Arch Occup Environ Health.* 2004;77:461-470.

80. Lund VJ. Malignancy of the nose and sinuses: epidemiological and aetiological considerations. *Rhinology.* 1991;29:57-68.

81. Baur X. Occupational medicine aspects of nasal diseases [in French]. *Laryngorhinootologie.* 1998;77:191-195.

82. Lin SC, Tai CC, Chan CC, Wang JD. Nasal septum lesions caused by chromium exposure among chromium electroplating workers. *Am J Ind Med.* 1994; 26:221-228.

83. Baletic N, Jakovljevic B, Marmut Z, et al. Chronic laryngitis in glassblowers. *Ind Health.* 2005;43:302-307.

84. Battista G, Comba P, Orsi D, et al. Nasal cancer in leather workers: an occupational disease. *J Cancer Res Clin Oncol.* 1995;121:1-6.

85. Ahman M, Soderman E, Cynkier I, Kolmodin-Hedman B. Work-related respiratory problems in industrial arts teachers. *Int Arch Occup Environ Health.* 1995; 67:111-118.

86. Easton DF, Peto J, Doll R. Cancers of the respiratory tract in mustard gas workers. *Br J Ind Med.* 1988;45:652-659.

CHAPTER 19

87. Savov A. Damages to the ears, nose and throat in copper production [in Bulgarian]. *Probl Khig.* 1991;16:149-153.
88. Wittczak T, Walusiak J, Palczynski C. "Sick building syndrome": a new problem of occupational medicine. *Med Pr.* 2001;52:369-373.
89. Kricker A, Armstrong BK, English DR. Sun exposure and non-melanocytic skin cancer. *Cancer Causes Control.* 1994;5:367-392.
90. Brown TT, Quain RD, Troxel AB, Gelfand JM. The epidemiology of sunburn in the US population in 2003. *J Am Acad Dermatol.* 2006;55:577-583.
91. Thieden E, Philipsen PA, Sandby-Moller J, Wulf HC. Sunburn related to UV radiation exposure, age, sex, occupation, and sun bed use based on time-stamped personal dosimetry and sun behavior diaries. *Arch Dermatol.* 2005;141:482-488.
92. Kimlin MG, Martinez N, Green AC, Whiteman DC. Anatomical distribution of solar ultraviolet exposures among cyclists. *J Photochem Photobiol B.* 2006; 85:23-7.
93. Michailov P, Dogramadjev I, Berowa N. UV radiation as occupational environmental damage (author's transl). *Derm Beruf Umwelt.* 1981;29:5-8.

Causation Related to Gender and Sex, Leukemia Related to Radiation, and Occupational Skin Lesions

William Ackerman, MD, and **Laurie Massa, MD**

Gender, Sex, and Occupational Causation

Gender is the socioculturally influenced trait such as masculinity or femininity. *Sex* refers to the genetically determined aspects of maleness and femaleness.[1] This section addresses gender and sex as possible causes or risks for an occupational injury. A medical literature search using the key words gender and work injury yielded 384 articles. There were no articles that identified gender as a direct cause of a work-related injury. However, 27 articles gave strong evidence of an association between gender or sex and the propensity to injury.

Individual Anatomic and Physiologic Male and Female Risk Factors

Women have more musculoskeletal disorders than do men.[2] This observation may be related in part to women having less opportunity to relax and exercise outside of work. Parenthood exacerbates this difference, with mothers reporting the least time to relax or exercise.[2] The sex-segregation of women into sedentary, repetitive, and routine work and the persisting gender imbalance in domestic work are interlinking factors that may explain gender differences in musculoskeletal disorders. Men in general have greater bone mineral content and bone area and are taller and heavier than women.[3] Men also have significantly higher bone mineral density than women at all regions of the body except at the femoral neck and lumbar spine. Men, furthermore, have significantly larger femoral neck shaft angles than do women. These factors, together with the subsequent higher rate of bone loss in women, may influence the incidence of bone fracture in later life.[3] Females exhibit greater knee laxity than males before and after exercise.[4] This finding may explain the increased incidence of anterior cruciate ligament injuries in females compared with males. Sex differences between men and women include lower extremity alignment, physiologic laxity, pelvis width, tibial rotation, and foot alignment.[5]

Work-Related Gender and Sex Risk Factors

Controversy exists with respect to gender and sex being major risk factors in injury epidemiology. Female workers have been reported to have a greater risk of specific injury or illness compared with male workers in various industries.[6] On the other hand, Ballau[7] reported that gender is not a major etiologic factor in accidents. Some investigators have correlated an increase in musculoskeletal injuries in females with anatomic inequities with specific emphasis on tendon anatomy.[8] Women with work histories of repetitive strain injury and who are affected by biopsychosocial distress have a higher frequency of these injuries than do men and workmates not affected by biopsychosocial distress.[9]

Health Care Occupational Injuries

In a retrospective case-control study, risk factors for four types of work-related injury in hospital employees were analyzed.[10] The results of this study demonstrated that strain injuries were related to increased age, increased body mass index (BMI), and maintenance, custodial, and direct-caregiver employment types. Repetitive-motion injuries were related to increased BMI and clerical and custodial employment occupations. Exposure and reaction injuries were related to increased age, increased BMI, and maintenance, custodial, and direct-caregiver employment occupations. Contact and assault injuries were related to increased age, increased BMI, and maintenance, custodial, and direct-caregiver employment types. All injury types were most often related to female gender and full-time employment status. Female nurses have been reported to be at risk for occupational musculoskeletal injuries while working in psychiatric hospitals. High rates of acute injuries and physical assaults were noted among nurses and certified nursing assistants working in long-term psychiatric care facilities compared with male health care workers.[11] A higher risk of assault was found among women and higher risks of injury and assault were observed among full-time employees than among per diem or pool agency workers. In addition, weekend shifts were found to have a higher rate of injuries and a lower rate of assaults than weekday shifts.

Military Occupational Hazards

Women in the military service experience an excess of work-related injuries compared with men.[12] An excess risk for women in the military exists when they undertake the same arduous training as men, and this fact highlights the conflict between health and safety legislation and equal opportunities legislation. For training, women were initially given lower entry and exit standards, but it became apparent that many women did not have the strength necessary for their work, which has been shown to be associated with overuse injuries.[13]

Sex differences were studied to assess the cause of low back pain in a population of military personnel who were expected to undertake high levels of sports, exercise, and physical military training.[14] Low back pain and injuries to the hip, thigh, and lower leg were more frequent in female soldiers.[15] There was a statistically significant increase in the rate of medical discharge for musculoskeletal disease and injury in female personnel in the British armed forces.[16] Mixed-sex training imposes particular ergonomic stresses on women, and that is a major risk factor for overuse injury. Female runners are reported to be more likely to sustain certain lower extremity injuries compared with their male counterparts.[17] The majority of the excess medical discharges that occurred in women younger than 22 years were a result of musculoskeletal disorders. The incidence of low back pain

CHAPTER 20

in female soldiers was also reported to be higher than in their male counterparts with an odds ratio of 3.17. Female soldiers are significantly more likely to have low back pain as a result of physical military training or their occupation.

In US Army personnel, eye injury rates were reported to be higher in men than in women.[18] These investigators hypothesized that differences in the use of protective eyewear between men and women may have contributed to differences in eye injury rates. The differences in eye injury rates may be behavioral. Male personnel frequently neglected to wear protective eyewear, whereas female soldiers had a higher frequency of using protective eyewear. The number of military female aviators is increasing as well. Women may be more susceptible to motion sickness, radiation, and decompression sickness than men but may be more resistant to immersion in cold water and altitude sickness.[19]

Athletics and Sex

Female runners demonstrate significantly greater peak hip adduction, hip internal rotation, and knee abduction angle compared with male runners.[20] A careful history of the frequency of recreational running should be obtained when any employee complains of knee or hip pain related to an alleged occupational injury. Knee instability, as such, and constant or recurrent knee instability were found to be positively associated with female sex and different features of occupational work. Knee instability is a commonly reported phenomenon among active female athletes and is independent of the type and the amount of sports activity but highly dependent on female sex and type and amount of occupational work.[20]

Injury and Gender

On occasion, an employee may sustain a cervical sprain or strain injury during employment. A study was done to attempt to identify prognostic factors for poor recovery in patients with whiplash-associated disorders who still had neck pain and accompanying complaints 2 weeks after their accidents.[21] Factors related to poor recovery were female gender, a low level of education, high initial neck pain, more severe disability, and higher levels of somatization and sleep difficulties. The intensity of the neck pain and work disability proved to be the most consistent predictors for poor recovery.

Age and sex can affect the severity of injury in some circumstances.[22] When all mechanisms were reviewed, examples of the impact of age were seen for women older than 65 years, who were more likely to sustain forearm and wrist fractures than were older men following a fall at work. For the individual mechanism of motor vehicle collision, there was a significant increase in the lower extremity and distal upper extremity fractures in older women. Similarly, older women were more likely to sustain lower leg fractures and distal upper extremity fractures than were older men. This finding raises the possibility that increased bone loss, as seen in older women, may be reflected in the injury patterns they sustained given the same mechanism. On the other hand, young males had the highest rate of traumatic fractures referred for orthopedic services.[23] Adolescents of both sexes had high rates of traumatic dislocations referred for orthopedic services.

Agricultural Injuries and Sex

Women continue to make significant contributions to farming. Differences in size and stature, increased physical strain, and low maximal oxygen uptake may predispose women to ergonomic-related injuries.[12] Sex differences are noted in the incidence of farm injuries.[24] The most common machinery mechanisms of fatal injuries were rollover accidents (32%) for males and run-over accidents (45%) for females. Injuries requiring hospitalization that were related to agricultural machinery showed similar patterns, with proportionally more men older than 60 years injured. The male-female ratio for non–machinery-related hospitalizations averaged 3:1. A greater percentage of males were struck by or caught against an object, whereas for females, animal-related injuries predominated. This study demonstrated that sex is an important factor to consider in the interpretation of fatal and nonfatal farm injuries. A greater number of males were injured, regardless of how the occurrence of injury was categorized, particularly when farm machinery was involved.

Effect of Sex on Heavy-Load Injuries

Differences in spinal load tolerance exist between sexes.[25] This study evaluated the differences in spine loading between men and women when exposed to similar workplace demands, using an electromyography-assisted model. Men had significantly greater compression forces than women.[26] The differences between men and women were even greater when lifting either of the heavier loads from the lower fixed shelf (>50% greater). Men produce the greater loads on their spines during lifting. The differences in spine loads seem to be a result of kinematic trade-offs and muscle coactivity differences in combination with unequal body masses between sexes. However, when the loads were put into context of the expected tolerances of the spine, women were found to be at increased risk of injuries, especially when lifting heavy loads or under asymmetric lifting conditions.

In non-heavy load injuries there is a higher prevalence of occupational low back injuries in men and a higher rate of repetitive-motion and neck injuries in women. Men had a significantly higher rate of lumbar injuries than did women, whereas women had a significantly higher rate of cervical injuries. Men returned to work and retained work at a 40-hour-per-week job at a higher rate at 1-year follow-up. Women evidenced a higher rate of health-care seeking behaviors from new providers.[27] Men and women experience different cognitive, emotional, and vocational outcomes following traumatic brain injuries.[28] With respect to cervical sprain and strain injuries, sex did not have a significant effect on the incidence of neck pain following low-velocity frontal impacts.[29] There is a higher incidence of reported upper-extremity musculoskeletal complaints in women. Mental stress may induce muscle tension and has been proposed to contribute to the development of work-related upper extremity disorders by driving low-threshold motor units into degenerative processes by overload.[30] In fertilizer plant workers, the prevalence of cervicobrachial and lumbosacral radicular syndromes is higher for women than for men.[31]

Manual Labor

Age-standardized odds ratios were computed by gender for five injury settings and four socioeconomic groups, using salaried employees as the reference group.[32] Compared with salaried employees, male manual workers showed an excess risk of injury in all settings except sports. Males from all socioeconomic groups showed significantly higher morbidity in production and education areas. Female manual workers showed significantly higher morbidity in production, education, and home settings. As for those who belong to an unspecified population, such as long-term unemployed students, they showed higher morbidity in home settings, transport, and other areas.

Musculoskeletal Injuries

There are striking gender disparities in the rates of carpal tunnel syndrome (CTS). Overall, three times more women have CTS than men. However, a study was performed to determine the injury rates of CTS for men and women in six high-risk occupations: (1) assembler, (2) laborer-nonconstruction, (3) packaging and filling machine operators, (4) janitors and cleaners, (5) butchers and meat cutters, and (6) data entry keyers.[33] The sixth occupational title, data entry keyers, which requires a single physical task, had a risk rate ratio of 1.06. This ratio suggests that an equal risk between genders exists when the occupational tasks are truly similar. Job task analysis may unmask potential biases that may wrongly attribute diagnoses to workplace risk factors. In a study involving traumatic amputations in the workplace, 50% of all amputations were in people younger than 25 years. Males accounted for five times as many cases as females.[34]

Causation

Causation is an identifiable factor (accident or exposure) that results in a medically identifiable medical condition. The medical literature does not support gender or sex as a cause of occupational injuries. However, the examples presented in this section suggest that gender and sex can be associated with an increased risk of injury in certain occupations.

Radiation and Leukemia

Established and suspected risk factors for leukemia can be classified as familial, genetic, environmental (e.g., benzene, high-dose ionizing radiation, chemotherapeutics, and electromagnetic fields), and lifestyle (e.g., smoking, obesity, and dietary intake).[35] Associations are also suggested between leukemia and the use of permanent black hair dye.[36] Residential petrochemical exposure is an environmental risk factor for leukemia as well.[37]

Work-Related, Nonradiation Risk Factors for Leukemia

Exposure to benzene, an important industrial chemical and component of gasoline, is a widely recognized cause of leukemia.[38] The occupational exposure to pesticide increases the risk of non-Hodgkin lymphoma and hairy cell leukemia.[39] The risk of developing leukemia is associated with radiation exposure.[40]

Radiation

Radiation absorbed by the body causes cell changes that may increase the risk of cancer and hereditary effects. A millisievert (mSv; Système International measure of radiation, which is different from the conventional standard, millirem [mrem]), is the unit used to measure the amount of radiation received by an individual. The amount of natural background radiation a person receives each year is between 2 and 4 mSv. The maximum amount of radiation people are allowed to receive in the workplace is regulated. An excessive dose may harm health and cause leukemia.

Radiation is classified as ionizing and nonionizing. *Ionizing radiation* consists of higher-energy electromagnetic waves (gamma) or heavy particles (beta and alpha). There is energy high enough to pull electrons from orbit. *Nonionizing radiation* consists of lower-energy electromagnetic waves and does not have enough energy to pull electrons from orbit but can excite the electrons. The composition of radiation can vary depending on what may be ionized. Examples of ionizing radiation include electrons, neutrons, atomic ions, photons, X-rays, and gamma rays. Visible light, near UV, infrared, microwaves, and radio waves are examples of nonionizing radiation.

A number of reports have suggested that strong electromagnetic fields may be a risk factor for leukemia as well, although other studies have failed to confirm these findings. The associations between exposure to ionizing radiation and the development of cancer are mostly based on populations exposed to relatively high levels of ionizing radiation, such as Japanese survivors of the atomic bomb and recipients of selected diagnostic or therapeutic medical procedures. Cancers associated with high-dose exposure include leukemia and thyroid, breast, bladder, colon, liver, lung, esophagus, ovarian, multiple myeloma, and stomach cancers.

Leukemia

Leukemia is a cancer of the blood or bone marrow and is characterized by an abnormal proliferation of white blood cells, or leukocytes. Damage to the bone marrow can occur by displacement of the normal marrow cells with increasing numbers of malignant cells. Possible causes of leukemia include natural and artificial ionizing radiation, hydrocarbon chemicals, some viruses, and genetic predispositions.[35] Ionizing radiation has many practical uses, but it is also dangerous to human health. Although researchers have studied the many cellular changes associated with leukemia, it is unknown why these changes occur. It is likely that certain risk factors are involved.

A literature search using the key words leukemia, causation, and radiation yielded 483 articles in medical journals. Leukemia begins as a mutation in the DNA within certain cells; one or more white blood cells experience DNA loss or damage. Those errors are copied and passed on to subsequent generations of cells. The abnormal leukemic cells remain in an immature blast form that never matures properly. These cells tend to multiply and accumulate within the body. Numerous risk factors may be responsible for DNA damage within the blood cells.

Occupational Risk Factors

With respect to the previously mentioned medical journals, 43 were related to occupation and 24 were published after 1996. The risk factors believed to have the strongest associations with leukemia include the following: age, older than

50 years, and radiation, which increases the risk of chronic myelogenous leukemia in people who have been exposed to high doses. Chemicals such as benzene increase the risk of acute leukemia among workers with long-term exposure.[41,42] Risk also is increased among workers exposed to herbicides and pesticides.[43,44]

The human T-cell leukemia virus I is related to acute T-cell leukemia. Leukemia has been reported in workers such as butchers, slaughterhouse workers, and veterinary professionals who are exposed to animal viruses.[45] Workers in the meat industry are exposed to viruses that can cause leukemia and lymphoma in cattle and chickens and also to carcinogenic chemical agents. Excess risks of tumors of the hematopoietic and lymphatic systems were observed throughout the meat industry, except in meatpacking plants. Slaughtering activities involving heavy exposure to oncogenic viruses were strongly associated with these tumors. Elevated risks have been observed in butchers and in workers who killed animals in chicken-slaughtering plants and workers in cattle, sheep, and pig abattoirs.

Among supermarket workers, wrapping meat was associated with increased risk of tumors of the hematopoietic and lymphatic systems, with elevated odds of lymphomas and tumors of the myeloid stem cells. On the other hand, meat cutting in supermarkets (almost exclusively a male activity) was associated with multiple myeloma; the odds ratio for men was 18.0, with no myeloma cases recorded in women. These associations persisted after limited control for exposures outside the industry that have also been observed to be associated with excess risk, such as exposure to pesticides, working or living on pig farms, and exposure to X-rays.

The findings provide evidence that workers in the meat industry may be at elevated risk of tumors of the hematopoietic and lymphatic systems. Cigarette smoking is also a risk factor for leukemia.[46]

A preliminary study published in 1980 reported that 9 cases of leukemia occurred among 3224 men who participated in military maneuvers during the 1957 nuclear test explosion "Smoky."[47] This number represents a significant increase from the expected incidence of 3.5 cases. The interval from the nuclear test to diagnosis ranged from 2 to 19 years (mean, 14.2 years). Film-badge records, which were available for eight of nine men, indicated increased gamma radiation exposure levels. A further follow-up of the health status of the men in these military maneuvers was completed through 1979 for 3072 (95.5%) of 3217 nuclear test participants.[48] In these participants, 112 cases of cancer were diagnosed, compared with 117.5 cases expected. During the same follow-up period, 64 persons died of cancer, compared with an expected 64.3 individuals. A statistically significant increased frequency of occurrence and mortality was found only for leukemia. Although uncertainty remains about the exact amount of radiation exposure that each worker received, the lack of a significant increase after 22 years in the incidence of or the mortality from any other cancer and the apparent lack of a dose effect by unit led to the consideration that the leukemia findings may be attributable to chance, factors other than radiation, or some combination of risk factors.

Another study was done to examine the effects of radiation exposure on uranium miners. [49] When using conditional logistic regression models, a dose-response relationship between leukemia risk and radon progeny could not be confirmed. Yet, a significantly elevated risk was seen in people with exposures of 400 mSv or more when combining gamma-radiation and long-lived radionuclides. A nested case-control study using conditional logistic regression was conducted to evaluate the exposure-response relationship between external exposure to ionizing radiation and leukemia mortality among civilian workers at the Portsmouth Naval Shipyard, Kittery, Maine. [50] The civilian workers received occupational radiation exposure while performing construction, overhaul, repair, and refueling activities on nuclear-powered submarines. A significant positive association was found between leukemia mortality and external radiation exposure.

A significant cancer risk could be induced by prolonged exposure to low-dose ionizing radiation in Chinese X-ray workers when the cumulative dose reached a certain level. [51] One of the most recent and extensive studies of worker exposure to radiation was reported by Cardis et al[52] in 2005. This study was done to provide direct estimates of the risk of cancer after exposure to protracted low doses of ionizing radiation. The excess relative risk for cancers other than leukemia was 0.97 per Sv. On the basis of these estimates, 1% to 2% of deaths due to cancer among workers in this cohort may be attributable to radiation. These estimates are higher than, but statistically compatible with, the risk estimates used for current radiation protection standards. The results suggest that there is a small excess risk of cancer, even at the low doses and dose rates typically received by nuclear workers in this study. The linear dose-response model suggests that any increase in dose, no matter how small, results in an incremental increase in risk. Under this model, about 1% of a population would develop cancer in its lifetime as a result of ionizing radiation from background levels of natural and manufactured sources. It should be mentioned that with respect to health care workers, no evidence indicates that current radiation exposures associated with medical use are harmful. [53]

Individual Risk Factors

Potential leukemia-causing chemicals in tobacco smoke include benzene, polonium-210, and polycyclic aromatic hydrocarbons.[41-43] Medications, such as growth hormones and phenylbutazone, have reportedly shown some associations with leukemia.[44] Obesity is also a risk factor, and an elevated BMI increases the risk of most of the adult leukemia subtypes.[54] Leukemias have been observed in recipients of organ transplants, and certain immunodeficiency syndromes are associated with leukemias.[55, 56] The interval between radiation exposure and the detection of cancer is known as the *latent period*. The cancers that may develop as a result of radiation exposure are indistinguishable from cancers that occur naturally or as a result of exposure to other chemical carcinogens. Furthermore, other chemical and physical hazards and lifestyle factors, such as smoking, alcohol consumption, and diet, significantly contribute to many of these same diseases.[57] To assess the health impacts of lower radiation doses, investigators rely on models of the process by which radiation causes cancer; several models have emerged that predict differing levels of risk.

In some instances, it is equivocal if leukemia is caused by individual or environmental factors. For example, it remains undetermined as to whether cosmic radiation causes leukemia in airline pilots.[58-61] Studies of atomic bomb survivors have provided some information on radiation exposure and cancer. Cancer results, although uncertain, are consistent with estimates of risk that are based on studies of atomic bomb survivors and suggest that the individuals face a small increase in the probability of developing leukemia and other cancers. Several major international studies such as those performed on the survivors of the atomic bomb, have shown a clear linkage between exposure to ionizing radiation and the occurrence of various cancer types, including leukemia.[62] Although these studies are mostly characterized by high-dose rates, studies on populations exposed after the Chernobyl accident are, in most cases, characterized by low-dose rates.

Nonionizing Radiation

Studies on the effects of nonionizing electromagnetic radiation on cell systems, animals, and human subjects report conflicting results: some support carcinogenic effects, and others reject the hypothesis that nonionizing electromagnetic radiation in the extremely low frequency fields and microwave range is carcinogenic.[63] The increased use of mobile cellular phones by the public has been associated with a wave of contradictory reports about the possible health effects of exposure to nonionizing electromagnetic radiation.[64] At the time of this writing, there was no evidence to suggest that cell phone use causes or increases the risk of leukemia.

CHAPTER 20

Occupational Skin Disease

Occupational skin disease is a significant public health concern.[65] Occupational exposure as a cause of dermatoses accounts for a surprisingly large number of occupational illnesses. The US Bureau of Labor Statistics (BLS), for example, reported that skin diseases accounted for a consistent 30% to 45% of all cases of occupational illnesses through the mid 1980s.[66] Occupational skin disease was evaluated by examining 14,703 workers' compensation cases reported for the year 1981 in three major industry divisions: agriculture, manufacturing, and construction. In 1993, BLS data estimated 60,200 cases of occupational skin diseases or disorders in the US workforce. In 1999, BLS data showed 44,600 total cases of occupational skin diseases or disorders, or an incidence of 49 cases per 100,000. In 1999, 12% of all occupational illnesses reported were skin diseases or disorders. Skin disease in the workplace can be divided into several categories, including irritant eczema, allergic contact eczema, urticaria, frictional dermatitis, skin cancer, and less commonly reported conditions such as folliculitis and nail disorders.

Irritant Eczema

Irritant eczema (IE) is the most commonly reported occupational skin disorder.[67] In a study by Lim and Goon[68] reported in 2007, 125 patients at the Contact and Occupational Dermatoses Clinic, National Skin Centre, Singapore, from January 2003 to December 2004 were given a diagnosis of an occupational skin disease. Of the cases, 62.4% were diagnosed as irritant dermatitis. The main irritants were wet work, oil, grease, and solvents. Several factors can increase the likelihood of developing IE. Irritant eczema is an extremely common disorder among people involved in wet work, such as nurses, physicians, and dishwashers. Frequent hand washing exacerbates the condition, especially in the winter when the air is drier. People with a history of atopic dermatitis are at higher risk,[69] as are older people whose epidermal barrier decreases with age.[70] Hand eczema is twice as common clinically among females as among males.[67] Several studies have looked at sex and irritant dermatitis. Experimentally, there is no higher reactivity in women than in men, but clinically, it is seen more often in women.[71] It is theorized that women have more wet work at home, caring for children, dishwashing, and cleaning, and, thus, are more prone to further irritation at work.[72,73]

Irritant eczema is defined by subjective and objective criteria. Subjectively, a worker complains of itching, pain, burning, or stinging within minutes to two weeks after environmental exposure. Many workers in the same environment will have similar complaints. Objectively, the worker often has edema, fissuring, erythema, and hyperkeratosis of the skin. Any area of the skin may be affected, but the most common area is the hand. Often the hands appear scalded or burned.

Vesicles may be present, but they often suggest allergy. The results of relevant patch testing are usually negative. A worker often states that the dermatitis improves on days off from work. Patch testing with the appropriate allergens can help differentiate allergy from irritation. Fiberglass workers are somewhat of an exception. They develop pruritis and pseudofolliculitis at exposed sites.[74] In these cases, a diagnosis can be made with biopsy or by a potassium hydroxide skin preparation to look for glass spicules.

Allergic Contact Dermatitis

Allergic contact dermatitis is another common occupational hazard and may result from many allergens. Common personal allergens are fragrance, nickel, formaldehyde, and neomycin,[75] but occupational allergens often vary by profession.[76] For example, the most common allergens of dental workers are glutaraldehyde, rubber, and composite resins.[77] In electronic workers, epoxy resins and acrylates are the most common allergens.[78] Certain occupations have their own sets of allergens to which workers react.[76]

In a study reported in 2006 from the United Kingdom, 7319 cases of work-related skin disease were reviewed that had been reported by dermatologists and occupational physicians.[79] Allergic contact dermatitis was most commonly due to rubber chemicals, soaps and cleaners, wet work, nickel, and acrylics. The most commonly affected workers were in the petrochemical, rubber, and plastics manufacturing industries. Machinists and workers in metal and automotive industries also were shown to be at a higher risk for contact dermatitis. Allergic contact dermatitis is marked by erythema, lichenification, and vesicles. The rash is frequently symmetrical and well demarcated. Allergic contact dermatitis is virtually indistinguishable from IE until patch testing reveals relevant allergens, although workers often complain of more itching with allergic contact dermatitis than with IE. Allergic contact dermatitis is a delayed hypersensitivity response that may take weeks to years of exposure to manifest clinically. Allergic contact dermatitis is more common in patients with a history of atopic dermatitis and in jobs with substantial amounts of frictional work.[80] Other risk factors described by these authors include wet work, sweating, and pressure from clothing, boots or objects in one's work place.

Environmental Work Factors

Work environments present a variety of opportunities for physical damage to the skin. Repetitive motions can cause hyperkeratosis, bruising, pressure urticaria, and tattooing from metals. Work with chemicals such as acids and alkalis, cement calcium salts, chromates, hydrofluoric acid, ethylene oxide, phenol, and

CHAPTER 20

phosphorus involves the risk of chemical burns. Vibration of the skin can lead to Raynaud phenomenon.[81] A cold environment can cause frostbite, pernio, cold urticaria, and cold panniculitis.[82-85]

Contact Urticaria

Contact urticaria usually refers to a wheal and flare-type reaction, which occurs within 20 to 30 minutes after exposure.[86] The most frequently documented cause of contact urticaria is latex, although the potential triggers are numerous. In the United Kingdom Study, contact urticaria was attributed most often to rubber and its derivatives, followed by foods and flour.[79] Patch or prick testing for allergies can be performed to aid in diagnosis.

Frictional Dermatitis

Frictional dermatitis is caused by repetitive trauma to the skin.[87] With constant friction, the skin responds by thickening and becoming lichenified and generally does not itch. Friction can also trigger psoriasis via the Koebner phenomenon, tattooing from exposure to metals, pressure urticaria, or blistering.[88] Friction also increases the likelihood of contact and irritant dermatitis.[87]

Skin Cancer

People in occupations with a significant amount of sun exposure, including lifeguards and road and construction workers, are at an increased risk for skin cancers. Basal cell and squamous cell carcinomas are the most common cancers diagnosed in the world each year.[89] Risk factors for skin cancer include fair skin, light hair, blue eyes, and a history of a significant amount of sun exposure.[90-92] Other risk factors include exposure to benzo[a]pyrene (hydrocarbons such as tar, coal, and soot), radiation, and arsenic.[93-95]

Inflammation

Folliculitis is most commonly reported in workers exposed to petrolatum, cutting oils and coolants.[79] At the sites of exposure, pustules, folliculitis, and furuncles are seen, especially where there is occlusion. Areas under a helmet or under tight pants can also develop acne, termed *acne mechanica* and thought to be due to rubbing and friction.[95-97]

Nail Disorders

Nail disorders can be divided into traumatic and chemical disorders.[98,99] The most common trauma-induced nail disorder is subungual hematoma due to bleeding under the nail plate. Long-term trauma can also lead to splinter hemorrhages, thickening of the nail, and onycholysis (separation of the nail from the nail plate). Contact allergens can also cause onycholysis, subungual hyperkeratosis, and nail dystrophy.

Causation

In Chapter 4 of this text, an approach to the determination of work-relatedness was presented. When considering occupational skin disease, evidence of the disease must first be established. This can usually be done by visualization of the skin lesion. A dermatologist should then define the disease. The epidemiologic evidence that supports the diagnosis must subsequently be presented and should support a relationship with the work environment. To establish occupational causation, the frequency, intensity, and duration of the risk exposure should be defined. Individual risk and nonoccupational factors should be identified. When the information presented has been determined to be valid, a conclusion of work-relatedness can be formulated.

CHAPTER 20

References

1. Money J. Gender: history, theory and usage of the term in sexology and its relationship to nature/nurture. *J Sex Marital Ther.* 1985;11:71-79.
2. Strazdins L, Bammer G. Women, work and musculoskeletal health. *Soc Sci Med.* 2004;58:997-1005.
3. Tuck SP, Pearce MS, Rawlings DJ, et al. Differences in bone mineral density and geometry in men and women: the Newcastle Thousand Families Study at 50 years old. *Br J Radiol.* 2005;78:493-498.
4. Pollard CD, Braun B, Hamill J. Influence of gender, estrogen and exercise on anterior knee laxity. *Clin Biomech (Bristol, Avon).* 2006;21:1060-1066.
5. Hutchinson MR, Ireland ML. Knee injuries in female athletes. *Sports Med.* 1995;19:288-302.
6. Islam SS, Velilla AM, Doyle EJ, Ducatman AM. Gender differences in work-related injury/illness: analysis of workers compensation claims. *Am J Ind Med.* 2001;39:84-91.
7. Ballau RL. Study shows that gender is not a major factor in accident etiology. *Occup Health Saf.* 1978;47:54-56, 58.

8. Trappe TA. Sex inequity in tendon metabolism [editorial]? *J Appl Physiol.* 2006;102:507.

9. Neves IR. Work, exclusion, pain, suffering, and gender relations: a survey of female workers treated for repetitive strain injury at a public health . *Cad Saude Publica.* 2006;22:1257-1265.

10. Thomas NI, Brown ND, Hodges LC, et al. Risk profiles for four types of work-related injury among hospital employees: a case-control study. *AAOHN J.* 2006;54:61-68.

11. Myers D, Kriebel D, Karasek R, et al. Injuries and assaults in a long-term psychiatric care facility: an epidemiologic study. *AAOHN J.* 2005;53:489-498.

12. McCoy CA, Carruth AK, Reed DB. Women in agriculture: risks for occupational injury within the context of gendered role. *J Agric Saf Health.* 2002;8:37-50.

13. Gemmell IM. Injuries among female army recruits: a conflict of legislation. *J R Soc Med.* 2002;95:23-27.

14. Strowbridge NF. Gender differences in the cause of low back pain in British soldiers. *J R Army Med Corps.* 2005;151:69-72.

15. Ferber R, Davis IM, Williams DS III. Gender differences in lower extremity mechanics during running. *Clin Biomech (Bristol, Avon).* 2003;18:350-357.

16. Geary KG, Irvine D, Croft AM. Does military service damage females? An analysis of medical discharge data in the British armed forces. *Occup Med (Lond).* 2002;52:85-90.

17. Strowbridge NF. Musculoskeletal injuries in female soldiers: analysis of cause and type of injury. *J R Army Med Corps.* 2002;148:256-258.

18. Smith GS, Lincoln AE, Wong TY, et al. Does occupation explain gender and other differences in work-related eye injury hospitalization rates? *J Occup Environ Med.* 2005;47:640-648.

19. Lyons TJ. Women in the fast jet cockpit: aeromedical considerations. *Aviat Space Environ Med.* 1992;63:809-818.

20. Hahn T, Foldspang A, Ingemann-Hansen T. Prevalence of knee instability in relation to sports activity. *Scand J Med Sci Sports.* 2001;11:233-238.

21. Hendriks EJ, Scholten-Peeters GG, van der Windt DA, et al. Prognostic factors for poor recovery in acute whiplash patients. *Pain.* 2005;114:408-416.

22. Tornetta P III, Hirsch EF, Howard R, McConnell T, Ross E. Skeletal injury patterns in older females. *Clin Orthop Relat Res.* 2004;(422):55-56.

23. Brinker MR, O'Connor DP. The incidence of fractures and dislocations referred for orthopaedic services in a capitated population. *J Bone Joint Surg Am.* 2004; 86:290-297.

24. Dimich-Ward H, Guernsey JR, Pickett W, et al. Gender differences in the occurrence of farm related injuries. *Occup Environ Med.* 2004;61:52-56.

25. Marras WS, Davis KG, Jorgensen M. Gender influences on spine loads during complex lifting. *Spine J.* 2003;3:93-99.

26. Marras WS. The case for cumulative trauma in low back disorders. *Spine J.* 2003;3:177-179.

27. McGeary DD, Mayer TG, Gatchel RJ, et al. Gender-related differences in treatment outcomes for patients with musculoskeletal disorders. *Spine J.* 2003;3:197-203.

28. Bounds TA, Schopp L, Johnstone B, et al. Gender differences in a sample of vocational rehabilitation clients with TBI. *NeuroRehabilitation.* 2003;18:189-196.

29. Kumar S, Narayan Y, Amell T. Analysis of low velocity frontal impacts. *Clin Biomech (Bristol, Avon)*. 2003;18:694-703.

30. Lundberg U. Psychophysiology of work: stress, gender, endocrine response, and work-related upper extremity disorders. *Am J Ind Med*. 2002;41:383-392.

31. Kostova V, Koleva M. Back disorders (low back pain, cervicobrachial and lumbosacral radicular syndromes) and some related risk factors. *J Neurol Sci*. 2001;192:17-25.

32. Laflamme L, Eilert-Petersson E. Injury risks and socioeconomic groups in different settings: differences in morbidity between men and between women at working ages. *Eur J Public Health*. 2001;11:309-313.

33. McDiarmid M, Oliver M, Ruser J, Gucer P. Male and female rate differences in carpal tunnel syndrome injuries: personal attributes or job tasks? *Environ Res*. 2000;83:23-32.

34. Olson DK, Gerberich SG. Traumatic amputations in the workplace. *J Occup Med*. 1986;28:480-485.

35. Ilhan G, Karakus S, Andic N. Risk factors and primary prevention of acute leukemia. *Asian Pac J Cancer Prev*. 2006;7:515-517.

36. Miligi L, Costantini AS, Benvenuti A, et al. Personal use of hair dyes and hematolymphopoietic malignancies. *Arch Environ Occup Health*. 2005;60:249-256.

37. Yu CL, Wang SF, Pan PC, et al. Residential exposure to petrochemicals and the risk of leukemia: using geographic information system tools to estimate individual-level residential exposure. *Am J Epidemiol*. 2006;164:200-207.

38. Smith MT, Jones RM, Smith AH. Benzene exposure and risk of non-Hodgkin lymphoma. *Cancer Epidemiol Biomarkers Prev*. 2007;16:385-391.

39. Penel N, Vansteene D. Cancers and pesticides: current data. *Bull Cancer*. 2007;94:15-22.

40. Boice JD, Cohen SS, Mumma MT, et al. Mortality among radiation workers at Rocketdyne (Atomics International), 1948-1999. *Radiat Res*. 2006;166:98-115.

41. Bollati V, Baccarelli A, Hou L, et al. Changes in DNA methylation patterns in subjects exposed to low-dose benzene. *Cancer Res*. 2007;67:876-880.

42. Yie XB, Fu H. Review of leukemia induced by benzene poisoning. *Zhonghua Lao Dong Wei Sheng Zhi Ye Bing Za Zhi*. 2005;23:392-395.

43. Miligi L, Costantini AS, Veraldi A, et al. Cancer and pesticides: an overview and some results of the Italian multicenter case-control study on hematolymphopoietic malignancies. *Ann N Y Acad Sci*. 2006;1076:366-377.

44. Thorpe N, Shirmohammadi A. Herbicides and nitrates in groundwater of Maryland and childhood cancers: a geographic information systems approach. *J Environ Sci Health C Environ Carcinog Ecotoxicol Rev*. 2005;23:261-278.

45. Metayer C, Johnson ES, Rice JC. Nested case-control study of tumors of the hemopoietic and lymphatic systems among workers in the meat industry. *Am J Epidemiol*. 1998;147:727-738.

46. Austin H, Cole P. Cigarette smoking and leukemia. *J Chronic Dis*. 1986; 39:417-421.

47. Caldwell GG, Kelley DB, Heath CW Jr. Leukemia among participants in military maneuvers at a nuclear bomb test; a preliminary report. *JAMA*. 1980;244: 1575-1578.

CHAPTER 20

48. Caldwell GG, Kelley D, Zack M, et al. Mortality and cancer frequency among military nuclear test (Smoky) participants, 1957 through 1979. *JAMA.* 1983;250:620-624.

49. Mohner M, Lindtner M, Otten H, Gille HG. Leukemia and exposure to ionizing radiation among German uranium miners. *Am J Ind Med.* 2006;49:238-248.

50. Kubale TL, Daniels RD, Yiin JH, et al. A nested case-control study of leukemia mortality and ionizing radiation at the Portsmouth Naval Shipyard. *Radiat Res.* 2005;164:810-819.

51. Wang JX, Zhang LA, Li BX, et al. Cancer risk assessment among medical X-ray workers in China. *Zhongguo Yi Xue Ke Xue Yuan Xue Bao.* 2001;23:65-68, 72.

52. Cardis E, Vrijheid M, Blettner M, et al. Risk of cancer after low doses of ionizing radiation: retrospective cohort study in 15 countries. *BMJ.* 2005;331:77. http://www.ncbi.nlm.nih.gov/entrez/query.fcgi?cmd=Retrieve&db=PubMed&dopt=Citation&list_uids=15987704 . Accessed July 9, 2007.

53. Yalow RS. Concerns with low-level ionizing radiation. *Mayo Clin Proc.* 1994;69:436-440.

54. Kasim K, Levallois P, Abdous B, et al. Lifestyle factors and the risk of adult leukemia in Canada. *Cancer Causes Control.* 2005;16:489-500.

55. Cheson BD. The gift that keeps on giving [letter]. *Clin Adv Hematol Oncol.* 2006;4:787.

56. Hoshida Y, Aozasa K. Malignancies in organ transplant recipients. *Pathol Int.* 2004;54:649-658.

57. Williams RR, Horm JW. Association of cancer sites with tobacco and alcohol consumption and socioeconomic status of patients: interview study from the Third National Cancer Survey. *J Natl Cancer Inst.* 1977;58:525-547.

58. Ott C, Huber S. The clinical significance of cosmic radiation in aviation. *Schweiz Rundsch Med Prax.* 2006;95:99-106.

59. Ballard T, Lagorio S, De Angelis G, Verdecchia A. Cancer incidence and mortality among flight personnel: a meta-analysis. *Aviat Space Environ Med.* 2000;71:216-224.

60. Gundestrup M, Storm HH. Radiation-induced acute myeloid leukemia and other cancers in commercial jet cockpit crew: a population-based cohort study. *Lancet.* 1999;354:2029-2031.

61. Irvine D, Davies DM. British Airways flightdeck mortality study, 1950-1992. *Aviat Space Environ Med.* 1999;70:548-555.

62. Kheifets L, Afifi AA, Shimkhada R. Public health impact of extremely low-frequency electromagnetic fields. *Environ Health Perspect.* 2006;114:1532-1537. http://www.ncbi.nlm.nih.gov/entrez/query.fcgi?cmd=Retrieve&db=PubMed&dopt=Citation&list_uids=15987704. Accessed July 9, 2007.

63. Salvatore JR, Weitberg AB. Non-ionizing electromagnetic radiation and cancer: is there a relationship? *R I Med J.* 1989;72:15-21.

64. Leventhal A, Karsenty E, Sadetzki S. Cellular phones and public health. *Harefuah.* 2004;143:614-618, 620.

65. Dickel H, Bruckner T, Bernhard-Klimt C, et al. Surveillance scheme for occupational skin disease in the Saarland, FRG: first report from BKH-S. *Contact Dermatitis.* 2002;46:197-206.

66. O'Malley M, Thun M, Morrison J, et al. Surveillance of occupational skin disease using the Supplementary Data System. *Am J Ind Med.* 1988;13:291-299.

CHAPTER 20

67. Meding B. Epidemiology of hand eczema in an industrial city. *Acta Derm Venereol Suppl (Stockh).* 1990;153:1-43.
68. Lim YL, Goon A. Occupational skin diseases in Singapore 2003-2004: an epidemiologic update. *Contact Dermatitis.* 2007;56:157-159.
69. Meding B, Swanbeck G. Occupational hand eczema in an industrial city. *Contact Dermatitis.* 1990;22:13-23.
70. Patil S, Maibach HI. Effect of age and sex on the elicitation of irritant contact dermatitis. *Contact Dermatitis.* 1994;30:257-264.
71. Meding B, Swanbeck G. Predictive factors for hand eczema. *Contact Dermatitis.* 1990;23:154-161.
72. Nilsson E. Individual and environmental risk factors for hand eczema in hospital workers. *Acta Derm Venereol Suppl (Stockh).* 1986;128:1-63.
73. Hogen D. The prognosis of contact dermatitis. *J Am Acad of Dermatol.* 1990;23:300-307.
74. Minamoto K, Nagano M, Inaoka T, Futatsuka M. Occupational dermatoses among fiberglass-reinforced plastics factory workers. *Contact Dermatitis.* 2002;46:339-347.
75. Tomar J, Jain VK, Aggarwal K, et al. Contact allergies to cosmetics: testing with 52 cosmetic ingredients and personal products. *J Dermatol.* 2005;32:951-955.
76. Lushniak BD. Occupational contact dermatitis. *Dermatol Ther.* 2004;17:272-277.
77. Hamann CP, DePaola LG, Rodgers PA. Occupation-related allergies in dentistry. *J Am Dent Assoc.* 2005;136:500-510.
78. Kiec-Swierczynska M, Krecisz B, Swierczynska-Machura D, Zaremba J. An epidemic of occupational contact dermatitis from an acrylic glue. *Contact Dermatitis.* 2005;52:121-125.
79. McDonald JC, Beck MH, Chen Y, Cherry NM. Incidence by occupation and industry of work-related skin diseases in the United Kingdom, 1996-2001. *Occup Med (Lond).* 2006;56:398-405.
80. Ponyai G, Temesvari E, Karpati S. Adulthood atopic dermatitis: epidemiology, clinical symptoms, provoking and prognostic factors. *Orv Hetil.* 2007;148:21-26.
81. Mason HJ, Poole K, Elms J. Upper limb disability in HAVS cases: how does it relate to the neurosensory or vascular elements of HAVS? *Occup Med (Lond).* 2005;55:389-392.
82. Ballanger F, Barbarot S, Masseau A, et al. Cutaneous lesions of the hands worsened by coldness. *Rev Med Interne.* 2005;26:751-753.
83. Henry F, Letot B, Pierard-Franchimont C, Pierard GE. Winter skin diseases. *Rev Med Liege.* 1999;54:864-866.
84. Spittell JA Jr, Spittell PC. Chronic pernio: another cause of blue toes. *Int Angiol.* 1992;11:46-50.
85. Geller M. Cold-induced cholinergic urticaria: case report. *Ann Allergy.* 1989;63:29-30.
86. Krogh V. The contact urticaria syndrome. [Letter]. *Semin Dermatol.* 1982;1:56.
87. McMullen E, Gawkrodger DJ. Physical friction is under-recognized as an irritant that can cause or contribute to contact dermatitis. *Br J Dermatol.* 2006;154:154-156.
88. Samitz MH. Repeated mechanical trauma to the skin: occupational aspects. *Am J Ind Med.* 1985;8:265-271.

CHAPTER 20

89. Marks R, Motley RJ. Skin cancer: recognition and treatment. *Drugs.* 1995; 50:48-61.

90. McDonald CJ. American Cancer Society perspective on the American College of Preventive Medicine's policy statements on skin cancer prevention and screening. *CA Cancer J Clin.* 1998;48:229-231.

91. Harmful effects of ultraviolet radiation. Council on Scientific Affairs. *JAMA.* 1989;262:380-384.

92. Kricker A, Armstrong BK, English DR, Heenan PJ. Pigmentary and cutaneous risk factors for non-melanocytic skin cancer: a case-control study. *Int J Cancer.* 1991;48:650-662.

93. Mun SA, Larin SA, Brailovskii VV, Lodzia AF, Zinchuk SF, Glushkov AN. Ambient air benz[a]pyrene and cancer morbidity in Kemerovo. *Gig Sanit.* 2006;(4):28-30.

94. Tseng CH. Arsenic methylation, urinary arsenic metabolites and human diseases: current perspective. *J Environ Sci Health C Environ Carcinog Ecotoxicol Rev.* 2007;25:1-22.

95. Aytas FI, Aslan N, Habiboglu R, et al. Radiation induced skin reactions in adult cancer patients. *Clin Oncol (R Coll Radiol).* 2007;19:S23-S24.

96. Mills OH Jr, Kligman A. Acne mechanica. *Arch Dermatol.* 1975;111:481-483.

97. Basler RS. Acne mechanica in athletes. *Cutis.* 1992;50:125-128.

98. Duhard-Brohan E. Mechanical nail pathology. *Rev Prat.* 2000;50:2251-2255.

99. Scher RK. Occupational nail disorders. *Dermatol Clin.* 1988;6:27-33.

Toxic Exposure Claims: A Framework for Causation Analysis

Gideon Letz, MD, and Mark H. Hyman, MD

This chapter provides a framework for analyzing causation issues involving occupational and environmental exposures to various agents. The most common context for this framework is in workers' compensation, but the same approach can be adapted to other dispute-resolution systems, including short- and long-term disability, Social Security Disability Insurance, service-related military personnel in the Veterans Administration, product liability, and personal injury lawsuits.

Compared with traumatic musculoskeletal injuries, causation analysis in cases involving toxic exposures is complicated by a number of factors (Table 21-1). Questions of causation related to toxic exposures most often involve relatively common conditions that are not uniquely associated with chemical exposures, such as asthma, hepatitis, end-stage renal disease, peripheral neuropathy, and many common forms of cancer. Only rarely does the diagnosis itself imply causation. Examples of imputed causation include silicosis and silica dust exposure in a foundry worker, mesothelioma in an asbestos worker, and angiosarcoma in a rubber worker exposed to vinyl chloride. Causation can also be obscured by long latency periods, 20+ years for some forms of cancer. Long latencies mean that the first clinical manifestations of disease can appear after retirement and when it is no longer possible to monitor environmental levels of toxic materials or even reconstruct workplace exposure conditions. Multiple confounding variables such as age, smoking history, and comorbid disease states can also obscure causation. This is commonly an issue in patients with occupational exposure to suspect human carcinogens and a significant history of tobacco use.

TABLE 21-1	Acute Trauma vs Occupational Disease
Acute Trauma	**Occupational Disease**
No latency	Latency varies from 0 to >20 y
Cause usually obvious	Causation often obscure
Rehabilitation usually without impairment	Permanent disability common
Not usually litigated	High litigation rate

There is a relatively poor correlation between claims data and actual incidence and prevalence of occupational disease.[1-3] True cases are often not identified because physicians do not carefully obtain work histories, there are often long latencies, or the disease state in question is common in the general population. On the other hand, many claims for occupational disease lack scientific evidence for causation.[4] Yet these unmerited claims may be settled in favor of the claimant owing to expediency or legal technicalities unrelated to the scientific evidence (Letz. G. Personal Communication). Other reasons that benefits may be awarded, despite lack of clear evidence include the following:

- Legal *presumptions* in state laws that are based on politics rather than scientific evidence (e.g., cancer and heart disease in police officers)
- Incentives created by lack of health insurance for employees to file workers' compensation claims and clinicians to support them, even without scientific evidence of work-relatedness
- Pressure to settle the claim rather than prolong the legal proceedings created by the high litigation rate in this type of claim

Three-Step Process for Analyzing Toxic Exposure Questions

A systematic approach is needed when analyzing causation issues to avoid wasting time, effort, and resources pursuing unreasonable hypotheses, while at the same time not missing the opportunity to find previously unrecognized hazards. There are three distinct steps in the reasoning and investigative process.[5] These steps can be summarized as "Does," "Can," and "Did."

Step 1: Establish or Verify the Diagnosis

The first step is to establish or verify the diagnosis (i.e., determine what is wrong with the patient; or *Does* the patient have the [disease]?). This step is accomplished by careful review of the available medical records and/or examination of the patient. Determining whether there is evidence of disease or illness is a clinical and pathologic process. Whether an exposure occurred is irrelevant until the presence of disease or illness has been established.

The following scenarios need to be considered:
1. In some situations, the diagnosis can be verified with objective clinical measurements using imaging or laboratory data that are standardized in terms of sensitivity and specificity. An example would be the presence of

CHAPTER 21

thyroid dysfunction (hypothyroidism). In some cases, the treating physician may use objective tests that have not been validated sufficiently in the peer-reviewed literature (e.g., some of the laboratory indicators of immune system dysregulation). In these cases, the issue about presence of disease must be resolved before going further in the investigation.

2. In other situations, the diagnosis has been made entirely on the basis of subjective, self-reported information from the patient, and there are no objective measures to confirm the diagnosis. This may be because there are no tests to objectively confirm the condition (e.g., chronic neuropathic pain syndromes) or because the appropriate testing has never been done (e.g., cognitive complaints without neuropsychological testing). In these cases, further testing may be required or the presence of disease or illness must be accepted on the basis of the clinical history in the absence of objective verification.

3. The most problematic cases involve controversial diagnoses such as multiple chemical sensitivity, chronic fatigue syndrome, and systemic candidiasis. Careful investigation of the cases reveals that most patients have evidence of a comorbid psychiatric disorder in the context of a personality structure showing high tendency toward somatization.[16] In this context, it is easy to understand how a chemical exposure incident can become the focus of ongoing symptoms and disability. Often the challenge is to sort out the psychosocial determinants of illness behavior from the pathophysiologic effects of a chemical exposure.[6]

It must be remembered that the presence of persistent symptoms associated with a history of exposure to a potentially toxic chemical does not necessarily equate to a pathophysiologic effect from that exposure. This is the common problem of differentiating simple *association* from the more rigorously defined *causation*.

Step 2: Determine Whether a Cause-Effect Relationship Exists

If a diagnosis has been established, the next step in the causation analysis process is to determine whether a cause-effect relationship between the exposure and the disease state is *plausible* (i.e., Can the agent cause what the patient has?). This is a question of how to research and evaluate the published literature and how to weigh the strength of the evidence found in peer-reviewed scientific articles. The ranking of evidence has been widely discussed in the published literature.[7] Randomized clinical trials are the "gold standard" for measuring the strength of evidence related to toxic effects of chemical agents. Unlike therapeutic drug trials, ethical standards have not allowed studies to be done with chemical agents that have no potential benefit for test subjects. Therefore, conclusions about the toxic effects of industrial chemicals depend on epidemiologic surveys of exposed vs. nonexposed populations and on animal data. In general, human data are considered more relevant than animal or in vitro data; prospective cohort studies are more relevant than retrospective case-control studies, which in turn are more relevant than case series and case reports.

An epidemiologic study may demonstrate an association that is *not* causal owing to chance, bias, or confounding. If the association is believed to be valid, i.e., the disease occurrence is not equal among exposed and unexposed populations and the association *cannot* be explained by chance, bias, or confounding, whether the data support a *cause-and-effect* relationship must be considered. Factors to be considered in regard to defining an association as causal were originally proposed by Hill[8] and include the following:

- The strength of the association
- Whether a dose-response relationship has been demonstrated
- The presence of other studies showing the same result (consistency across studies and design types)
- Demonstrated biological plausibility (i.e., mechanism of action)
- An appropriate time sequence (whether cause precedes effect)

Resources that should be considered in formulating an opinion based on the literature would include online sites such as the National Library of Medicine sites (http://www.nlm.nih.gov; Haz-Map, http://www.hazmap.nlm.nih.gov/ index.html; and Environmental Health and Toxicology, http://www.sis.nlm. nih.gov/enviro.html); the Report on Carcinogens from the National Toxicology Program (http://www.ntp.niehs.nih.gov); the Centers for Disease Control and Prevention sites (http://www.cdc.gov; Agency for Toxic Substances and Disease Registry, http://www.atsdr.cdc.gov; and exposure reports, http://www.cdc.gov/ exposurereport/report.htm); the International Agency for Research on Cancer (http://www.iarc.fr); the Reprorisk System (http://www.micromedex.com); and the Environmental Protection Agency (http://www.epa.gov). Printed texts should also be consulted,[9] as should standard textbooks.

Step 3: Implement the Hazard Evaluation Process

Only when the diagnosis has been established *and* there is credible evidence that a cause-effect relationship *could* exist based on the available literature, is an investigation into the specific exposure situation in order (i.e., *Did* the agent cause the problem?). This is the *hazard evaluation process* and is a multidisciplinary endeavor involving medical, toxicologic, and industrial hygiene resources.[10] The decision to proceed with a comprehensive investigation should be reserved for situations in which there is documented illness or disease that can be reasonably related to environmental factors (steps 1 and 2). This process will decrease unnecessary anxiety among coworkers and allow efficient use of limited health and safety resources. The hazard evaluation process can be organized into a number of distinct tasks:

Attention to the Occupational History

Are the symptoms associated with presence at work and do they improve during time away from work, e.g., weekends and vacations? Are symptoms related to specific activities in the workplace? Are other workers similarly affected? Is there evidence of exposure to dust, fumes, or vapors?

Characterization of the Latent Period

The time between first exposure and clinical manifestation of toxic effects can vary from no interval to many years. Some effects may go unnoticed for years until an irreversible loss of function has occurred, such as end-stage renal disease. There may be progression of tissue damage long after exposure ceases, as seen with asbestosis, although this is relatively rare. Most toxic agents do not cause delayed reactions; thus, if no effects are observed at the time of exposure, there is no increased risk of illness months or years later. Allergic reactions are particularly problematic in this respect. Depending on environmental levels and individual susceptibility, reactions can vary from immediate at the time of first exposure, to delayed onset months or years after the first exposure. It is rare for asthma of recent onset, however, to be related to exposure that occurred uneventfully many years before. [17]

Identification of Toxic Agents

Identification of toxic agents can be a difficult and time-consuming task and may be only by inference when the exposures have occurred in the past and the worksite is no longer operational or changes in environmental controls or processes have made current monitoring irrelevant. If the workplace is operational, Material Safety Data Sheets are mandated by the Occupational Safety and Health Administration (OSHA) to be available at the worksite for each potentially hazardous material that may be encountered. Although the Material Safety Data Sheets give basic toxicity information, the information is often incomplete and sometimes inaccurate. [11]

Review of Available Toxicologic Information

Once potentially harmful materials have been identified, a toxicologic profile of each ingredient needs to be developed, which is best accomplished by using standard reference texts; data from the texts can be easily updated with online literature searches when necessary. Of note is the fact that many commonly used chemicals have not been adequately characterized from a toxicologic standpoint, especially in reference to carcinogenesis, toxic effects on reproduction, and other chronic effects.

Estimation of Exposure Dose

The diagnosis of illness or disease caused by exposure to toxic agents involves the synthesis of information in addition to the usual clinical data obtained from the history, physical examination, and laboratory studies. Once a diagnosis has been established that is *possibly* related to a toxic exposure, an effort must be made to characterize the *exposure dose* of the chemical alleged to be the causative agent.

For most volatile chemicals, dusts, and fumes, data derived from timed air sampling provide the best evidence of exposure dose. Unfortunately, such information is rarely available; however, there are often important clues that can be obtained with a careful history that will be useful in estimating exposure:

- Length of time in the area where exposure occurred or time involved with specific processes or tasks when exposure was likely
- Presence or absence of engineering controls such as exhaust ventilation systems
- Use of and fit testing of personal protective equipment
- General work practices (e.g., eating or smoking in the work area)
- The presence of visible dust or fumes in the environment
- The presence of odors

In addition, the presence or absence of acute symptoms such as mucous membrane irritation or central nervous system (CNS) depression may allow estimation of exposure dose even when evaluating an illness months or years after the exposure has ceased. This is particularly important if the suspected work operation has been shut down or is not accessible.

For agents that are well characterized in terms of acute toxicity, such as organic solvents that cause CNS depression, a history of the expected symptoms may be adequate to conclude a cause-effect relationship. But for agents that produce delayed or chronic effects without much acute toxicity, the absence of acute symptoms at the time of exposure is not helpful in ruling out the presence of hazardous conditions in the past.

The physical properties of a given substance such as vapor pressure may be useful in estimating probable airborne concentrations and, therefore, potential for respiratory exposure. Lipid solubility is important in predicting the potential for dermal absorption.

Development of a Dose-Response Model

This is the most critical phase of the hazard evaluation process. It involves the synthesis of clinical, industrial hygiene, and toxicologic information to determine whether the estimated dose was sufficient to explain observed clinical effects known to be associated with the agent in question. The available information may be ambiguous or incomplete; for example, there may be inadequate data to reasonably estimate environmental levels of toxicants, or the observed clinical condition may not be consistent with existing toxicologic information.

Whether one is evaluating the cause of illness in an individual claimant or the safety of a particular work environment, consideration of the dose-response model is essential. As stated by Paracelsus (1493-1541): "All substances are poisons. The right dose differentiates a poison from a remedy.[18]" Misunderstandings, erroneous judgments, and inappropriate actions in reference to a suspected toxic exposure are usually traceable to disregard for dose-response considerations. [17] Highly toxic materials can be used safely in the presence of appropriate engineering controls and/or use of personal protective equipment, whereas exposure to materials of low toxicity can be hazardous under unusual conditions such as working in confined spaces and not using adequate personal protective equipment.

Biological Monitoring and the Establishment of Chemical Disease

The advancements in the development of sensitive and precise analytic methods to measure chemicals and drugs in blood, urine, and other body fluids and tissue have provided useful information in the diagnosis of chemically induced disease. Available laboratory procedures for toxicologic analyses vary widely in accuracy, sensitivity, specificity, and cost. However, for a number of chemical agents, the ability to detect and measure trace amounts of chemicals in body fluids or tissue has outstripped the ability of clinicians to interpret the human health implications of the measured values, particularly in regard to the persistent organochlorines such as polychlorinated biphenyls, DDT, and other halogenated compounds.

In selected circumstances, however, toxicologic analyses can be an important adjunct to the history, physical examination, and routine laboratory testing in the diagnosis of disease secondary to chemical exposures. Whether done as a part of a causation evaluation or in the course of medical surveillance of potentially exposed populations, the following theoretical and practical limitations should be considered:

- Rational interpretation of results is possible only when sufficient information is available on the mechanism of toxicity and the pharmacokinetics of the substance being measured.
- Levels of specific chemicals can be interpreted only by comparing them with reference values in unexposed or asymptomatic populations. For a few chemicals such as lead and mercury, information is available correlating levels of the chemicals in body fluids or tissue with the risk of adverse effect. However, for the vast majority of chemical agents, no health-based reference values are available. This is particularly important for organochlorine compounds that persist in tissue for long periods. These substances have received much attention because trace amounts are being detected in humans and animals worldwide. For these compounds, the acute toxic effects generally are minimal. However, there are many unanswered questions about their potential long-term or delayed effects secondary to long-term, low-level (in the parts per billion range) exposure. Although such data may be important in epidemiologic studies designed to address public health concerns, the measured levels in a given person are not particularly useful in medical diagnosis or disability evaluations and are rarely useful in documenting past exposure levels.
- Ideally, it is considered that the measured level of a chemical in tissue or body fluid is a function of its rate of absorption, distribution, metabolism, and elimination. Unfortunately, a number of methodological considerations can affect the measured level apart from analytic errors. Some of these are summarized in Table 21-2.

CHAPTER 21

TABLE 21-2	Methodological Sources of Error in Laboratory Data*

I. Physiologic sources of variation
  A. Hydration
  B. Posture
  C. Activity level
  D. Pregnancy
  E. Pre-existing disease
  F. Use of tourniquet for venipuncture
  G. Time since last meal
II. Kinetic sources of variation
  A. Timing of sample in reference to last exposure
  B. Tissue sampled (blood, urine, alveolar air)
  C. Skin absorption affecting local venous blood levels
III. Variation associated with specimen storage and collection
  A. Factors that cause spuriously *high* results
    1. External contamination from workplace air, skin, or clothing
    2. Contamination from specimen container or additives
    3. Contamination during laboratory analysis
  B. Factors that cause spuriously *low* results
    1. chemical decomposition (influenced by temperature, pH, time to analysis)
    2. Absorption to container
    3. Evaporative loss
IV. Nonoccupational environmental exposures
    1. Smoking
    2. Alcohol
    3. Diet
    4. Leisure-time activities (hobbies, home maintenance)

* From Letz.[10] TABLE 3-4. Methodologic Sources of Error In the interpretation of Toxicologic Analyses (Nonanalytic Errors)

Despite the pitfalls that must be considered, enough information about toxicologic, kinetic, and population reference values exists to make biological monitoring feasible for a number of common industrial chemicals.[12,13] The following case examples are presented to illustrate the practical application of the three basic steps in the evaluation and investigation of alleged illness related to toxic exposures:

Case 1

A 56-year-old secretary employed at an architect's office complained of head-aches and went to her family doctor for evaluation. The headaches seemed to be worse during the week and improved on the weekends. Otherwise, her history and physical examination findings were unremarkable except for an enlarged thyroid gland. Laboratory results revealed a high level of thyroid stimulating hormone and a borderline low level of thyroxine. The diagnosis was Hashimoto disease, and thyroid replacement therapy was started.

She was responsible for operation and maintenance of a blueprint machine in the office and was often bothered by the odor of ammonia from the machine. She subsequently filed a claim alleging that her thyroid disease was related to exposure to ammonia vapor.

Step 1: What DOES the patient have?

Careful review of the medical records confirmed the diagnosis of Hashimoto disease and did not reveal any other abnormalities to explain her headaches. She was taking no medications other than thyroid replacement and occasional ibuprofen for headache.

Step 2: CAN the agent (ammonia) cause the disorder in question (thyroid disease)?

Review of the literature failed to identify *any* human or animal data that would suggest a possible relationship between exposure to ammonia and risk of any thyroid disease. In fact, the physical and chemical properties of ammonia make it extremely unlikely that inhalational exposure could result in any type of systemic toxicity because ammonia is such a potent upper respiratory and mucous membrane irritant that unless the person were trapped in a confined space, the irritant effects would preclude systemic absorption of a significant amount of ammonia. Surveys of workers exposed on a long-term basis to low-level ammonia concentrations indicated that the maximum concentration not resulting in significant complaints is 25 ppm. Tolerance to usually irritating concentrations of ammonia may occur by "adaptation" in workers exposed on a long-term basis.[14] No measurements of ammonia levels in the office environment were available.

CHAPTER 21

Step 3: DID *the exposure in question (ammonia) cause the disorder (thyroid disease) in this case?*

In this situation, no further investigation of the work environment is necessary to conclude that there is no causal relationship between the claimant's thyroid condition and exposure to ammonia vapor. The actual concentrations of ammonia in her work environment are not needed to develop this conclusion because a cause-effect relationship is not likely at *any* exposure dose. Of note however, is the possibility that her headache symptoms could be related to the ammonia vapor because it is known that any degree of mucous membrane irritation or offensive odor can result in headache symptoms. An industrial hygiene investigation would not be necessary to develop a sound conclusion.

Case 2

A worker at a pesticide storage and distribution facility was cleaning the inside of a tank through a porthole on the top of the tank with a high-pressure water sprayer. He could not remove some residual material on the inside wall of the tank and climbed inside to complete the operation. Less than 5 minutes later, he complained of feeling ill and collapsed. A supervisor was called to the scene, and he also climbed inside the tank in an attempt to rescue his coworker. The first man was inside the tank for 45 minutes before being rescued by fire crews using self-contained breathing apparatus. The supervisor rescued at the same time was in the tank for approximately 30 minutes. Both victims were decontaminated at the scene by washing with a fire hose, and both were noted to have a strong chemical odor during transport to the hospital. The first worker died 12 hours later with metabolic acidosis, CNS depression, and laboratory evidence of liver damage. The supervisor died 64 hours later with intractable metabolic acidosis and hepatic and renal failure.[15]

Step 1: What DOES the patient have?

In this case, the question is modified slightly to "What was the cause of death?" It is clear from the medical facts reflected in the paramedic, emergency department, and hospital records that both men died of refractory metabolic acidosis and multiple organ system failure after a brief, confined-space exposure. Although this unfortunate incident graphically demonstrates the severe hazards of working in confined spaces without adequate personal protection, it was also important to determine the exact cause of death because there were obvious liability issues that would be litigated.

The OSHA investigators arrived at the scene 2 hours after the accident and collected samples of the liquid material in the bottom of the tank through a drainage valve. The material was subsequently analyzed and found to contain high concentrations of nitrates and phosphates and from 0.1% to 0.3% ethylene dibromide (EDB), a highly toxic fumigant. Air sampling was done inside the tank approximately 20 hours after the accident, and EDB was the only toxin detected, at concentrations ranging from 15 to 40 ppm.

Step 2: CAN the agent (EDB) cause the disorder (death after a brief, confined-space exposure) in question?

Review of the literature revealed two published cases of acute poisoning and death from EDB: One early case involved the accidental use of EDB instead of *ethyl bromide* as an anesthetic gas. Death occurred of uterine hemorrhaging after 44 hours. Autopsy revealed advanced states of parenchymatous degeneration of the heart, liver, and kidneys and hemorrhages in the respiratory tract. The second case involved intentional ingestion of EDB capsules that were formulated as a soil fumigant. The calculated dose was 140 mg/kg of EDB, and, 54 hours after ingestion, the patient died of extensive hepatic and renal damage. Acute exposure of experimental animals to lethal inhalational doses resulted in pathologic effects similar to those described in humans. At a high enough dose, it is obvious that EDB can cause lethal effects in humans secondary to multiple organ system failure, particularly liver and kidney.

Step 3: DID the exposure in question (EDB) cause the disorder (acute lethal poisoning) in this case?

Initially, the only information available was that the victims had become ill while cleaning a tank that contained fertilizer and/or pesticides. The key clinical question was the differential diagnosis of metabolic acidosis after exposure to unknown chemicals. However, it became known relatively early that EDB was the most likely toxin. Subsequently, data from a variety of sources confirmed that there had been significant exposure to EDB:

- Industrial hygiene monitoring at the scene demonstrated EDB in the air and liquid inside the tank.
- Serum bromide concentrations were elevated before death and postmortem.
- Postmortem tissue concentrations of EDB were measurable in both victims.
- The EDB concentration was measurable in the breathing zone of the pathologists who performed the autopsy on case 2!

- Skin lesions developed 24 hours after exposure in the second victim. The delayed onset and morphologic features of the lesions were exactly analogous to previous reports of dermal effects observed in workers exposed to EDB.

Calculation of the exact absorbed dose of EDB was not possible. The victims could have inhaled or swallowed EDB, but absorption by the dermal route was significant given that they both collapsed on the bottom of the tank that contained a solution of EDB. The airborne concentrations of EDB measured 20 hours after the incident would not produce acute toxic effects in animals, although the concentration could have been much higher when the men were inside the tank. It is also possible that their initial collapse was secondary to lack of oxygen in the confined space rather than the toxic effect of EDB itself.

Case 3

A 31-year-old worker at a small sign-painting shop worked 4 hours on New Year's Eve at his usual job, which involved plastic sign preparation and painting. After work, he went hiking in the nearby hills and subsequently complained of nausea and vomited. He fell asleep at home, and when he could not be easily aroused, a friend took him to the emergency department. On examination he appeared mildly "drunk," but there was no history of ethanol ingestion. He had horizontal nystagmus, but otherwise, his physical examination findings were normal. Initial blood gases and chemistry results were within normal limits, with a calculated anion gap of 21.

He was admitted for observation and given 2 to 3 L of fluid because of orthostatic vital signs. During the next 24 hours, severe metabolic acidosis developed, with a pH of 7.19, a P_{CO_2} of 14, and an elevated anion gap of 45. A coworker provided a list of chemicals used at his worksite, which included isopropanol, acetone, and methanol. An initial toxicology screen revealed a methanol level of 372 mg/L (37 mg %). He was treated with hemodialysis. After the first hemodialysis treatment, the methanol level was 205 mg/L, and it was undetectable after the second treatment. His hospital course was uncomplicated, his altered mental status resolved. Visual signs and symptoms are known to occur in some patients with severe methanol poisoning, but never developed.

An OSHA investigation revealed that a few weeks before the incident, a chemical salesman had suggested substitution of methanol for isopropanol, which was used as a cleaning agent because it would evaporate faster in the cold winter months. No information on the potential hazards of working with methanol was provided. The patient was using copious amounts of methanol without respiratory or skin protection before his illness.

The patient has been seen numerous times since resolution of the acute poisoning episode in a period of 9 months. He has complained of persistent fatigue with occasional palpitations and paresthesias. However, a complete internal medicine evaluation found no abnormalities, and he was released for work without restrictions. As of 1 year after exposure, he had not returned to work owing to his generalized fatigue.

Step 1: What DOES the patient have?

In this case, there is no doubt that the *acute* illness was related to methanol toxicity from dermal and inhalational exposure at work. But are his persistent symptoms also secondary to the methanol poisoning? Is he malingering, or does he have physical or psychological sequelae that can be legitimately related to methanol poisoning?

There is obviously a need for additional information to resolve this case. An internal medicine evaluation undoubtedly did not include a thorough neuropsychological evaluation to detect subtle cognitive deficits, an anxiety or a depressive disorder, or a psychosomatic disorder that might explain the symptoms of fatigue. There was probably no detailed assessment of possible psychosocial barriers to recovery. Such an evaluation would be necessary to establish the diagnosis and exclude the possibility of malingering.

Step 2: CAN the agent (methanol) cause the disorder (generalized fatigue following a severe poisoning) in question?

We must rely on the published information about methanol poisoning, in particular the potential for persistent symptoms and possible psychological sequelae following a severe poisoning episode. The only documented long-term effects of acute methanol poisoning are related to the visual system (e.g., blurred vision and constricted visual fields) and include irreversible blindness. There are no reports of other persistent CNS effects after recovery from the acute illness.

Step 3: DID the exposure in question (methanol poisoning) cause the disorder (chronic fatigue) in this case?

Even with the incomplete information about the possibility of a psychiatric diagnosis or significant psychosocial barriers to recovery, it can be concluded that the persistent disability is unrelated to the pathophysiologic effects of methanol poisoning. The presence or absence of psychiatric impairment that might explain the persistent disability cannot be addressed without additional information.

Additional information about exposure is irrelevant because the patient has not returned to work. Cessation of methanol use at this worksite was recommended, however, to prevent further injuries.

Summary

The framework outlined herein will facilitate logical, easily understandable reasoning. The use of this model will ensure that conclusions are formulated objectively, consistently, and according to scientifically sound guidelines. When the conclusion can be clearly and logically presented, it is more likely to be understood by lay audiences, legal colleagues, and claims administrators or judges who may have limited technical knowledge or experience with toxicologic information.

References

1. Brandt-Rauf SI. Workers' compensation and occupational disease: the case of cancer. *Occup Med.* 1987;2:189-195.
2. Brown TC. The mythology of occupational disease compensation. *J Public Health Policy.* 1985;6:371-378.
3. Azaroff LS, Levenstein C, Wegman DH. Occupational injury and illness surveillance: conceptual filters explain underreporting. *Am J Public Health.* 2002; 92:1421-1429.
4. Boden LI. Workers' compensation in the United States: high costs, low benefits. *Annu Rev Public Health.* 1995;16:189-218.
5. Gots RE. Medical causation and expert testimony. *Regul Toxicol Pharmacol.* 1986; 6:95-102.
6. Weiser SR. Psychosocial aspects of occupational musculoskeletal disorders. *In,* M Nordin, GBJ Andersson, MH Pope, eds., *Musculoskeletal Disorders in the Workplace: Principles and Practice.* St Louis, MO: CV Mosby; 1997:51-61.
7. Mulrow C, Langhorne P, Grimshaw J. Integrating heterogeneous pieces of evidence in systematic reviews. *Ann Intern Med.* 1997;127:989-995.
8. Hill AB. The environment and disease: association or causation? *Proc R Soc Med.* 1965;58:295-300.
9. American Conference of Governmental Industrial Hygienists. 2007 TLVs and BEIs. ACGIH Signature Press. Cincinnati, Ohio: 2007.
10. Letz G. *The Diagnosis of Occupational Disease.* In: G Hathaway, NH Proctor, JP Hughes, ML Fischman, eds., Chemical Hazards of the Workplace, 3rd edition, New York, NY: Van Nostrand Reinhold, 1991: chap 3.

11. Letz G, Wugofski L, Cone JE, Patterson R, Harris KE, Grammer LC. Trimellitic anhydride exposure in a 55-gallon drum manufacturing plant: clinical, immunologic, and industrial hygiene evaluation. *Am J Ind Med.* 1987;12:407-417.

12. Baselt RC. Disposition of Toxic Drugs and Chemicals in Man, 6th ed. Foster City, CA: Chemical Toxicology Institute, 2002.

13. Lauwerys RR and Hoet P. Industrial Chemical Exposure: Guidelines for Biological Monitoring, 3rd edition. Washington D.C.: Lewis Publishers, 2001.

14. Hathaway G, Proctor NH, Hughes JP, Fischman ML. *Proctor and Hughes' Chemical Hazards of the Workplace.* 3rd ed. New York, NY: Van Nostrand Reinhold; 1991.

15. Letz GA, Pond SM, Osterloh JD, Wade RL, Becker CE. Two fatalities after acute occupational exposure to ethylene dibromide. *JAMA.* 1984; 252: 2428-2431.

16. Natelson BH, Chronic fatigue syndrome. JAMA. 2001;285:2557-2559. Wessely S. Chronic fatigue syndrome-trials and tribulations. JAMA.2001; 286;378:1378-1379.

17. Guidotti Tl. Principles of occupational toxicology. In Zenz C, Dickerson OB and Horvath EP. eds. *Occupational Medicine.* 3rd ed. St. Louis, MO: Mosby, 1994: 70-84.

18. Paracelsus. Wikipedia. http://en.wikipedia.org/wiki/Paracelsus#_note-1. Accessed Oct. 10, 2007.

CHAPTER 21

22

Putting It All Together: Causation Analysis as Illustrated by Example

Roger M. Belcourt, MD, MPH, and J. Mark Melhorn, MD

After reading this book, how does a health care provider put the whole process together to develop an answer to the questions of causation? Educators suggest that examples provide one of the best ways to learn new skills. To that end, the following example is provided.

Many occupational health care providers experience discomfort approaching the determination of causation because it does not seem consistent with patient advocacy and the historical physician-patient relationship. Lack of training or experience may also be partly to blame; it is often easier and less time-consuming to accept a person's analysis of what caused the illness or injury in question. This statement is not intended to minimize the importance of soliciting the person's beliefs about the cause of his or her medical condition. However, relying solely on the person's beliefs has inherent dangers.

In the case of occupational medicine, there is an increased likelihood of misclassification (occupational vs. nonoccupational), misdiagnosis, and potential public health ramifications. For example, no physician would accept the belief of a 50-year-old man with diabetes that his shortness of breath was due to deconditioning without first ruling out cardiac and pulmonary disease. Knowing the correct cause (medical causation analysis) of the shortness of breath would significantly influence the treatment chosen. Similarly, the blanket acceptance of carpal tunnel syndrome as an occupational event without a careful analysis of potential nonoccupational causative and/or contributing conditions (e.g., hypothyroidism, diabetes, and autoimmune disease) might result in incomplete medical management. Finally, a missed opportunity of establishing a sentinel event could result in morbidity to other workers.

Presumption of causation is a legal term that generally "trumps" medical causation analysis. For example, Nevada is one of several states with a presumption of occupational causation for heart and lung disease in police and firefighters. Applying a medical causation model to such a case is nonsensical and nonproductive. Consideration of the components of legal causation, i.e., cause in fact and proximate cause, are "part and parcel" of tort law, including medical malpractice.

An Example of Occupational Causation Analysis

A 32-year-old woman sought care at the Best Occupational Medical Center because of a 2-week history of bilateral shoulder pain with intermittent paresthesias and numbness into both upper extremities down to her fingertips. She is employed in a "Mom-and-Pop" dry cleaning business and has worked there for 5 years. She attributed her symptoms to grasping and hanging garments on the elevated rails. Her symptoms seemed to be worse toward the end of the shift and were greatly improved after a weekend off or after a vacation.

Additional preliminary history revealed that she was 28 weeks pregnant. She and her husband of 4 years had been trying to conceive for 3 years; they had believed they were an infertile couple. She experienced quickening at 20 weeks, and an ultrasound at that time was unremarkable.

Her medical history was remarkable for neck pain following a motor vehicle accident at the age of 18 years in which her car was rear-ended by a car traveling 35 mph. She related that X-ray results at the time were reported as normal. Treatment included medications, physical therapy, and chiropractic treatments. She recovered uneventfully after 6 or 8 weeks and, except an occasional stiff neck, she has had no further symptoms.

The review of systems was remarkable for a 10-lb weight gain during pregnancy and for lightheadedness and occasional frank vertigo. Indeed, she had fainted at work a month ago. Although she has had these symptoms intermittently for the previous 4 years, she was reassured by her obstetrician that these were common with pregnancy. She also reported nocturnal numbness and paresthesias into the radial aspect of both hands that had become worse during the past 2 months. She described palpitations associated with anxiety, usually while at work; she attributed these to the stresses associated with doing her job.

Her only medication was prenatal vitamins. She did not smoke cigarettes or drink alcohol.

The physical examination revealed the following: height, 5 ft 2 in; weight, 140 lb; temperature, 99.2°F; pulse, 88 beats per minute; and blood pressure, 102/58 mm Hg. Additional findings are shown in Table 22-1.

CHAPTER 22

TABLE 22-1	Physical Examination Findings
System	**Findings**
General	Well-developed, well-nourished woman appearing slightly older than stated age; right hand preference
Skin	Mild eczematous eruption on finger tips (flexor touchpads) and, to a lesser extent, over the palmar surfaces of both hands
Neck	Full range of motion, negative Spurling maneuver (axial load on head with neck extension to test for atlantoaxial instability); thyroid generally prominent without palpable nodules
Shoulders	Full range of motion; painful arc noted on the right from 100° to 140°; impingement sign positive on the right, negative on the left; apprehension sign negative bilaterally; thoracic outlet signs negative bilaterally
Heart	Regular rate and rhythm with grade 2/6 systolic ejection murmur at the left lower sternal border
Lungs	Clear to auscultation
Abdomen	No hepatosplenomegaly; fundal height, 25 cm
Neurologic	Equivocally positive Romberg test result; finger to nose testing occasionally positive (occasional finger not touching the nose or moving beyond the tip of nose)
Extremities	Finkelstein maneuver negative bilaterally; Phalen maneuver positive at 20 seconds on the right and 20 seconds on the left with paresthesias into the median nerve distribution; reverse Phalen maneuver positive at 20 seconds on the right and 35 seconds on the left; Tinel sign negative bilaterally; percussion of median nerve caused numbness; no ulnar or radial nerve symptoms

The initial diagnoses list included the following:
1. Possible tendinitis or impingement (pain in right shoulder)
2. Bilateral carpal tunnel syndrome
3. Pregnancy
4. Thyromegaly
5. Cervical strain (whiplash), old, possible mild residual, but asymptomatic
6. Previous syncopal episode
7. Mild hand dermatitis
8. Anxiety
9. Palpitations

No radiographs were obtained because of her pregnancy. Work restrictions, acetaminophen, and physical therapy were prescribed. She was given nighttime rigid splinting for her wrists.

Review of History and Physical Examination Process

In the preceding history, there are deficiencies. However, it is not atypical for the average occupational or primary care setting. The woman had symptoms suggestive of an environmental exposure; however, these were not elaborated on or pursued. Her occupation as an employee of a dry cleaning business was mentioned but not explored. Had the medical provider recognized this key issue, it would have been appropriate to inquire about the industrial process and perhaps schedule a workplace walk-through. Any environmental controls or lack thereof should be documented. A more thorough search for alternative causes of symptomatology should be undertaken, including hobbies, second occupations, and "recreational" drug use. A query should be undertaken of recent changes in work practices, i.e., significant overtime, process changes, and similar symptoms in coworkers.

A problem list in which symptoms and known diagnoses are included is a useful tool in causation analysis. As more data are obtained, each symptom can be matched to a specific diagnosis. It is recognized that there are many interested parties clamoring for a diagnosis and immediate assignment of all symptoms to a specific diagnosis. A provisional diagnosis can be supplied; however, a system that permits diagnostic modification as the analysis of causation proceeds is helpful. An example is the diagnosis pain in limb, International Classification of Diseases, Ninth Revision, Clinical Modification, code 729.5.[1] It is also useful, when appropriate, to request, with consent, prior medical records, concurrent medical records (in this case, from the obstetrician), and any prior radiographs and laboratory study results.

Discussion

The target of our analysis is focused primarily on the production of disease (injury) and less so on the issues of impairment and disability. This analysis, to the greatest extent possible, seeks to be more explicit than implicit.[2] The question of future impairment will be briefly dealt with later in this chapter.

Initial analysis of this case might lead to the assignment of single (direct) causation to the woman's shoulder complaints. At first glance, it would be reasonable to postulate that grasping several garments and raising them above shoulder level repetitively during a shift could lead to shoulder tendinitis. Although this hypothesis is not unreasonable, differing opinions could be made. For example, if the woman happened to have a type 3 acromion, elements of competing causation (see subsequent text) could be introduced into the analysis. Elements of direct causation are often illustrated by obvious cause and effect, ie, dropping a heavy object onto one's foot. The kinetic energy imparted to the extremity directly causes the observed physical findings (e.g., swelling and/or metatarsal fracture). However, as is common in occupational medical practice, "gray zones" often are present.

Included in this case is an illustration of what can be termed a *multiple cause* type of causation. Work-related and non–work-related factors may combine to form a "web" of causation. Without further characterizing the woman's upper extremity complaints, it would be plausible to postulate that the remote motor vehicle accident had, over time, caused sufficient degenerative changes and that she now has evidence of cervical disc disease resulting in a C6 radicular pattern of symptoms. In addition, personal risk factors may enter this web in that her relatively short stature may require more above-shoulder work than would be experienced by a taller employee.

The provisional diagnosis of carpal tunnel syndrome illustrates the elements of *competing causation,* which exists when independent work-related and non–work-related factors can be combined to elicit an observable health effect. Pregnancy and thyroid disease are known to be associated with the development of carpal tunnel syndrome. Conflicting information regarding high force and highly repetitive job activities and their association with carpal tunnel syndrome is present in the literature. Because three potential agents are present in this case and are truly independent of one another, they are said to be competitive.

An underpinning of this case is the reference to the woman's employment in a Mom-and-Pop dry cleaning establishment, which introduces a greater potential for exposure to perchloroethylene (also called PERC and PCE) than does employment in a large dry cleaning plant (see later text). Dry cleaners are the single largest users of perchloroethylene. Perchloroethylene is an organic solvent with known human toxic effects. Exposure to perchloroethylene can occur in the workplace or in the environment following release to air, water, land, or groundwater. Perchloroethylene enters the body when inhaled with contaminated air or when consumed with contaminated food or water. Once in the body, perchloroethylene can remain, stored in fat tissue. Symptoms associated with exposure include depression of the central nervous system; damage to the liver and kidneys; impaired memory; confusion; dizziness; headache; drowsiness; and eye, nose, and throat irritation. Peripheral neuropathy has also rarely been reported. Because perchloroethylene is a halogenated hydrocarbon, cardiac excitability and arrhythmias are known *sequelae.* Repeated dermal exposure may result in dermatitis.

Further review of the woman's history and review of systems reveals symptoms such as lightheadedness, vertigo, a syncopal episode, and palpitations and, possibly, peripheral neuropathy. She also had difficulty becoming pregnant, a possible sign of chronic disease (exposure). The physical examination demonstrated an "equivocally positive" Romberg test result and potential contact dermatitis. We have added more factors into the constellation of symptoms, thus adding to our web of causation. At this point in this case, we do not know with certainty whether exposure is an agent competing with the potential causative forces of upper extremity paresthesias or is an independent agent in the production of a distinct, coincidental occupational disease.

Additional knowledge of the workplace environment reveals that, like many smaller dry cleaning companies, a wet-to-dry or transfer-type machine is used, which only cleans and extracts. An additional step (manual transfer of the clothing to a second machine that dries) introduces not only additional handling by the worker, but also the potential for greater release of perchloroethylene into the work environment. Consideration of the potential workplace exposure to perchloroethylene should lead the occupational physician to consider that other workers may have similar exposure. From a public health perspective, this case should be handled as a *sentinel event,* which is a case of injury or illness that signals a need for immediate intervention or serves as a warning of hazardous conditions or process breakdown. The index case (first individual identified) should be tested for perchloroethylene. All fellow employees with significant potential exposure should be brought in for examination and confirmatory testing completed, as appropriate.

In our clinical example, an industrial hygienist confirmed elevated levels of perchloroethylene in the ambient air of the dry cleaning establishment that were well above the Occupational Safety and Health Administration permissible exposure limit and the American Council for Governmental Industrial Hygienists threshold limit value. Elevated blood levels were also found in our index case. Nerve conduction testing and an electromyogram demonstrated bilateral carpal tunnel syndrome, more on the right side than on the left. The woman had a mildly elevated thyroid stimulating hormone (TSH) level, and a chemistry panel showed a mild elevation in transaminase levels.

Our diagnosis list has been modified to include the following:
1. Bilateral shoulder tendinitis
2. Bilateral carpal tunnel syndrome, electrodiagnostically confirmed
3. Pregnancy
4. Hypothyroidism
5. Cervical strain (whiplash), remote with mild residual
6. Perchloroethylene exposure and toxicity indicated by the following: history of syncopal episode, mild dermatitis on the hands, anxiety, palpitations, and elevated liver function test results.

Criteria for the Evaluation of Causation Using Epidemiologic Evidence

As outlined in Chapter 4, Methodology, a six-part process, is most helpful in establishing causation.[3] This approach can be further refined for application to individual clinical cases by adding the five Hill criteria[4] to part 2 as follows:
1. Evidence of disease. What is the disease? Is the diagnosis correct? Does the evidence (e.g., history, physical examination, and supporting studies) support or fail to support the diagnosis?
2. Epidemiologic data. What is the epidemiologic evidence for that disease or condition? Do the data support a relationship with work? Modifications using the Hill criteria are as follows: (A) Temporality: It is logically necessary for a cause to precede an effect in time? (B) Strength of association: The stronger the relationship between the cause and effect, the less likely it is that the relationship is due to an extraneous variable. (C) Biological gradient, or dose-response relationship: There should be a direct relationship between the degree of exposure to the risk factor and the magnitude of the observed result. (D) Consonance with literature: There is consistency of the association across studies, subjects, and time in keeping with a body of knowledge. and (E) Biological credibility, or the plausibility of the exposure-disease relationship in question: Are the mechanism and duration of the exposure consistent with expectations, knowing the nature of the disease process?
3. Evidence of exposure. What evidence, predominantly objective, is there that the level of occupational environmental exposure (e.g., frequency, intensity, and duration) could cause the disease?
4. Other relevant factors. What other relevant factors are present in this case? Are there individual risk factors other than the occupational environmental exposure that could contribute to the development of the

disease? For example, if the diagnosis is carpal tunnel syndrome, is the worker pregnant, obese, or diabetic?

5. Validity of evidence. Are there confounding or conflicting data to suggest information obtained in the preceding parts of the process is inaccurate?
6. Evaluation and conclusions

A table is constructed for each diagnosis. The columns are the five Hill criteria, and the rows are the possible contributing diagnoses. A scale of 1 (lowest) and 4 (strongest) is used to determine contribution. The scale is arbitrary but should be based on the information obtained as described in Chapter 4. This assignment of numeric values is merely a tool to ensure that the thought process in this analysis is complete as it relates to the epidemiologic criteria. The tabular format gives a "global" picture of the component parts. The tables should be thought of as scratch pads that can be altered as more data emerge.

For diagnosis 1, shoulder tendinitis, the table would be created as follows:

Shoulder Tendinitis	Temporality	Strength of Association	Biological Gradient	Consonance With Literature	Biological Credibility
Occupational	4	2	3	2	3
Cervical strain	3	2	1	3	2
Type 3 acromion	4	3	2	3	4

Review of the shoulder tendinitis indicates a tendency toward its being included as an occupational diagnosis. Only if subsequent radiographs indicate a type 3 acromion would this hypothesis rise to a level of prominence in our analysis.

For diagnosis 2, carpal tunnel syndrome, the table would be created as follows:

Carpal Tunnel Syndrome	Temporality	Strength of Association	Biological Gradient	Consonance With Literature	Biological Credibility
Occupational	3	3	2	3	3
Hypothyroidism	2	2	2	3	3
Pregnancy	3	3	3	4	4
Cervical strain	1	1	2	2	2
Perchloroethylene	3	1	1	1	1

CHAPTER 22

Our initial analysis suggests that pregnancy is the most likely agent in the production of carpal tunnel symptoms. Hypothyroidism and the occupational grasping causes are weighted lower and in an equivalent manner. Of note is that these three potential causes of carpal tunnel syndrome are competing causation, and, thus, we would expect that an epidemiologic causation analysis would yield not too dissimilar results in terms of the overall strength of the association.

For diagnosis 3, pregnancy, and diagnosis 4, hypothyroidism, causation is not an issue. For diagnosis 5, cervical strain (whiplash), causation is not an occupational issue; the cause was a motor vehicle crash.

For diagnosis 6, perchloroethylene exposure and toxicity, the table would be created as follows:

Perchloroethylene Exposure	Temporality	Strength of Association	Biological Gradient	Consonance With Literature	Biological Credibility
Occupational	4	3	3	4	4
Hypothyroidism	2	2	2	3	3
Pregnancy	3	3	3	4	4
Cervical strain	1	1	2	2	2

The woman's symptomatology, previously attributed to pregnancy can now be linked to potential perchloroethylene toxicity, based on a thorough case-investigation, which demonstrated elevated levels of perchloroethylene in the indoor air environment and an elevated level of perchloroethylene in her serum.

Summary of Example

At this point, the evidence favors occupational exposure to perchloroethylene as the cause of the woman's symptomatology; carpal tunnel syndrome may be aggravated by pregnancy, hypothyroidism, perchloroethylene exposure, and tasks at work; and possible tendinitis of the shoulder that may be aggravated by perchloroethylene exposure and tasks at work.

Consideration of Likelihood

When available evidence does not support an *absolute* link between the exposure and the effect, the evaluator's opinion should be described in terms of the *likelihood* of causation.[5] The degree of certainty should be supported primarily by evidence, but should also be a product of logic and informed judgment. Useful legal terms include *more likely than not* and *probable,* which, in most cases, mean a probability of 51% or more. *Unlikely* and *possible* mean a probability of 50% or less. It is always useful to define these terms when using them. Other legal terms often identified in the occupational literature include *recurrence* and *aggravation.* Recurrence of an ongoing condition arises from the same cause as the preexisting condition, whereas aggravation of the preexisting condition involves a new event that makes an existing condition worse. Evaluators should use these terms carefully because they often have specific legal ramifications, and recurrence might lead to treatment different from that when aggravation is the case.

Definitive Causation

Definitive assessment of causation is made by reviewing all appropriate and obtainable documentation available. The individual or employer may be asked to provide additional history; private medical records; post hire and/or replacement employment histories, examinations, and test results; as well as surveillance data that may have been assimilated (baseline and postremediation, if appropriate). In our clinical case example, preliminary, epidemiologic, and some definitive causation features were applied at various stages in the workup. It is important, particularly in this multifactorial case, that the issues (particularly when a potential sentinel event is present) are addressed quickly and definitively. The case also illustrates that causation is a process, not necessarily a single event. In our clinical example, determination of the cause of shoulder complaints was less important than finding the perchloroethylene exposure, which may adversely affect not only the woman, but also her coworkers.

Determining that a problem is not work-related may avoid inappropriate limitations of work. In this case study, allowing the woman to undergo exogenous thyroid treatment and waiting for the delivery of a hopefully healthy infant may "cure" the carpal tunnel syndrome.

Consideration of the health status of the woman's child, at delivery and in the child's development, merits discussion. If an abnormality was found in the infant during the postnatal period or during childhood development, perchloroethylene could be considered a potential causal factor. Depending on the type of abnormality and the degree of severity, there could be issues of future compensation in this case.

CHAPTER 22

Barriers to the Progression of Causation Analysis

It is our belief that the performance of causation analysis can readily be accomplished by the majority of occupational medical providers. Education into the basics and importance of establishing causation in occupational medicine needs to continue, perhaps with greater emphasis on physician training programs.

In many state jurisdictions, providers are asked to make a determination of causation at the initial visit. This practice is contrary to the progressive nature of causation determination and risks misclassification of a greater percentage of cases as occupational when, in fact, they are not. In Nevada, for example, once a claim is accepted, it is nearly impossible for the decision to be reversed.

In several states, a provision of "lifetime medical treatment" is granted at claim closure. The further establishment of causation in these cases is hindered by an ever-present mindset that it is a foregone conclusion that, in all cases, the original injury is responsible for all subsequent disease or illness experienced by the person. In the California experience in particular, this bias toward misclassification is becoming terribly burdensome to the state. Were an evidence-based method applied to these cases, not only would more appropriate treatment be given, but also better outcomes for the person and society would be within reach.

From the occupational medical perspective, it is advisable for medical providers to state their uncertainty about causation when a question exists. Because many state forms limit providers to a "yes" or "no" response, it is our suggestion that providers fill in neither box but use a "?" as their answer. Until the state forms are modified, this type of response is the only interim solution we can put forth.

Several claims examiners have shared their opinion of their job as: "My job is to open and close claims." Obviously, the opening of the claim allows treatment to begin and benefits to be paid. The risk, of course, is that once this step occurs, it may be functionally irreversible. When claim acceptance is "in limbo," medical providers become concerned about the provision of services that may well be denied and claimants become worried about billings for which they may ultimately be responsible. Frequently, group health plans deny payment for services considered occupationally related and, thus, are not covered. This practice effectively leaves the claimant in an occupational "no man's land." In such a difficult situation, the greatest pressures are often placed on the claims examiner and can foster bad claims decisions. In some cases, consideration for shared risk among all the parties is appropriate. This can be accomplished by considering apportionment of the risk. The greatest need is to establish an investigational phase in which evidence-based treatment can proceed and workup of causation can be appropriately undertaken. The cost to society of misclassification of conditions as occupational greatly exceeds that of establishing a formalized investigative period before appropriate determination. Unfortunately, change is slow.

Future Considerations

Reduction or prevention of injuries and illnesses will require a change in our approach to risk. Risk of injuries and illnesses is a combination of individual risk and activity (environment/workplace) risk. Individual risk is based on age and inherited characteristics while activity risk is based on tasks performed by the individual. Occupational medicine providers are in an ideal position to work with employers proactively to increase safety (reduce workplace risk) and to reduce individual risk in an effort to diminish the antagonistic environment that results from workers' comp claims and litigation.

References

1. Melhorn JM. Occupational orthopaedics. *J Bone Joint Surg Am.* 2000;82A:902-904.
2. Hadler NM. *Occupational Musculoskeletal Disorders.* Philadelphia, PA: Lippincott; 2005:259-295.
3. Glass LS. *Occupational Medicine Practice Guidelines ACOEM: Evaluation and Management of Common Health Problems and Functional Recovery in Workers.* Beverly Farms, MA: OEM Press; 2004.
4. Hill AB. The environment and disease: association or causation? *Proc R Soc Med.* 1865;58:295-300.
5. Harber P, Shusterman D. Medical causation analysis heuristics. *J Occup Environ Med.* 1996;38:577-586.
6. Melhorn JM, Wilkinson LK, O'Malley MD: Successful management of musculoskeletal disorders. J Hum Ecolog Risk Assessment 7:1801-1810, 2001.
7. Melhorn JM: Rediscovering occupational orthopaedics for the next millennium. J Bone Joint Surg Am 81A:587-591, 1998.
8. Boden LI: Workers' compensation in the United States: high costs, low benefits. Annu Rev Public Health 16:189-218, 1995.

CHAPTER 22

INDEX

Ionizing radiation, *See* Radiation
Irrebuttable presumption, *See*
  Presumptions, irrebuttable
Irritable bowel syndrome, 360-361, 363
Irritant eczema, *See* Eczema

J

J-curve paradigm, nonlinear, low back
  pain, 123
Joint arthritis, rheumatoid, 309
Joint disease, degenerative, *See*
  Osteoarthritis
Joint injury, 69
Joint pain, 94
Joint trauma, osteoarthritis, 308
Jones Act, *26*

K

Kansas, aggravation rule, 25
Kappa statistic, 21
Kidney
  failure, 350, 351
  vesicoureteral reflux, 348
Knee
  injuries, women runners, 390
  meniscal disorders, 213-215, *214-215*
  osteoarthritis, 205-209, *206-209*
  osteoarthritis, *306*
Koch postulates of infection, 116

L

Laboratory data errors, *416*
Latent period, 412
Latex, contact urticaria, 400
Law
  causation as concept in, 14
  presumption of causation, 426

proximate cause, legal presumptions,
  16-18
hearing loss and, 376
tort law variations, 6
work-relatedness causation
  thresholds in state laws, *27-29*
Lead
  peripheral neuropathies, 292, 294
  renal disease and, 350
Lead time bias, 38
Leg, 203-219
  dragging, 95
  paresis (malingering, Hoover test),
    99-101
Legal causation, *See* Causation
Length bias, 38
Leukemia, radiation and, 393-397
Liability, 105
Lifting, 121
  heavy-load injuries, 391-392
Likelihood, 435
Likelihood ratio, description, 20-21
Limb, lower, *See* Foot; Heel; Hip; Knee;
  Leg
Limb, upper, *See* Arm; Elbow; Fingers;
  Hand; Shoulder; Thumb; Wrist
Literature reviews, causal association
  documented in, 35
Longshore and Harbor Workers'
  Compensation Act, *26*
Lorenz, Edward, 115
Low back pain, *See* Back pain, low
Lower limb, *See* Foot; Heel; Hip;
  Knee; Leg
Lumbar fusions, xv
Lumbar spinal stenosis, 129-130
Lumbosacral motion, 93
Lung cancer, 274-275
Lung disorders, 263-285
Lung disorders, fibrotic, 272-274
Lupus erythematosus, systemic, 310-312

M

Pulmonary disease, chronic obstructive, 274

Pulmonary disorders, 263-285
occupational, 266
occupational risk factor assessment, 277
risk factors, 265-266
smoking as chief risk factor, 265-266

R

Radiation
ionizing, 393, 396
ionizing, and multiple sclerosis, 290
nonionizing, 397

Radiation exposure
cataracts and, 377, 378
leukemia and, 393-397
measurement, 7

Radiculopathy, disc herniation and, 126-129

Radiologic diagnosis, 116

RADS, *See* Asthma

Railroad workers' cases, 109

Randomized controlled trials, 23

Range of motion, 69

Reactive airways dysfunction syndrome (RADS), *See* Asthma

Reasonable degree of medical certainty, *26-29*

Reasonable degree of medical probability, *26-29*

Reasoning, false, (*post hoc ergo propter hoc*), 16

Rebuttable presumption, *See* Presumptions, rebuttable

Recurrence, 435
definition, 8

Reflex sympathetic dystrophy, *See* Complex regional pain syndrome

Renal cell carcinoma, 350

Renal failure, 350, 351

Repetitive injury, *See* Injury, repetitive

Report writing, 103-111
expert witness testimony, 107-111

Research
assessment of study methods, 35, 37
blinding, *53, 54-55*
literature reviews, 35
psychosocial factors, *57*, 59
spinal disorder causation, 117-118
study biases, 37-38, *55-56*
study design identification, 36
study design pyramid (relative value of studies), *36*
study design quality scoring, 49-60, *52-58*
study design weighting factors, *57*
study impact rating, *58*
study limitations, other considerations, 58-59
study participation and dropout rates, *52-53*
study types described, 23-24

Residuals, 97

Respiratory problems, *See* Pulmonary disorders

Retrospective cohort, *57*

Reversibility, 39

Review, systematic, 24

Rheumatoid arthritis, 308-310

Rheumatologic disease, 305-320

Risk
absolute, 22
description of, 9

Risk factors
negative, *19*
non-occupational factors, 59
positive, *19*
probability concept in, 18
psychosocial factors, 59
work organization factors, 59
workers' compensation, 18

Risk, relative, 22

Rotator cuff tears, *See* Shoulder

Rubber glove test, 91

Rural areas, 289

S

Sacroiliac joint pain, 119
Schmorl nodes, 132
Scoliosis, 131
Scoot test, 95
Sensitivity, 19, *19*
Sensory patterns, 88
Sentinel event, 431
Sexual dysfunction, 352
Sexual function, 349
Sham motion, 87
Sham testing, 86-87
Shipyard workers, noise exposure, *65*
Shoe industry, nose and throat problems, 380
Shoulder
    rotator cuff tears, 184-190, *186-189*
    tendinitis (example of causation analysis), *433*
    tendinitis, impingement syndrome, 184-190, *186-189*
Sick building syndrome, 266, 379, 381
Sick house syndrome, 379
Silica, 273
    autoimmune diseases and, 310
    kidney damage, 351
Silicon, 272
Situational depression, 327
Skin
    inflammation, 400
    sun exposure, 381, 400
Skin cancer, 400
Skin diseases, occupational, 398-401
Skull, thin, *See* Thin skull principle, 124
SLE, *See* Lupus erythematosus, systemic
Sleep apnea, obstructive, 276
Smoking
    cataracts and, 377
    pulmonary risk factors, 265-266
Solvents
    hearing loss and, 375, 376
    lower urinary tract disease, 351-352

multiple sclerosis, 290
perchloroethylene, 430-432, *434*, 435
peripheral neuropathies, 292, 293
upper urinary tract disease, 350-351
Somatic syndromes, *See* Functional somatic syndromes
Somatoform disorders, 335-336
Sound levels, *See* Noise
Specificity, 39
    definition of, 19, *19*
Spinal disorders, 113-140
    cervical myelopathy, 130-132
    data sources, 117-118
    degeneration, 118
    environmental causation, 118
    injury model, 132
    low back pain, 114-126
    lumbar spinal stenosis, 129-130
    radiculopathy with disc herniation, 126-129
    scientific cause (etiology), 116-118
    trauma, 118
Spinal imaging, 96
Spine, fragile, principle of, 124
Spondylolisthesis, 131
Spondylolysis, 131
Spondylosis, 130
Sports medicine paradigm, low back pain, 122
Sports, women runners, 390
State laws
    tort law variations, 6
    work-relatedness causation thresholds, *27-29*
Statistical significance, 18, 38
Statistics
    biostatistics, 18
    definition of concepts, terms, 19-22
    probability, 18
Stomach, gastritis, 358-359
Strength testing, 91

Updated and enhanced: Guides Sixth offers the most current guidelines for correct impairment evaluation

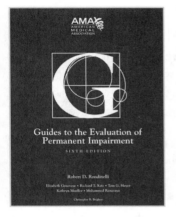

The new, revised *Guides to the Evaluation of Permanent Impairment*, sixth edition, from the AMA, emphasizes the fundamental skills used by physicians to evaluate and communicate patient impairments by performing objective clinical tests and incorporating patient's clinical and functional history.

Standardized methodology is applied to each chapter in order to enhance the relevancy of impairment ratings, improved internal consistency and promote application to the rating process. This structured method enables busy physicians to become proficient with rating multiple organ systems efficiently.

Guides to the Evaluation of Permanent Impairment, sixth edition
Hardcover, 8 1/2" x 11", 630 pages

Order #: OP025407	ISBN: 978-1-57947-888-9
Price: $189	**AMA member price: $139**

Put the new Sixth edition into practice, over 65 in-depth cases to help foster correct usage

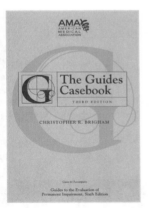

Apply the principles of the new *Guides Sixth* with this must-have companion book, offering more than 65 in-depth cases that cover an array of different systems and diagnoses. Each case shows insight into the sixth edition principles and methodology while pointing out updates and differences from prior editions. As a bonus feature, continuing medical education credits have been added.

The Guides Casebook, third edition
Softbound, 6"x 9", 400 pages

Order #: OP210007	ISBN: 978-1-57947-890-2
Price: $79.95	**AMA member price: $59.95**

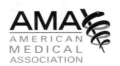

Tackle patient return-to-work and stay-at-work issues with ease!

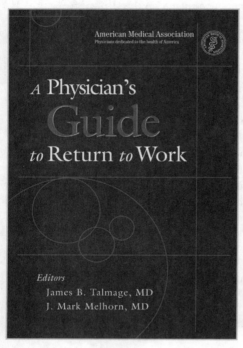

Own the guide book that gives comprehensive insight and tools on how to think through and solve return-to-work and stay-at-work issues that are best for patients.

Includes:

☐ Common questions faced by physicians, insurers, attorneys, employers and workers' compensation managers answered with the most current data

☐ Step-by-step guidance to negotiate return-to-work issues

☐ Discusses the implications of medication, work aspects and driving
☐ Health consequences of unemployment
☐ Specific examples and case studies help appropriate disability ranges to a specific diagnosis

A Physician's Guide to Return to Work
Softbound, 6" x 9", 356 pages, 50 tables

Order #: OP324005	ISBN: 978-1-57947-628-1
Price: $59.95	AMA member price: $44.95

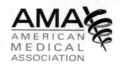